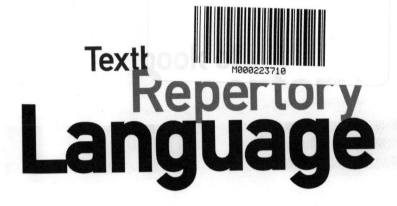

Textbook of Repertory Language

for the Essential Synthesis

Textbook of Repertory Language

for the Essential Synthesis

Dr. Frederik Schroyens and Peter Vint

Homeopathic Book Publishers

London

British Library Cataloguing in Publication Data
Textbook of Repertory Language, for the Essential Synthesis
Homeopathic Repertory
Frederik Schroyens, Dr. and Peter Vint

London, Homeopathic Book Publishers 2012

ISBN 978-0-9557151-1-2

Published by Homeopathic Book Publishers

Layout and Typesetting: E. Warnier, MK Partners, Braives (Belgium)
Cover design: Marie di Francesco
Printed in India by B. Jain Publishers

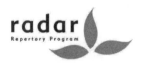
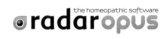

Homeopathic Software by Archibel SA
Rue Fontaine St Pierre 1E – 5330 Assesse – Belgium
Website: www.archibel.com/synthesisbook.html

Table of contents

Foreword for the Essential Synthesis

by Dr. Frederik Schroyens

The Essential Synthesis is a repertory offering that information which has proved to be essential.

The homeopathic community has for a long time been demanding to include new information in the repertories as fast as possible. While we have not been yielding uncritically to that request, our primary dedication has always been to offer quality. Of course, each edition of Synthesis did offer more new information and countless corrections.

In that evolution, it has been our goal to add more classical, verified information as well as more contemporary information. Throughout this has been a very difficult balancing act, because no two homeopaths would agree about what needs to be done.

Especially after the publication of edition 9.1 (2004), homeopathic colleagues requested me to put more emphasis on reliable information. Teachers were strongly voicing their opinion with their students in mind. This edition of Synthesis is the reply to that demand.

Back to basis?

Before explaining more, let me point out an interesting coincidence in the evolution of our community. Over the last few years, a new motto is appearing, which could be summarized as "back to basics". If you look at the themes of upcoming congresses, you cannot miss it:

- The annual LIGA Congress in Mexico is held with the slogan *"Returning to Hahnemann"* (August 2007)
- In Ettlingen (Germany) a international congress is being organized, reviving the pioneer's association "International Hahnemann Congress" to "advance the scientific development

of homeopathy *on the basis of its founding principles.*" (September 2007)

* The North American Academy of Veterinary Homeopathy holds its annual conference around the theme *"The Legacy of Hahnemann"* (October 2007)
* The journal Homeopathic Links has been the voice for most of the progressive ideas and is celebrating its 20 years with a Congress, end of October 2007. I am entranced that a goal of this congress is to "clarify how the different strands of development are *linked with the fundamentals of classical homeopathy*".

I believe that the better slogan would be "back to essentials" as basics are those elements which are easy, evident and not in need of explanation. Essentials on the other hand tend to be forgotten, but need to be focused on again and again if we want to remain successful.

The Essential View

How did we achieve that?

You may know that Synthesis, as a software, offers different views of the Repertory. Depending upon your repertory view you may see more or less information, with more or less reliability. The Quantum View displays more conservative information and therefore excludes two types of information:

* hypothetical information such as based on theoretical approaches and also dream provings and meditation provings.
* more recent provings or contemporary information which has not yet been repeatedly confirmed in the clinic.

We have carefully reviewed the Quantum View so to adhere very strictly to these criteria. So carefully that we decided to give it another name: the Essential View, basis for the Essential Synthesis. In other words: to obtain the Essential Synthesis, information has been removed from the Full Synthesis. The Essential Synthesis offers you those author references, those remedies and those symptoms which have proven their value and reliability repeatedly.

Full Synthesis comes with information from 905 author references, the Quantum View still considers 662 and the Essential Synthesis selects the 583 most reliable author references. Full Synthesis describes 2.375 remedies, the Essential Synthesis assists you to prescribe any of 1.990 remedies.

For the fine tuning of this concept, I relied as usually on a whole team of people and I want to thank especially: Dale Emerson (Belgium), Erik Van Woensel (Netherlands), Kim Elia (USA), Nishant and Kuldeep Jain (India), Peter Vint (Germany), Phil Edmonds (England), René Otter (Netherlands) and Reinhard Rosé (Germany) for the hard work and the following colleagues for the inspiring communications: Anthony Bickley (England), Barbara Turk (England), Bernhard Bloesy (Germany), George Vithoulkas (Greece), Jochen Rohwer (Germany), Marc Brunson (Belgium), Mike Andrews (England), Misha Norland (England), Nick Avery (England), Rob Willemse (Netherlands) and Robert Schore (USA).

The Treasure

Even if there is less information now, there is some most important new information compared to Synthesis 9.1. The Essential Synthesis contains Kent's Treasure, as it is really a trimmed down version of the *Synthesis Treasure Edition* (version 9.2 for those who prefer numbers).

The Treasure of Kent indicates the information J.T. Kent annotated in his personal copy of his own Repertory. The story of how this information became available can be found in an article further in this Textbook. Let me summarize it by stating that I believe that this is probably the best clinical information of one of the best homeopaths ever which now becomes available in print.

The author references related to the Treasure are k1a1, k1b1, k1b2 and k9. You will find the precise explanation on the CD. More important is to honor Ahmed Currim (USA) for his persistence and generosity to share this work of excellence with us. A long time has elapsed between our initial conversations in Toronto (Canada) and at his home in Fairfield, CT (USA) and the final set up of the job during the LIGA Congress in Berlin (2005). But now, with the help of Paul Debruyn (Belgium) the job has been done with accuracy.

Some 11.368 additions and corrections noted by Kent in his personal copies of different editions of his Repertory have been integrated as well as 333 handwritten additions as noted by Kent in his copy of Hering's "Guiding Symptoms".

Content of the Textbook

We have printed a separate Textbook in order to make the Repertory part as small as possible. The users of Synthesis 8.1 very much appreciated this in the past.
The actual textbook contains:
- The foreword by the editor
- For the first time, we have a chapter with **veterinary information** printed. It contains all veterinary interesting symptoms and all remedies of a veterinary origin. There is also a list of veterinary concepts leading to the related symptoms. This list has proven most useful for the beginning veterinary homeopaths in the software and becomes now available in the printed format.
- A limited list of remedy abbreviations (only those remedies present in the book). There is no list of author abbreviations as the book does not contain any.
- An index of keywords referring to page numbers in Synthesis

- Then again something new: we have added a very extended **list of localizations**. In the alphabetical list you can search for a localization and you will find in which chapter symptoms of this localization can be found. Sometimes the answer will be more than one chapter, which will help you to not overlook the symptoms you need.
- Finally, an article by Dr. Ahmed Currim explaining in detail the history and the value of the Treasure.

Content of the CD

The CD offers a read only version of the **Essential Synthesis** with all author references and all cross references.

We printed a maximum of 3 cross references, referring to the biggest rubrics, so that the book gives the most practical proposals first.

What will strike you is that **no author references** have been printed. I have always stated that, as in any scientific publication, source referencing is a must. In fact I did not change my opinion. The CD brings you all the source referencing you can possibly want.

All authors in the book have a minimum reliability so that immediate checking of the source becomes less needed.

In this regard I want to emphasize that we printed the **remedies copied to the superrubrics** in the pain sections and in the mind section, as we did in Synthesis 9.1. Therefore the Essential Synthesis will offer you instant access to the hitherto hidden times, sides, modalities, localizations, etc. which became visible because of restructuring the Repertory[1].

---

1 *You find a more detailed explanation of this major advantage in the Editor's foreword to Edition 9.1.*

We did not print rubrics which contain only Boger Bönninghausen remedies, such as "Mind - Morning". Similarly, we did not print the typical Boger Bönninghausen chapters "Neck", "Male and female genitialia/sex" nor "Urinary organs". We printed the b-bg remedies in other rubrics if they were completing an existing rubric.

The CD also contains the usual **"Textbook for Repertory Language"**, including an explanation of 1.500 key symptoms, full catalogues of remedies and author references, a families database, a relationship of remedies database, etc.

A Repertorization grid can be printed as many times as you wish to facilitate your manual repertorizations.

Content and form

I did not yet mention another concern which the Essential Synthesis addresses. As the different editions became larger, so did the number of people requesting a lighter repertory.
With edition 9.1 we addressed this among others with a smaller font, which made the book harder to use for a number of homeopaths. Now we have increased the font again one step and also the removal of the author references will make the remedy abbreviations more readable.

Still the concern is there to have a manageable book: one the student can easily take to school, the homeopath can take to the bedside or to the seminar.

By addressing the first concern, we do have a smaller and lighter book. In addition, we have further fine tuned our lay out with the help of Peter Vint (Germany) and Emmanuel Warnier (who has been working with us since Synthesis 5).

Synthesis 8.1 was weighing 2,020 kg (4,45 lb), Synthesis 9.1: 2,330 kg (5,14 lb). Now we are proud to offer you a very manageable book of a smaller size and yet weighing just about 1,300 kg (2,9 lb). The care that has been taken to optimize the form is also illustrated by the size of our test chapter "Chest". The first version counted 104 pages, the final one 91 pages.

Thank you very much to the B. Jain family for the nice printing work and for making a **thumb index** affordable. Many thanks also to the proof reading team with An Aerts and Gerd Van Brandt (Belgium) for the tedious but crucial work.

At last, but not least, I want to say that the Essential Synthesis is an **additional version** to the Full Synthesis 9.1 which has been printed already. The software users have had this choice for a long time. It seems that now the time has come that also book users can choose to either use the Full Synthesis or the Essential Synthesis. You will choose the Full Synthesis if you want to use modern provings and contemporary clinical experiences.

For a long time an increasing part of the homeopathic community has been pushing the repertory editors with a "the more, the better" cry. Fortunately, it took only a mouse click to remove unwanted information from the software version. Now the Essential Synthesis book comes with the "less is more" motto: a repertory stripped down to its essential information! We wish you a good reception of our work and efficient results in your practice.

Dr. Frederik Schroyens
Gent, August 4, 2007

INTRODUCTION

This *"Textbook of Repertory Language"* is the successor of the *"Blueprint for a new Repertory"*. The Blueprint, as the name indicated, was a plan of action explaining the development of Synthesis. Successive versions accompanied all editions of Synthesis until version 8.

In each of those Blueprint versions, the first line read: "This concept is a proposal". Over the years and in the course of many different versions, Synthesis has evolved into an *accepted* proposal. In many schools all over the world Synthesis is the preferred Repertory. It has been translated into many languages and has been reprinted more often than any other contemporary repertory.

As a result, Synthesis is probably the most widely used repertory nowadays. A lot of feedback has been integrated; a lot of brilliant thinking by many homeopaths has led Synthesis to where it stands now. Even though the development of Synthesis will continue, the time is ripe to present to the homeopathic community , which thought processes went into its creation.

This is the goal of the Textbook.

Here is some specific information about different parts of this Textbook, as adapted for the Essential Synthesis.

One important goal of the Essential Synthesis is to offer only the very practical information in a very manageable size and weight. We have followed that concept for the Textbook as well. As a result we have not printed any section unless it was relevant for daily practice.

- ◆ The main part of the Textbook for Repertory Language, which presented the *"Rules of Repertory Language"* was not reprinted. It can be found on the CD. Also, it has not changed in comparison to version 9.1.

- The same situation for the *"Explanation of Key Symptoms"*, the *"Families of remedies"*, *" Relationships of remedies "Information about new remedies"*: they are not printed, but can be found on the CD.

- A *"Veterinary chapter"* is an important innovation. There are two lists.
  - The first one is a list of all symptoms most often relevant for veterinary practice. If the symptom contains remedies, these are specifically based on veterinary practice. If the symptom is followed by a number, this refers to a page number in the Repertory and leads you to the human rubric to be used.
  - The second one is a list of veterinary concepts. These express symptoms and behavior typical for certain animals and are followed by the human symptoms which may apply in those cases. A goldmine for the beginning vet homeopath!

- A limited *"Catalogue of remedies"* has been printed with only those remedies present in the Essential Synthesis. The abbreviations are followed by the Synthesis name of the remedy. Synonyms follow between brackets, if applicable. The full catalogue of remedies can be found on the CD.

- The *"Catalogue of authors"* can only be found on the CD as the author references can only be found on the CD as well.

- An *"Index of words"* follows with page numbers referring to the main Repertory.

- Then we have a list of *"Localizations"* which is offered in two ways.
  - First a list of each localization per chapter. This order corresponds to the way that the localizations are sorted in the repertory and will help you to find certain localizations more easily.

- Second, a list of all single localizations with reference to the abbreviated chapter(s) where they can be found.

- At last we have included the full article reporting about the *"History of Kent's Repertory and Treasure"*, written by Dr. Ahmed Currim (USA). This article will be most interesting to understand the value of the current Essential Synthesis.

It is our wish that our work will assist you in finding a treasure for all your patients, the best fitting remedy.

Dr. Frederik Schroyens   Peter Vint

Gent, August 4, 2007

Mind

ABRUPT (see pg 1)

ABSENTMINDED:
- air; in open (see pg 1)
- epileptic convulsions:
  - before (see pg 1)
- menses; during (see pg 1)
- old age; in (see pg 1)
- periodical:
  - short lasting attacks of absentmindedness (see pg 1)
- spoken to; when:
- vertigo; during (see pg 1)

ABSORBED (see pg 1)
- daytime (see pg 1)
- morning (see pg 1)
- afternoon (see pg 1)
- evening (see pg 1)
- become of him; as to what would (see pg 1)
- eating:
  - after (see pg 1)
- menses, during (see pg 1)

ACTIVITY:
- desires activity (see pg 2): med$_{frc}$ **Phos**$_{frc}$ tub$_{frc}$
  - evening (see pg 2)
  - alternating with:
    - dullness (see pg 2)
    - indifference (see pg 2)
    - lassitude (see pg 2)
    - prostration; mental (see pg 2)
    - weakness (see pg 2)
  - perspiration; during (see pg 2)
- restless (see pg 3): med$_{frc}$ phos$_{frc}$
- sleeplessness; with (see pg 3)

ADMONITION:
- agg. (see pg 3): lach$_{frc}$ lyc$_{frc}$ plb$_{frc}$ verat$_{frc}$

ADULTEROUS (see pg 3)

AFFECTIONATE (see pg 3): *Calc*$_{ffd}$ calen$_{fmx}$ *Caust*$_{klp}$ *Ign*$_{klp}$ lyc$_{ffd}$ *Phos*$_{ffd}$ **Puls**$_{ffd,fmx,klp}$ thuj$_{ffd}$
- alternating with:
  - sadness (see pg 3)
- aversion to tenderness: ph-ac$_{brm}$
- estrus:
  - after:
  - before:
  - during: sep$_{brm}$
- false pregnancy; during: asaf$_{brm}$
- returns affection (see pg 3)
- too friendly; dog breeds usually suspicious are: puls$_{brm}$

AGILITY, mental (see pg 3)

AILMENTS FROM:
- abused; after being (see pg 3): arn$_{elg}$ **Nat-m**$_{dyc}$ *Staph*$_{dyc}$

Ailments from – **abused**; after being: ...
  - **demanding** too much while training or breaking in a horse:
  - **emotionally**:
  - **kept** not in accordance with their natural needs; after being:
- **anger** (see pg 3): **STAPH**$_{klp}$
  - suppressed (see pg 4): carc$_{klp}$ *Ign*$_{frc}$ *Nat-m*$_{brm}$ ph-ac$_{brm}$ **Staph**$_{brm,frc,klp}$
- **anticipation** (see pg 4)
- **anxiety** (see pg 4)
- **castration**: staph$_{dyc}$
- **contradiction** (see pg 4)
- **death** of loved ones (see pg 4): **Ign**$_{hnb,klp}$ **Ph-ac**$_{brm}$ sulph$_{brm}$
- **discords**:
  - parents; between one's (see pg 4): phos$_{frc}$
  - people; between: lyc$_{brm}$
- **egotism** (see pg 4)
- **embarrassment** (see pg 4)
- **excitement**:
  - emotional (see pg 5): lyc$_{ffd}$ *Nat-m*$_{ffd}$
  - suppressed (see pg 5)
- **friendship**; deceived (see pg 5)
- **fright** (see pg 5)
- **grief** (see pg 5): carc$_{klp}$ **IGN**$_{klp}$ **NAT-M**$_{klp}$ *Puls*$_{klp}$ **Staph**$_{klp}$
  - recent (see pg 5): ign$_{frc}$
- **homesickness** (see pg 5): *Ign*$_{hnb,klp}$ nat-m$_{brm}$
- **honor**; wounded (see pg 5)
- **hurry** (see pg 5)
- **indignation** (see pg 5)
- **injuries**, accidents; mental symptoms from (see pg 5): phos$_{hnb}$
- **jealousy** (see pg 5): lyc$_{frc}$ Nux-v$_{frc}$
- **joy**:
  - excessive (see pg 5)
- **love**; disappointed (see pg 5)
- **mental** exertion (see pg 6)
- **mental** shock; from (see pg 6)
- **mortification** (see pg 6)
- **music** (see pg 6)
- **noise** (see pg 6)
- **punishment** (see pg 6)
- **quarrelling** (see pg 6)
- **remorse** (see pg 6)
- **reprimands** (see pg 6)
- **reproaches** (see pg 6)
- **rudeness** of others (see pg 6): *Calc*$_{ffd}$
- **sexual** excesses (see pg 6)
- **sexual** excitement (see pg 6)
- **shame** (see pg 6)
- **starting**:
- **surprises** (see pg 7)
- **violence** (see pg 7)
- **warmth** and security at home; lack of:
  - children; in: lac-c$_{hnb}$
- **weaning** too early:

AIR; in open:

- **amel.** (see pg 7)
- **desire:**
AMATIVENESS:
- **want** of amativeness:
AMUSEMENT:
- **aversion** to (see pg 8): $Bar\text{-}c_{klp}$ $calc_{klp}$
- **desire** for:
  · **toy** shops; wants to go to: $phos_{brm}$
ANGER (see pg 8): Aur_{klp} $Lyc_{fmx,hnb}$ $Phos_{fmx}$ $Staph_{klp}$
- **abused**; after being:
  · **demanding** too much while training or breaking in a horse:
  · **kept** not in accordance with their natural needs; after being: $nat\text{-}m_{klp}$
  · **physically:**
  · **sexually:**
- **activity**; with great physical:
- **animals**; towards:
  · **other** breed; of:
  · **other** species; of:
    ⁞ **certain** animals of another species; towards:
  · **same** breed; of:
  · **same** species; of:
    ⁞ **certain** animals of the same species; towards:
- **beside** oneself; being (see pg 9)
- **breed**; towards:
  · **other:**
  · **same**; of the:
- **caressing**; from (see pg 9)
- **castration**; after:
- **causeless** (see pg 9)
- **children**; in (see pg 9)
- **children**; towards:
  · **other's** children; towards:
  · **own** children; towards one's: $nat\text{-}m_{klp}$
- **chill:**
  · **during** (see pg 9)
- **coition:**
  · **after** (see pg 9)
- **cold**; after taking (see pg 9)
- **combing** or cleaning; on: $merc_{brm}$ sep_{brm}
  · **places**; wants to be combed only when sitting in certain: $sulph_{brm}$
- **consoled**; when (see pg 9)
- **contradiction**; from (see pg 9): $Lyc_{ffd,hnb}$ $Nux\text{-}v_{ffd}$ $sulph_{brm}$ $tarent_{brm}$
- **cough:**
- **delivery**; during:
- **dominant** animals; in:
- **easily** (see pg 9): $bell_{gl3}$ $Nux\text{-}v_{gl3}$
- **epileptic** convulsions:
  · **before:**
- **excitement**; after emotional: $nux\text{-}v_{brm}$

Anger: ...
- **fever:**
  · **during** (see pg 9)
- **himself**; with (see pg 9): $merc_{frc}$ $nux\text{-}v_{frc}$ $phos_{frc}$ tub_{frc}
- **hungry**; when: $calc\text{-}p_{brm}$ lyc_{brm} $sulph_{brm}$
- **interruption**; from (see pg 10)
- **jealousy**; with (see pg 10): $hyos_{bnfl.es,frc,itm}$ $lach_{bnfl.es,frc,itm}$ lyc_{frc} $nux\text{-}v_{frc}$ $puls_{itm}$
- **leukorrhea** ceases; as soon as:
- **light:**
  · **bright:**
    ⁞ **agg.** (see pg 10)
- **love**; from disappointed (see pg 10)
- **menses:**
  · **before** (see pg 10)
  · **during** (see pg 10)
- **mental** exertion:
  · **after** (see pg 10)
- **milk** of mother:
  · **suppression** of milk; anger causes:
  · **vomits** from anger of mother; child (see pg 10)
- **noise**; at (see pg 10)
- **odors:**
  · **agg.** (see pg 10)
- **ovariectomy**; after:
- **pains:**
  · **about** (see pg 10)
  · **agg.** (see pg 10): $cham_{brm}$
- **paralysis** from anger:
- **past** events; about (see pg 10)
- **persons:**
  · **certain**; to:
- **pregnancy**; during:
- **reproaches**; from (see pg 10): $phos_{frc}$
- **sex:**
  · **opposite** sex; to the:
  · **own** sex; to one's:
- **spitefulness**; with:
- **stool:**
  · **before** (see pg 10)
- **sudden** (see pg 10): lyc_{fmx} $phos_{fmx}$ $puls_{fmx}$
  · **animal**; towards another:
    ⁞ **family**; of the same: ign_{brm}
  · **touched**; when: lyc_{fmx}
    ⁞ **Abdomen**; at: lyc_{fmx}
- **suffocative** attack; with:
- **talk**; when hearing other people (see pg 10)
- **touched**; when (see pg 10)
- **travelling**; while: sep_{brm}
- **trifles**; at (see pg 10)
- **veterinarian**; towards the: $bell_{brm}$ lyc_{brm} $stram_{brm}$
- **vex** others; inclined to (see pg 10): $phos_{frc}$

- **violent** (see pg 10)
- **waking**; on (see pg 11)
- **worm** complaints; in:

ANGUISH:
- **daytime** (see pg 11)
- **morning** (see pg 11)
- **forenoon** (see pg 11)
- **noon** (see pg 11)
- **afternoon** (see pg 11)
- **evening** (see pg 11)
- **night** (see pg 11)
  - **midnight**:
- **air**; in open:
  - **amel**. (see pg 11)
- **alone**, when (see pg 11)
- **alternating** with:
  - **prostration**:
    ⋮ fever; during: bell$_{qqh}$
- **amenorrhea**; during:
- **anger**, from (see pg 11)
- **cardiac** (see pg 11)
- **chill**, during (see pg 11)
- **crowded** room (see pg 11)
- **driving** from place to place (see pg 11)
- **eating**:
  - **after** (see pg 11)
  - **during** (see pg 11)
- **fainting** after anguish:
- **fever**; during (see pg 11): acon$_{qqh}$
- **friend**; from losing his (see pg 11)
- **heat**:
  - **during** heat; anguish (see pg 11)
- **lamenting**, moaning (see pg 11)
- **light**:
  - **room** full of light (see pg 11)
- **lying**:
  - **must** lie down (see pg 11)
- **menses**:
  - **before** (see pg 11)
  - **during** (see pg 11)
- **motion** amel. (see pg 11)
- **palpitation**, with (see pg 12)
- **perspiration**:
  - **cold** perspiration; with:
    ⋮ **Forehead**; on:
  - **during** (see pg 12)
    ⋮ **night** (see pg 12)
- **respiration**, preventing (see pg 12)
- **restlessness**; with (see pg 12)
- **shock** from injury, in (see pg 12)
- **stool**:
  - **before** (see pg 12)
  - **during** (see pg 12)
  - **urging**; with ineffectual:

Anguish: ...
- **tossing** about, with (see pg 12)
- **uremia**, in:
- **vomiting**, with (see pg 12)
- **waking**, on (see pg 12)
- **walking** in open air (see pg 12)
- **weather**; in stormy:
- **weeping**, with (see pg 12)

ANIMALS:
- **aversion**:
  - **breed**; aversion to animals of the same:
- **love** for animals:
  - **dogs** (see pg 12): merc$_{brm}$
  - **other** species; only for:
    ⋮ **cats**:
    ⋮ **dogs**:
    ⋮ **horses**:
  - **weaker** animals: calc$_{hnb}$

ANIMATION:
- **agg.** (see pg 12)
- **alternating** with:
  - **absentmindedness** (see pg 12)

ANOREXIA NERVOSA (see pg 12): ign$_{klp}$
- **animal** home; when in: nat-m$_{brm}$
- **grief**; from: puls$_{brm}$
- **owner** is absent; when: thuj$_{brm}$

ANSWERING:
- **abruptly** (see pg 12)
- **aversion** to answer (see pg 12)
- **dictatorial** (see pg 12)
- **difficult** (see pg 12)
- **hesitating** (see pg 13)
- **nodding**; by (see pg 13)
- **offensive** (see pg 13)
- **rapidly** (see pg 13)
- **refusing** to answer (see pg 13)
- **slowly** (see pg 13)
- **stupor** returns quickly after answering (see pg 13)
- **vaguely** (see pg 13)

ANTISOCIAL (see pg 14)

ANXIETY (see pg 14): **Lyc**$_{gl3}$ *Nat-m*$_{gl3}$ **Puls**$_{gl3}$ **Sulph**$_{gl3}$
- **daytime** (see pg 14)
- **morning** (see pg 14)
- **forenoon** (see pg 14)
- **noon** (see pg 14)
- **afternoon** (see pg 14)
- **evening** (see pg 14)
- **abdomen**; with distension of (see pg 15)
- **air**; in open:
  - **amel**. (see pg 15): iod$_{qqh}$
- **alone**; when (see pg 15): bamb-a$_{hnb}$ gels$_{pkj1}$ ign$_{pkj1}$ lac-c$_{hnb}$ **Phos**$_{fmx,hnb}$

- anger:
  - **after** (see pg 16)
  - **during** (see pg 16)
    : **anguish**; with:
- **anticipation**; from (see pg 16)
- **ascending** stairs; on (see pg 16)
- **barking**; when other dogs are: nat-m$_{brm}$
- **bathing** the feet; after (see pg 16)
- **beside** oneself from anxiety; being (see pg 16)
- **causeless** (see pg 16)
- **children**:
  - **about** his (see pg 16)
  - **in** (see pg 16)
- **chill**:
  - **after** (see pg 16)
  - **before** (see pg 16)
  - **during** (see pg 16)
- **closing** eyes; on (see pg 16)
- **coition**:
  - **after** (see pg 16)
  - **during** (see pg 16): phos$_{frc}$
- **cold**:
  - **becoming**, from (see pg 16)
  - **drinks**:
    : **amel**. (see pg 16)
    : **ice-cold** drinks:
- **coldness**:
  - **during** (see pg 16)
- **company**; when in (see pg 17)
- **continence** prolonged; from (see pg 17)
- **convulsions**:
  - **before** (see pg 17)
  - **between**:
- **cough**:
  - **after**:
  - **before** (see pg 17)
  - **during** (see pg 17)
- **crowd**; in a (see pg 17)
- **dark**; in (see pg 17)
- **dentition**; during (see pg 17)
- **diarrhea**:
  - **suppressed**; from (see pg 17)
- **drinking**:
  - **after** (see pg 17)
  - **cold** water amel. (see pg 17)
- **driving** from place to place (see pg 17)
- **eating**:
  - **after** (see pg 17)
  - **amel**. (see pg 17)
  - **before** (see pg 17)
  - **while** (see pg 17)
- **epistaxis** amel. (see pg 17)
- **eructations**:
  - **amel**. (see pg 17)
  - **ending** with (see pg 17)
- **excitement**; from (see pg 17)
- **exercise**:
  - **amel**. (see pg 18)
  - **from** (see pg 18)

- **faintness**:
  - **with** faintness (see pg 18)
- **fasting**; when (see pg 18)
- **fear**; with (see pg 18)
- **fever**:
  - **during** (see pg 18)
- **fits**:
  - **before** (see pg 18)
  - **with** fits (see pg 18)
- **followed** by:
  - **indifference** (see pg 18)
- **foot**-bath; after a (see pg 18)
- **friends** at home; about his (see pg 18)
- **fright**:
  - **after** (see pg 18)
- **head**:
  - **congestion** to; with (see pg 18)
  - **heat** of; with (see pg 18)
  - **perspiration** on forehead; with (see pg 18)
- **house**, in (see pg 19)
- **hungry**, when (see pg 19)
- **hurry**, with (see pg 19)
- **hysterical** (see pg 19)
- **joyful** things; from most:
- **looking** steadily (see pg 19)
- **lying** (see pg 19)
- **masturbation**, from (see pg 19)
- **menopause**; during (see pg 19)
- **menses**:
  - **after** (see pg 19)
  - **before** (see pg 19)
  - **during** (see pg 19)
- **mental** exertion, from (see pg 19)
- **moaning**; with (see pg 19)
- **motion**:
  - **agg**. (see pg 19)
  - **amel**. (see pg 19)
- **music**, from (see pg 19)
- **new** things; when seeing (see pg 19): nat-m$_{brm}$
- **noise**, from (see pg 19)
- **nursing**:
  - **after** (see pg 20)
  - **during** (see pg 20)
- **others**, for (see pg 20)
- **pains**, from the (see pg 20): bell$_{pkjl}$
- **paralyzed**, as if (see pg 20)
- **periodical** (see pg 20)
- **perspiration**:
  - **amel**. (see pg 20)
  - **during** (see pg 20)
- **pollutions**; after (see pg 20)
- **pregnancy**, in (see pg 20)
- **pressure**; from:
  - **Chest**; on (see pg 20)
  - **Epigastrium**; in (see pg 20)
- **pulsation** in the abdomen, with (see pg 20)
- **rest**, during (see pg 20)
- **riding**, while (see pg 20)

- **rising**:
  - **after** (see pg 20)
  - **lying**, from (see pg 20)
- **room**, on entering a (see pg 20)
- **sedentary** life; from (see pg 20)
- **sexual** desire; from suppressed (see pg 20)
- **sitting** (see pg 20)
- **sleep**:
  - **before** (see pg 20)
  - **during** (see pg 20)
  - **going** to, on (see pg 20)
  - **loss** of (see pg 20)
  - **starting** from, on (see pg 21)
- **still**; when keeping (see pg 21)
- **stool**:
  - **after** (see pg 21)
  - **before** (see pg 21)
  - **during** (see pg 21)
- **strangers**, in the presence of (see pg 21)
- **sudden** (see pg 21)
- **suicidal** disposition, with (see pg 21)
- **swoon**, after (see pg 21)
- **touched**; anxiety from being (see pg 21)
- **trifles**, about (see pg 21)
- **tunnel**:
  - **train** is in a tunnel; when the (see pg 21)
- **urination**:
  - **after** (see pg 21)
  - **before** (see pg 21)
  - **during** (see pg 21)
- **vaccination**; after:
  - **rabies**; against: lyss-vc$_{brm}$
- **vexation**:
  - **after** (see pg 21)
- **vomiting**, on (see pg 21)
- **waking**, on (see pg 21)
- **warmth**:
  - **from** (see pg 21)
- **weariness**; with (see pg 22)
- **weather**:
  - **stormy** weather; during (see pg 22): *Lyc*$_{ffd}$ nat-m$_{brm}$ nux-v$_{brm}$ phos$_{ffd}$

APPROACHED by persons; being:
- **aversion** to (see pg 22): bar-c$_{frc}$

ATTACHED:
- **owners**; very attached to the: sulph$_{brm}$

ATTACK others, desire to (see pg 23)
- **doorbell** rings; when the: lach$_{brl}$
- **face**; when looked into the: lyc$_{hnb}$
- **nervous** excitement; from:
- **owner**; the (see pg 23): nux-v$_{brm}$ sep$_{brm}$ valer$_{lkk}$
  - **scolded**; after being: lach$_{lkk}$
- **people**: arn$_{elg}$

AUDACITY (see pg 23): nux-v$_{frc}$

AVARICE (see pg 23)

AVERSION:
- **affection** for anybody:
  - **pregnancy**; has no affection during (see pg 23)
- **around** him; to those (see pg 23)
- **children**, to (see pg 23)
  - **others**; of: nat-m$_{klp}$
  - **own**; her (see pg 23)
  - **sadness**; from:
- **everything**, to (see pg 23)
- **family**; to members of (see pg 23)
- **fetching** objects; to: sil$_{brm}$
- **friends**, to (see pg 23)
- **mother**, to (see pg 23)
- **night**; of (see pg 23)
- **parents**, to:
- **persons**:
  - **all**, to (see pg 23)
  - **certain**, to (see pg 24)
    : **bed**; lying next to him in (see pg 24): lyc$_{brm}$
- **places**; to certain (see pg 24)
- **water**, to (see pg 24)
  - **puddles**; wants to avoid pools or: calc-p$_{brm}$
- **women**; to (see pg 24)

AWKWARD:
- **bashfulness**; from (see pg 24)
- **children**, in (see pg 24)
- **drops** things (see pg 24)
- **haste**, from (see pg 24)
- **pregnancy**, during:
- **strikes** against things (see pg 24): calc$_{frc}$
- **young** animals; in:

BARKING (see pg 24)
- **anger**; from: nux-v$_{brm}$
- **approached**; when being:
  - **people**; by: calc-p$_{brm}$
- **aversion** to: phos$_{brm}$ zinc$_{sld}$
- **incessant**: cham$_{brm}$
  - **dog** is passing; when a: sulph$_{brm}$
- **moon**:
  - **full**:
    : at the moon; barking:
    : **during**:
- **other** dogs are barking; when:

BED:
- **owner's** bed; one's:
  - **aversion** to sleep in the owner's bed: merc$_{brm}$ phos$_{brm}$ sep$_{brm}$ sulph$_{brm}$
  - **desire** to sleep on owner's bed: calc-p$_{brm}$
    : **dark**; only in the: sulph$_{brm}$
  - **pillow**; sleeps on the owner's: agar$_{brm}$
  - **under** owner's bed: nat-m$_{brm}$

BEHAVIOR PROBLEMS:
- **castration**; after:
- **orchiectomy**; after:
- **ovariectomy**; after:
- **ovariohysterectomy**; after: acon$_{klp}$ staph$_{klp}$

BITING (see pg 25): Bell$_{gl3}$ cham$_{gl3}$

- **about** him; bites (see pg 25)
- **arms**; bites his own (see pg 25): merc$_{frc}$ nux-v$_{frc}$ phos$_{frc}$ tub$_{frc}$
- **cars** passing by: cham$_{brm}$
- **children**; her own:
- **convulsions**; during (see pg 25)
- **delirium**, during (see pg 25)
- **dogs**:
  - **unfamiliar** to him: sep$_{brm}$
- **fingers** (see pg 25): carc$_{klp}$
- **hands** (see pg 25)
- **nails** (see pg 25): ign$_{brm}$ *Lyc*$_{ffd}$ *Sil*$_{hnb}$
- **objects** (see pg 25)
- **paws**: lyc$_{brm}$ puls$_{brm}$
- **people** (see pg 26): cham$_{brm}$ cic$_{brm}$ hyos$_{brm}$ ign$_{brm}$ lyc$_{brm}$ nux-v$_{brm}$ sep$_{brm}$ stram$_{brm}$
  - **approached**; when being:
    : **bed**; while lying in:
    : **bed**; while lying in the owner's bed:
  - **approaching**; when someone is:
    : **owner's** bed; the:
    : **sleeping** place; the:
  - **attacking** from behind: ign$_{brm}$
  - **disturbs** him; bites everyone who (see pg 26)
  - **owners**:
    : **trifles**; because of: lac-c$_{brm}$
  - **pain**; from having: cham$_{brm}$
  - **strangers**: lyc$_{brm}$
  - **veterinarian**; the: lyc$_{brm}$ nux-v$_{brm}$ phos$_{brm}$ stram$_{hnb}$
- **suddenly** (see pg 26): stram$_{hnb}$
- **territorial** behavior; from: lyc$_{brm}$
- **worm** affections; in (see pg 26)

BRANCHES:
- **bark** of the branches; desire to remove the:
- **carry**; must:
- **chew** branches vigorously; must: sep$_{brm}$

BREAKING things (see pg 26)

BROODING:
- **corner**; brooding or moping in a (see pg 26)

BULIMIA (see pg 27): phos$_{frc}$

BUSY:
- **fruitlessly** (see pg 27)

CALLING:
- **baby**:
  - **after** weaning it; mother keep calling for her: ign$_{elg}$

CAPRICIOUSNESS (see pg 27)

CAREFREE (see pg 27): sulph$_{frc}$

CAREFULNESS (see pg 27)

CARESSED; being:
- **aversion** to (see pg 28): calc-p$_{brm}$ nux-v$_{brm}$ phos$_{frc}$ puls$_{frc}$ sep$_{brm}$ sulph$_{brm}$
  - **evening**: sep$_{brm}$
  - **strangers**; being caressed by: calc-p$_{brm}$ nat-m$_{brm}$
  - **Abdomen**; on the: sep$_{brm}$

Caressed; being – aversion to: ...
  - **Head**; on the: calc-f$_{hnb}$ lach$_{klp}$
- **desire** to be caressed (see pg 28): calc$_{klp}$ carc$_{klp}$ phos$_{klp}$ puls$_{klp}$
  - **all** the time: puls$_{hnb}$
    : **vet**; even by the: puls$_{hnb}$
  - **Abdomen**; on the:
  - **Everywhere**:
  - **Head**; on the:

CARESSING:
- **husband** and child, then pushes them away; caresses (see pg 28)

CARRIED:
- **aversion** to be carried (see pg 28)
- **desire** to be carried (see pg 28)

CAUTIOUS (see pg 28): nat-m$_{brm}$
- **anxious** (see pg 28)

CHANGE:
- **aversion** to (see pg 29): ars$_{frc}$ *Bry*$_{klp}$ calc$_{frc}$
  - **house** or flat; in the: ars$_{brm,dyc}$ calc$_{hnb}$
- **desire** for (see pg 29): merc$_{qqh}$ tub$_{frc}$

CHAOTIC (see pg 29): lach$_{frc}$

CHARACTER, lack of (see pg 29): puls$_{frc}$

CHASING:
- **cars**:
- **cats**:
  - **other** cats out of one's own garden; chasing: phos$_{brm}$
- **cyclists**:
- **joggers**:

CHEERFUL:
- **daytime** (see pg 29)
- **morning** (see pg 29)
- **noon**:
- **afternoon** (see pg 29)
- **evening** (see pg 30)
- **night** (see pg 30)
- **air**, in open (see pg 30)
- **alternating** with:
  - **grief** (see pg 30)
  - **laziness** (see pg 30)
  - **palpitation** (see pg 30)
  - **quiet** disposition (see pg 30)
  - **sadness** (see pg 30)
  - **seriousness** (see pg 30)
  - **sympathy**; want of (see pg 30)
  - **timidity** (see pg 30)
  - **weeping** (see pg 30)
- **causeless** (see pg 30)
- **chill**, during (see pg 30)
- **coition**; after (see pg 30)
- **collar** against scratching; in spite of wearing a: nat-m$_{brm}$

- **company**, in (see pg 30)
- **constipated**, when (see pg 30)
- **convulsions**; after (see pg 30)
- **dancing**, laughing, singing; with (see pg 30)
- **destructiveness**; with (see pg 30)
- **dreams**; after (see pg 30)
- **eating**:
  - **after** (see pg 30)
  - **when** (see pg 30)
- **fearful**; but (see pg 31)
- **foolish**, and (see pg 31)
- **heart** disease; with (see pg 31)
- **heat**, during (see pg 31)
- **hysterical** (see pg 31)
- **itching** eruption; though there is an:
- **loquacious** (see pg 31): lach$_{frc}$
- **menses**:
  - **before** (see pg 31)
  - **during** (see pg 31)
- **music**, from (see pg 31)
- **never** (see pg 31)
- **pain**:
  - **after** (see pg 31)
  - **during** (see pg 31)
- **paroxysms**, in (see pg 31)
- **perspiration**, during (see pg 31)
- **quarrelsome**, and (see pg 31)
- **room**; in the:
  - **amel.** (see pg 31)
- **sadness**:
  - **after** (see pg 31)
  - **with** (see pg 31)
- **stool**:
  - **after** (see pg 31)
- **thunders** and lightens; when it (see pg 31)
- **urination**:
  - **after** (see pg 31)
- **waking**, on (see pg 31)
- **walking** in the open air and afterwards (see pg 31)

CHILDISH behavior (see pg 31): sulph$_{fmx}$
- **delivery**; after (see pg 31)
- **old** people; in (see pg 31)

CHILDREN:
- **flies** from her or his own children (see pg 31)

CLAIRVOYANCE (see pg 31): *Acon* $_{frc}$ lach$_{frc}$ *Phos* $_{frc}$

CLEANNESS:
- **mania** for:
  - **branches**, wooden sticks; cleaning: sep$_{brm}$
  - **defecating** always at the same place: ars$_{ags,hnb}$
  - **dung** on the paddock; disturbed by: ars$_{brm}$
  - **litter**-box:
    : **covering** stool of all cats in the: ars$_{elg}$ nat-m$_{brm}$ sulph$_{elg}$
    : **evade** contact with the paws; trying to: lyc$_{brm}$

Cleanness – mania for: ...
- **oneself**; obsessively cleaning:

CLIMBING:
- **aversion** to:
  - **trees**; aversion to climbing: nat-m$_{brm}$ sulph$_{brm}$
- **desire** to:
  - **walls**:

CLINGING:
- **children**; in:
  - **awakens** terrified, knows no one, screams, clings to those near; child (see pg 32)
  - **grasps** the nurse when carried; child (see pg 32)
  - **mother**; child clings to the (see pg 32)
- **convulsions**:
  - **before** (see pg 32)
- **persons** or furniture; to (see pg 32)
- **restlessness**, with (see pg 32)

CLOSING EYES:
- **amel.** (see pg 32)

COMMUNICATIVE (see pg 34)

COMPANY:
- **agg.** (see pg 34)
- **aversion** to (see pg 34): **NAT-M**$_{dyc,klp}$ *Puls*$_{brm}$
  - **alone** amel.; when (see pg 34): sulph$_{brm}$
  - **bear** anybody, cannot (see pg 34)
  - **country** away from people; wants to get into the (see pg 34)
  - **delivery**; after:
  - **desire** for solitude (see pg 34)
  - **fear** of being alone; yet (see pg 34): ign$_{brm}$ lyc$_{brm,ffd}$
  - **fever**; during: bry$_{qqh}$
  - **friends**, of intimate (see pg 34)
  - **heat**, during (see pg 34)
  - **loathing** of company:
  - **menses**, during (see pg 34)
  - **owner**; only tolerates company of: merc$_{brm}$
  - **perspiration**, during (see pg 34)
  - **pregnancy**, during (see pg 34)
  - **room**; likes to be alone in a: nat-m$_{brm}$
  - **sight** of people; avoids the (see pg 34): sulph$_{frc}$
  - **strangers**, aversion to the presence of (see pg 34)
    : **urination**; during (see pg 34): **NAT-M** $_{ffd}$
- **desire** for (see pg 34)
  - **morning**:
    : **walking**; after: nat-m$_{brm}$
  - **evening** (see pg 35)
  - **night** (see pg 35)
  - **alone** agg.; when (see pg 35)
    : **fear** of people; yet (see pg 35)
    : **fever**; during: stram$_{qqh}$

- **desire** for: ...
  - **alternating** with:
    - ∶ aversion to company:
  - **amel.** in company (see pg 35)
  - **big** animals; of:
  - **friend**, of a (see pg 35)
  - **menses**, during (see pg 35)
  - **pregnancy**; during: nat-m$_{fmx}$
  - **small** animals; of:
    - ∶ **breeds**; of other:
    - ∶ **species**; of other: calc$_{hnb}$
  - **treats** those who approach him outrageously; yet (see pg 35)
  - **watched** constantly; wants to be (see pg 35)

COMPLAINING:
- **disease**, of (see pg 35)
- **menopause**; during:
- **offenses**; of long past (see pg 35)
- **pain**, of (see pg 35)
- **pitiful** (see pg 35)
- **pregnancy**, during (see pg 35)
- **sleep**, in (see pg 35)
- **trifles**, of (see pg 35)
- **waking**, on (see pg 35)

COMPREHENSION:
- **easy** (see pg 35)

CONCENTRATION:
- **active** (see pg 35)
- **difficult**:
  - **air**; in open:
    - ∶ **amel.** (see pg 36)
  - **attention**, cannot fix (see pg 36)
  - **aversion** to (see pg 36)
  - **eating**:
    - ∶ **agg.**:
    - ∶ **amel.** (see pg 36)

CONFIDENCE:
- **want** of self-confidence:
  - **support**; desires (see pg 37): puls$_{frc}$

CONFIDENT (see pg 37): ferr$_{frc,qqh}$ lach$_{frc}$ merc$_{frc}$ nux-v$_{frc}$ sep$_{frc}$
- **alternating** with:
  - **timidity** (see pg 37)

CONFOUNDING:
- **objects** and ideas (see pg 37)

CONFUSION of mind:
- **epileptic** convulsions:
  - **after** (see pg 39)
  - **before** (see pg 39)
- **epistaxis**; amel. (see pg 39)
- **excitement**; amel. (see pg 39)
- **heat**, during (see pg 39)
- **injury** to head:
  - **after** (see pg 39)
- **knows** not where he is (see pg 39)
- **loses** his way in well-known streets (see pg 39)

Confusion of mind: ...
- **menses**:
  - **after** (see pg 39)
  - **before** (see pg 39)
  - **during** (see pg 39)
- **mental** exertion:
  - **from** (see pg 39)
- **noise**:
  - **agg.** (see pg 39)
- **old** age, in (see pg 39)
- **pain**; during paroxysms of (see pg 39)
- **pregnancy**, during (see pg 40)
- **sun**; in the (see pg 40)
- **vertigo**, with (see pg 40)
- **vexation**:
  - **after** (see pg 40)
- **vomiting** amel. (see pg 40)
- **waking**, on (see pg 40)

CONSCIENTIOUS about trifles (see pg 40): caps$_{brm}$ Sep$_{brm}$

CONSOLATION:
- **agg.** (see pg 41)
  - **sympathy** agg. (see pg 41)
- **amel.** (see pg 41): syph$_{brm}$

CONTEMPTUOUS:
- **everything**; of (see pg 41)

CONTENT:
- **alternating** with:
  - **sadness** (see pg 41)
- **quiet**; and (see pg 41)

CONTRADICTION:
- **agg.** (see pg 41)
- **disposition** to contradict (see pg 41)
  - **owner**; the: tarent$_{brm}$
- **intolerant** of contradiction (see pg 41)

CONTRARY (see pg 41)

COQUETTISH:
- **not** enough (see pg 42)
- **too** much (see pg 42)

COURAGEOUS (see pg 42): merc$_{brm}$ nux-v$_{frc}$
- **alternating** with:
  - **discouragement**:
  - **fear** (see pg 42)
- **foolish** boldness: merc$_{frc}$ nux-v$_{frc}$

COWARDICE (see pg 42): Lyc$_{ffd}$ phos$_{ffd}$

CRETINISM (see pg 42)

CRUELTY:
- **loves** to make people and animals suffer (see pg 42)
- **seeing** or hearing cruelty; cannot bear (see pg 43)

CURIOUS (see pg 43): puls$_{fmx}$

CUT, mutilate or slit; desire to:

In this chapter only remedies from veterinary authors are printed

- **others** (see pg 43)

DANGER:
- **lack** of reaction to danger (see pg 43)
- **no** sense of danger; has (see pg 43)

DARKNESS:
- **agg.** (see pg 43)
- **amel.**:
- **aversion** to (see pg 43)
- **desire** for (see pg 43)

DECEITFUL (see pg 44): **Lach** hnb

DEFIANT (see pg 44)

DELIRIUM:
- **night** (see pg 45)
- **abortion**:
  · **after** (see pg 45)
- **absurd** things, does (see pg 45)
- **air** amel.; in open (see pg 45)
- **angry** (see pg 45)
- **anxious** (see pg 45)
- **apathetic** (see pg 45)
- **aroused**, on being (see pg 45)
- **bite**, desire to (see pg 46)
- **carotids** pulsating, with (see pg 46)
- **changeable** (see pg 46)
- **chill**, during (see pg 46)
- **closing** the eyes, on (see pg 46)
- **cold**:
  · **catching**; after:
- **coldness**, with (see pg 46)
- **collapse**, with (see pg 46)
- **coma** vigil; with (see pg 46)
- **congestion**, with (see pg 46)
- **convulsions**:
  · **after** (see pg 46)
  · **before** (see pg 46)
  · **during** (see pg 46)
- **dark**, in (see pg 46)
- **depletion**; after (see pg 46)
- **eating**:
  · **amel.** (see pg 46)
- **encephalitis**; with (see pg 46)
- **envy**, with (see pg 46)
- **epilepsy**:
  · **after** (see pg 46)
  · **during** (see pg 46)
- **erotic** (see pg 46)
- **escapes** in abortion; she:
- **eyes**; with brilliant (see pg 46)
- **fear**; with (see pg 46)
- **fever**:
  · **during** (see pg 46): **Bell** qqh *Bry* qqh **Calc** qqh
    mur-ac qqh
- **fierce** (see pg 46)
- **frightful** (see pg 47)
- **furious** (see pg 47)
- **gather** objects off the wall, tries to (see pg 47)

Delirium: ...
- **gay**, cheerful (see pg 47)
- **grinding** teeth; with:
- **groping** as if in dark (see pg 47)
- **heat**:
  · **agg.** (see pg 47)
- **hemorrhage**:
  · **after** (see pg 47)
- **hot** head, with:
- **hysterical**, almost (see pg 47)
- **injuries** to head; after (see pg 47)
- **intermittent** (see pg 47)
- **jealousy**, from (see pg 47)
- **jerking**, with (see pg 47)
- **jumping**, with (see pg 47)
- **lips** move as if talking (see pg 47)
- **lochia**, during (see pg 47)
- **look** fixed on one point (see pg 47)
- **loquacious** (see pg 47)
- **maniacal** (see pg 47)
- **meningitis** cerebrospinalis (see pg 47)
- **menses**:
  · **before** (see pg 47)
  · **during** (see pg 47)
- **mild** (see pg 47)
- **moving**:
  · **constantly** from place to place; moving:
  · **queer**; moving (see pg 47)
- **muttering** (see pg 47)
- **noisy** (see pg 47)
- **nonsense**, with eyes open (see pg 47)
- **pains**:
  · **from** (see pg 47)
  · **with** the (see pg 48)
- **paroxysmal** (see pg 48)
- **periodical** (see pg 48)
- **perspiration**:
  · **amel.** (see pg 48)
  · **with** (see pg 48)
- **pupils**, with dilated (see pg 48)
- **quarrelsome** (see pg 48)
- **quiet** (see pg 48)
- **rabid** (see pg 48)
- **raging** (see pg 48)
- **rambling** (see pg 48)
- **recognizes** no one (see pg 48)
- **restless** (see pg 48)
- **rolling** on floor (see pg 48)
- **running**, with (see pg 48)
- **sad** (see pg 48)
- **sepsis**, from (see pg 48)
- **shy**, hides himself (see pg 48)

- **silent** (see pg 48)
- **sleep**:
  - **after** (see pg 48)
  - **during** (see pg 48)
- **sleepiness**, with (see pg 48)
- **sleeplessness**:
  - **from** (see pg 48)
  - **with** (see pg 48)
- **sopor**, with (see pg 48)
- **stupid** (see pg 48)
- **terror**, expressive of (see pg 48)
- **thirst**, with (see pg 48)
- **trembling**, with (see pg 48)
- **urinating**:
  - **floor**; tries to urinate on the (see pg 48)
- **vertigo**:
  - **after** (see pg 48)
  - **with** (see pg 48)
- **vexation**, from (see pg 49)
- **violent** (see pg 49)
- **waking**, on (see pg 49)
- **warm** room agg. (see pg 49)
- **water**, jumping into (see pg 49)
- **wild** (see pg 49)

DELIVERY:
- **after** (see pg 49)

DELUSIONS (see pg 49)
- **nursing**; she is:
  - **child**; her:
    - **pregnancy**; during imaginary:
  - **poor**; he is (see pg 72): Sep_{brm}

DEMENTIA:
- **epileptics**, of (see pg 83)
- **masturbation**, with (see pg 83)
- **paretic** (see pg 83)
- **sadness**, with (see pg 83)
- **senilis** (see pg 83)
- **sexual** excesses; from (see pg 83)

DEPENDENT of others (see pg 83): $Puls_{frc}$ sil_{frc}

DESTRUCTIVENESS (see pg 85): $calc-p_{qqh}$
- **car**; when alone in the: $phos_{hnb}$
- **home**; in (see pg 85): $lach_{lkk}$
  - **alone**; when: $bamb-a_{hnb}$

DETACHED (see pg 85)

DEVELOPMENT of children:
- **arrested** (see pg 85): sil_{frc}
- **slow**:
  - **lifting** of leg for urinating in male dogs; late: $calc_{ffd}$ lyc_{ffd}

DICTATORIAL (see pg 85): $nux-v_{frc}$
- **power**, love of:
  - **territorial** claim: lyc_{brm}

DIRTY:
- **defecating**:
  - **bath**; in the: lyc_{brm} $sulph_{brm}$

Dirty – defecating: ...
  - **crib**; into their:
  - **everywhere**:
    - **owners** looking; when:
  - **food**; on their:
  - **grief**; from:
  - **indoors** (see pg 85): $phos_{brm}$
    - **alone**; when: $calc_{klp}$ $puls_{klp}$
    - **only**: $calc_{hnb}$ sep_{brm} $stram_{klp}$
    - **owners** looking; when:
      - **vexation**; from: ign_{hnb}
    - **raining**; when it is:
  - **jealousy**; from:
  - **mud**; always walking in the:
  - **pain**; during:
  - **resentment**; from:
  - **young** animals; in:
- **drinking**; when:
  - **wetting** and dirtying everything: $calc-p_{brm}$ $sulph_{brm}$
- **eating**; when: $calc-p_{brm}$ lyc_{brm} $nat-m_{brm}$ $sulph_{brm}$
- **everything**; dirtying (see pg 85)
- **mud**; always walking in the:
- **plays**:
- **sitting** or lying in feces (see pg 86): $calc_{brm}$
- **skin**, with dirty (see pg 86)
- **urinating** and defecating:
  - **bath**; in the: ign_{brm}
  - **crib**; into their: $sulph_{brm}$
  - **everywhere** (see pg 86): ars_{elg} bry_{brm} $canth_{elg}$ $puls_{elg}$ $staph_{elg}$
    - **children** (see pg 86)
    - **owners** are looking; when:
  - **food**; on their: $merc_{brm}$
  - **grief**; from:
  - **house**; after moving to another: $staph_{elg}$
  - **indoors** (see pg 86): $lach_{lkk}$ lyc_{brm}
    - **alone**; when: $calc_{klp}$ $puls_{klp}$
    - **only**:
    - **raining**; when:
  - **jealousy**; from:
  - **mud**; always walking in the: $sulph_{brm}$
  - **pain**; during:
  - **resentment**; from:
  - **young** animals; in:
- **urinating** deliberately:
  - **afraid** of; at objects he is: $stram_{pfg}$
  - **basket**; in the:
  - **bell** is ringing; when the: sep_{brm}
  - **crib**; into their:
  - **everywhere**: lyc_{brm} $merc_{brm}$ $nat-m_{brm}$ $sulph_{brm}$
    - **owners** looking; when: $merc_{brm}$
  - **female** lifts her leg:
  - **food**; on their:
  - **grief**; from: $carc_{klp}$ ign_{klp} $puls_{klp}$ $staph_{klp}$
  - **himself**; at: $sulph_{brm}$
  - **indoors**: $acon_{klp}$ $ambr_{klp}$ $anac_{klp}$ arn_{klp} ars_{klp} aur_{klp} $bar-c_{klp}$ $bell_{klp}$ bry_{klp} $calc_{klp}$ $calc-p_{klp}$ $caps_{klp}$ $carc_{brm,klp}$ $caust_{klp}$ $cham_{klp}$ $chin_{klp}$ $coloc_{klp}$ con_{klp} $gels_{klp}$ $graph_{klp}$

In this chapter only remedies from veterinary authors are printed

- **urinating** deliberately – **indoors**: ...
  hyos$_{klp}$ ign$_{klp}$ kali-p$_{klp}$ lac-f$_{klp}$ lach$_{klp}$ merc$_{brm,klp}$
  nat-m$_{klp}$ nit-ac$_{klp}$ nux-v$_{klp}$ op$_{klp}$ ph-ac$_{klp}$ phos$_{klp}$
  pic-ac$_{klp}$ plat$_{klp}$ pluv$_{brm}$ puls$_{klp}$ sep$_{klp}$ staph$_{klp}$ stram$_{klp}$
  sulph$_{klp}$ tarent$_{klp}$ thuj$_{klp}$ verat$_{klp}$ zinc$_{klp}$
  - **alone**; when: calc$_{klp}$ ign$_{klp}$ puls$_{klp}$
  - **only**: carc$_{brm}$
  - **owners** looking; when: plat$_{hnb,klp}$
  - **raining**; when it is: sep$_{brm}$
  - **unobserved**; when: aur$_{brm}$ calc$_{klp}$ ign$_{brm,klp}$ puls$_{klp}$
  - **jealousy**; from: hyos$_{klp}$
  - **litter**-box; besides the: ign$_{brm}$
  - **male** does not lift his leg:
  - **mud**; always walking in the:
  - **pain**; during:
  - **people**; at: sulph$_{brm}$
  - **protest**; as a:
  - **resentment**; from:
  - **urine** spraying in the house or flat: lyc$_{brm}$
  - **young** animals; in: bar-c$_{klp}$ calc$_{klp}$

DISCOMFORT:
- **bathing**, after (see pg 86)
- **chill**, during (see pg 86)
- **eating**, after (see pg 86): lyc$_{frc}$ nux-v$_{frc}$
- **heat**, during (see pg 86)
- **walking**, after (see pg 86)

DISCONTENTED:
- **always** (see pg 86)
- **children** (see pg 86)
- **everything**, with (see pg 86)
- **himself**, with (see pg 86)
- **menses**, during (see pg 87): sep$_{frc}$
- **others**; with (see pg 87)
- **surroundings**, with (see pg 87)
- **weather**:
  - **rainy** weather; during (see pg 87)

DISOBEDIENCE (see pg 88): nat-m$_{brm}$ *Syph*$_{brm}$
- **delicacies**; after:
  - **not** amel.: nat-m$_{brm}$

DISTURBED; averse to being (see pg 88): ars$_{qqh}$
Bry$_{qqh}$ chin$_{qqh}$ *Cocc*$_{qqh}$ gels$_{qqh}$

DOUBTFUL (see pg 88)

DRINKING:
- **bubblers** or fountains; aversion to drink from: sulph$_{brm}$

DULLNESS (see pg 89)
- **daytime** (see pg 90)
- **morning** (see pg 90)
- **noon** (see pg 90)
- **afternoon** (see pg 90)
- **evening** (see pg 90)
- **night** (see pg 90)
- **air**:
  - **open** air; in (see pg 90)
  - **wet** air:
    - **from** (see pg 90)

Dullness: ...
- **alone**, when (see pg 90)
- **castration**; after:
- **children**, in (see pg 90)
- **chill**, during (see pg 91)
- **company**, in (see pg 91)
- **diabetes**, in (see pg 91)
- **emotions**, from (see pg 91)
- **epilepsy**:
  - **before** (see pg 91)
- **eruptions**; from suppressed (see pg 91)
- **excitement**; from:
- **gassing**, by (see pg 91)
- **heat**:
  - **after** (see pg 91)
  - **during** (see pg 91)
- **injuries** of head, after (see pg 91)
- **mental** exertion, from (see pg 91)
- **mortification**, after (see pg 91)
- **motion**:
  - **agg.** (see pg 91)
  - **amel.** (see pg 91)
- **old** people, of (see pg 91)
- **ovariectomy**; after:
- **pain**; with (see pg 91)
- **palpitation**, with (see pg 91)
- **paroxysmal** (see pg 91)
- **periodical** (see pg 91)
- **perspiration**, during (see pg 91)
- **sexual** excesses, after (see pg 91)
- **sleepiness**, with (see pg 91)
- **toothache**, from (see pg 92)
- **urine** amel.; copious flow of (see pg 92)
- **vertigo**; during (see pg 92)
- **vexation**; after (see pg 92)
- **vomiting** amel. (see pg 92)
- **waking**, on (see pg 92)
- **walking**:
  - **after** walking rapidly (see pg 92)
  - **air**; in open:
    - **amel.** (see pg 92)
  - **amel.**:
- **warm** room, on entering a (see pg 92)
- **weather**; in cold (see pg 92)

DWELLS:
- **disappointments**, on (see pg 92)
- **grief** from past offenses:
- **offenses** come back to him; long forgotten:
- **past** disagreeable occurrences, on (see pg 92): calc-p$_{brm}$ coloc$_{brm}$
  - **night** (see pg 92)

EATING:
- **after**:
  - **agg.** (see pg 93)
- **refuses** to eat (see pg 93)
  - **animal** home; when in:
  - **unusual** place; if feeding dish is at: ars$_{brm}$
    sulph$_{brm}$

- **when:**
  - **amel.** (see pg 93)

EGOTISM (see pg 93)

ELATED:
- **alternating** with:
  - **sadness** (see pg 94)

EMBITTERED (see pg 94): ign$_{hnb}$

EMBRACES:
- **everyone** (see pg 94): puls$_{frc}$

ENNUI (see pg 94): arg-n$_{dyc1}$ lil-t$_{dyc1}$

ENVY:
- **avidity**, and (see pg 94)
- **food**; about: aur$_{hnb}$
- **hate**, and (see pg 94)

EPISTAXIS:
- **amel.** (see pg 94)

ERUPTIONS; mental symptoms after suppressed (see pg 94)

ESCAPE, attempts to (see pg 94): calc-p$_{frc,qqh}$
- **night** (see pg 94): sulph$_{frc}$
- **anxiety** at night, with:
- **family** and children; attempts to escape from her (see pg 95)
- **fever**, during (see pg 95)
- **jumps** up suddenly from bed (see pg 95)
- **mania** puerperalis, in:
- **meningitis** cerebrospinalis, in (see pg 95)
- **pregnancy**; during:
- **restrained** with difficulty, is (see pg 95)
- **run** away, to (see pg 95)
  - **female** in estrus; to find a: cann-i$_{hnb}$
- **strangers**; in the presence of: lyc$_{brm}$
- **street**; into (see pg 95)
- **waking**; on:
- **window**, from (see pg 95)

ESTRANGED:
- **children**; flies from her own (see pg 95): sep$_{frc}$
- **family**; from his:
  - **strangers**, but not with his entourage and his family; being kind with (see pg 95)

EUPHORIA:
- **alternating** with:
  - **sadness** (see pg 95)

EXCITEMENT:
- **morning** (see pg 96)
- **noon** (see pg 96)
- **evening** (see pg 96)
- **night** (see pg 96)
- **agg.** (see pg 96)
- **anticipating** events, when (see pg 96)
- **bath**, during (see pg 96)
- **cardiac** symptoms, with (see pg 96)
- **coition**, after (see pg 96)
- **company**, in (see pg 96)
- **contradiction**, from slightest (see pg 96)

Excitement: ...
- **convulsions:**
  - **after** (see pg 96)
  - **with** (see pg 96)
- **cough:**
  - **during** (see pg 96)
- **darkness**; in:
- **epilepsy**; before (see pg 96)
- **excretions**; from suppression of (see pg 96)
- **exertion**, after (see pg 97)
- **feverish** (see pg 97)
- **heat:**
  - **during** heat; excitement (see pg 97): arn$_{qqh}$ ars$_{qqh}$ merc$_{frc,qqh}$ *Rhus-t*$_{qqh}$
  - puerperal heat:
- **hemorrhage**, after (see pg 97)
- **hydrocephalus**, in (see pg 97)
- **hysterical** (see pg 97)
- **joy**, from (see pg 97)
- **leukorrhea**; after suppressed (see pg 97)
- **menopause**; during (see pg 97)
- **menses:**
  - **after** (see pg 97)
  - **before** (see pg 97)
  - **during** (see pg 97)
- **music**, from (see pg 97)
- **nervous** (see pg 97)
- **pain**, during (see pg 97)
- **palpitation**, with violent (see pg 97)
- **perspiration**, during (see pg 97)
- **pregnancy**, during (see pg 97)
- **sadness**, after (see pg 97)
- **trembling**, with (see pg 97)
- **trifles**, over (see pg 98)
- **veterinarian**; when seeing the: phos$_{brm}$
- **water** poured out, from hearing (see pg 98)

EXERTION:
- **physical:**
  - **amel.** (see pg 98)
  - **aversion** (see pg 98)
  - **desire** (see pg 98)

EXHILARATION:
- **air**, in open (see pg 98)
- **alternating** with:
  - **discouragement** (see pg 98)
  - **grief** (see pg 98)
  - **sadness** (see pg 98)
  - **timidity** (see pg 98)
- **coition**, after (see pg 98)
- **diarrhea**, during (see pg 98)
- **followed** by:
  - **exhaustion** (see pg 98)

- **perspiration**, during (see pg 98)
- **sadness**, after (see pg 98)
- **walking** in open air, while (see pg 98)

EYES:
- **downcast**:
  - walks with the eyes downcast:

FASTIDIOUS (see pg 100): lach$_{frc}$
- **food**; about:
- **time**; always wants everything to happen at the same: sulph$_{brm}$

FEAR (see pg 100): **Calc-p**$_{brm}$ *Nat-m*$_{brm}$
- **afternoon** (see pg 100)
- **night** (see pg 101)
- **air**:
  - **open**; in (see pg 101): calc$_{brl}$
- **alone**, of being (see pg 101): **Ars**$_{klp}$ caust$_{brm}$ *Lac-c*$_{hnb}$ **Phos**$_{klp}$ *Puls*$_{klp}$
  - **garden**; in the: sil$_{brm}$
  - **ground** floor; on the: rhus-t$_{brm}$
  - **new** environment; in a:
  - **strange**, unknown environment; in a: phos$_{brm}$
- **animals**, of (see pg 101): brom$_{pkj1}$ calc$_{brm}$
  - **own** species; fear of:
- **approaching**; of (see pg 102)
- **ascending**, of (see pg 102): acon$_{mmj1}$ arg-n$_{mmj1}$ gels$_{mmj1}$ ign$_{mmj1}$ lyc$_{mmj1}$ op$_{mmj1}$ puls$_{mmj1}$ rhus-t$_{mmj1}$
- **attacked**; fear of being (see pg 102)
- **balloons**; of: rhus-t$_{brm}$
- **birds** (see pg 102)
- **black**:
  - **everything** (see pg 102)
- **brilliant** objects or cannot endure them; fear of (see pg 102)
- **bugs**; of (see pg 102)
- **cage**; of carrying: arg-n$_{lkk}$
- **carried**, fear of being (see pg 102)
- **cars** and vehicles in the street; of (see pg 102): thuj$_{brl}$
- **cats**; of (see pg 102)
  - **eating**, running away from fear of cats; when: ign$_{brm}$
  - **indoors**, but outdoors beating other cats; when another cat comes: carc$_{brm}$
  - **watching** other cats through the window; when: nat-m$_{brm}$
- **cattle**; of: calc$_{brm}$
- **causeless** (see pg 102)
- **change**; of any sudden: ars$_{frc}$ calc$_{frc}$
- **chickens** (see pg 102)
- **children**, in (see pg 102)
- **children** in animals; fear of: calc-p$_{brm}$ phos$_{brm}$
- **chill**, during (see pg 102)
- **chronic** (see pg 103)
- **closing** eyes, on (see pg 103)
- **cockroaches**; of (see pg 103)
- **coition**:
  - **during**:
- **company**, of (see pg 103)
- **competitions**; of: nux-v$_{brm}$

Fear: ...
- **continuous** (see pg 103)
- **control**; losing (see pg 103): calc$_{frc}$
- **crossing**:
  - **bridge**; a (see pg 103)
    : **look** through; one can: carc$_{brm}$
  - **street** (see pg 103)
- **crowd**, in a (see pg 103): Acon$_{klp}$ calc$_{klp}$ *Lyc*$_{klp}$ staph$_{klp}$ stram$_{klp}$
- **dark** colors; of people dressed in:
- **dark**; of (see pg 103): *Calc*$_{ffd}$ *Lyc*$_{ffd}$ nat-m$_{brm}$ nux-v$_{brm}$ *Phos*$_{ffd}$ sil$_{fmx}$ **STRAM**$_{klp}$
- **diarrhea**:
  - **fear**; with (see pg 104)
- **doctors** (see pg 105)
- **dogs**, of (see pg 105): calc-p$_{brm}$ lyc$_{brm}$
  - **black** dogs; of (see pg 105): nat-m$_{brm}$
  - **growling** dogs; of: lyc$_{brm}$
  - **male** dogs; of: lyc$_{brm}$ phos$_{brm}$ sulph$_{brm}$
    : **female** dogs; in:
    : **male** dogs; in:
  - **unknown** dogs; of: sil$_{brm}$
- **door**:
  - **closed**; lest the door should be (see pg 105)
  - **opened**; when the door is (see pg 105)
- **downward** motion, of (see pg 105)
- **drinking**; of (see pg 105)
- **electrical** wires; fear of: med$_{brm}$
- **elevators**; of (see pg 105)
- **escape**; with desire to (see pg 105): calc$_{frc}$
- **everything**, constant of (see pg 105)
- **extravagance**, of (see pg 106)
- **falling**, of (see pg 106)
- **fever**:
  - **during** fever (see pg 106): acon$_{qqh}$
- **fireworks**; of:
- **flies**, of (see pg 106): calc$_{frc}$
- **flying**; of (see pg 106)
  - **airplane**; in (see pg 106)
- **frogs**; of (see pg 106)
- **full** of fear (see pg 106): calc$_{frc}$
- **going** out, of (see pg 107): bar-ar$_{sxj,vkw}$ lyc$_{brm}$ med$_{brm}$ nat-m$_{brm}$ op$_{elg}$ sep$_{brm}$ stram$_{klp}$ sulph$_{brm}$
- **green** stripes; on seeing (see pg 107)
- **gun**; thunder of a (see pg 107): acon$_{brm}$ borx$_{hnb}$ ign$_{brm}$ lyc$_{brm}$ nat-m$_{brm}$ nux-v$_{brm}$ phos$_{brm}$ puls$_{brm}$ sep$_{brm}$ sulph$_{brm}$
- **heat**:
  - **during** (see pg 107)
  - **from**:
- **high** places, of (see pg 107)
- **home**; of coming: ther$_{brm}$
- **horses**; of:
  - **herd** of horses; in a: led$_{brm}$ nux-v$_{brm}$
- **hungry**, when (see pg 107)
- **insects**; of (see pg 108): sulph$_{brm}$

- **knives**; of (see pg 108)
- **labor**:
  - **after** (see pg 108)
  - **during** (see pg 108)
- **lifelong**:
- **light**:
  - **bright**: tarent$_{brm}$
- **lightning**, of (see pg 108)
- **men**; of [=male persons] (see pg 109)
- **men**; of [old rubric] (see pg 109)
- **menses**:
  - **after** (see pg 109)
  - **before** (see pg 109)
  - **during** (see pg 109)
  - **suppressed** menses from fear (see pg 109)
- **mental** exertion:
  - **of** mental exertion (see pg 109)
- **mice** (see pg 109)
- **mirrors** in room, of (see pg 109): syph$_{brm}$
- **motion**, of (see pg 109)
- **movements** by people; of quick: calc-p$_{brm}$ lyc$_{brm}$
- **music**, from (see pg 109)
  - **piano**; from listening to a: verat$_{lkk}$
- **narrow** place, in (see pg 109)
- **near**; of those standing (see pg 109)
- **new** persons; of (see pg 109)
- **new** situations: acon$_{klp}$ arg-n$_{elg,klp}$ calc$_{klp}$ lyc$_{brm,klp}$ stram$_{elg}$
- **noise**, from (see pg 109): ign$_{klp}$ *Lyc*$_{brm}$ puls$_{brm}$ sulph$_{brm}$ tarent$_{brm}$
  - **rushing** water; of:
    - **shower**; hearing the: sulph$_{brm}$
  - **trucks**; of: calc$_{brm}$
- **odors**: tarent$_{brm}$
- **open** spaces; fear of (see pg 110)
- **operation**, of each (see pg 110): acon$_{frc}$
- **pain**:
  - **during** (see pg 110)
    - **Abdomen**; in (see pg 110): plb$_{brm}$
- **palpitation**, with (see pg 110)
- **people**; of (see pg 110): *Cic*$_{brm}$ *Puls*$_{fmx}$ stram$_{brm}$
- **pregnancy**, during:
- **quarrels**; of:
  - **owners**; of disputes between the: lyc$_{brm,hnb}$
- **raised**, fear of being:
- **rats** (see pg 110)
- **recurrent** (see pg 111)
- **red**, anything (see pg 111)
- **riding** in a carriage, when (see pg 111)
- **robbers**, of (see pg 111)
- **room**, on entering (see pg 111)
- **run** over; fear of being:
- **sadness**, with (see pg 111)
- **scorpions**; of (see pg 111)
- **sex**; of opposite (see pg 111): puls$_{frc,pkj1}$
- **shadows** (see pg 111)
  - **his** own shadow; of (see pg 111): stram$_{brm}$

Fear: ...
- **sighing**, with (see pg 111)
- **snakes**, of (see pg 111)
- **solitude**, of (see pg 111)
- **spiders**, of (see pg 111)
- **spoken** to, when (see pg 111)
- **starting**, with (see pg 111)
- **starving**, of (see pg 111)
- **strangers**, of (see pg 112)
- **struck**:
  - **approaching** him; of being struck by those (see pg 112): Arn$_{elg}$
- **sudden** (see pg 112): gels$_{dyc1}$ phos$_{dyc1}$ stram$_{dyc1}$
- **telephone**, of (see pg 112)
- **things**; of real and unreal (see pg 112): calc$_{frc}$
- **thunderstorm**, of (see pg 113): acon$_{dyc1}$ *Borx*$_{klp}$ caps$_{brm}$ hyos$_{dyc1}$ *Lyc*$_{ffd}$ *Nat-m*$_{brm}$ **PHOS**$_{ffd,klp}$ puls$_{brm}$ *Sep*$_{brm}$
  - **before** (see pg 113): gels$_{pkj1}$
- **touched**; of being:
  - **chest** wall; on (see pg 113)
  - **sore** parts; on (see pg 113)
- **train**; while travelling by: cham$_{brm}$
- **tremulous** (see pg 113)
- **trifles**, of (see pg 113): calc$_{ffd}$ caps$_{brm}$ *Lyc*$_{ffd,klp}$ nux-v$_{brm}$
- **tunnels**; of (see pg 113): **STRAM**$_{brm}$
- **unfamiliar** objects (see pg 113): acon$_{brm}$ ars$_{dyc}$ calc$_{brm}$ cupr$_{sld}$ hyos$_{dyc}$
- **urinating**, after (see pg 113)
- **vertigo**; of (see pg 113)
- **vexation**; after (see pg 113)
- **voices**; of:
  - **loud**: phos$_{brm}$
- **waking**, on (see pg 113)
- **warm** room:
  - **of** (see pg 113)
- **washed**; of being (see pg 113)
- **wasps**; of (see pg 113)
- **water**, of (see pg 113)
  - **legs** in the water; goes only with: phos$_{hnb}$
- **wind**, of (see pg 113): arn$_{elg}$ lyc$_{brm,ffd}$ nux-v$_{brm}$ phos$_{ffd}$

FEARLESS (see pg 114): *Ign*$_{fmx}$ sil$_{fmx}$

FECES:
- **covering** feces:
  - **not** covering feces in litter box: lyc$_{brm}$
- **licks** up cow-dung, mud, saliva (see pg 114)
- **passed** on the floor (see pg 114)
- **swallows** feces:
  - **animals**; of (see pg 114): calc$_{frc}$ lyc$_{frc}$ nux-v$_{frc}$ sep$_{brm}$
    - **different** species; of:
    - **same** species; of the: calc$_{brm}$ sulph$_{brm}$
  - **human** feces: syph$_{brm}$
  - **own**; his (see pg 114): calc$_{frc}$ merc$_{brm}$ sulph$_{brm}$ tritic$_{sxj}$

FEIGNING:
- **fainting** (see pg 114)
- **pregnancy** (see pg 114)
- **sick**; to be (see pg 114)

FIGHT, wants to (see pg 114)

FLATTERED:
- **aversion** to be (see pg 114)
- **desire** to be (see pg 114)

FLATTERING (see pg 114)

FOOLISH behavior (see pg 115)

FORSAKEN feeling (see pg 116): *Calc-s* frc
- **morning** (see pg 116)
- **evening** (see pg 116)
- **air** amel.; in open (see pg 116)
- **beloved** by his parents, wife, friends; feeling of not being (see pg 116)
- **waking**, on (see pg 116)
- **weaning**; when:

FORSAKING:
- **children**; his own (see pg 116): sep frc

FRIGHTENED easily:
- **noon** (see pg 117)
- **evening** (see pg 117)
- **night** (see pg 117)
- **chill**, during (see pg 117)
- **closing** the eyes (see pg 117)
- **fever**, during (see pg 117)
- **going** to sleep; on (see pg 117)
- **menses**:
  - **before** (see pg 117)
- **pains**, from (see pg 117)
- **pollutions**, after (see pg 117)
- **shadow**, his own (see pg 117): stram brm
- **touch**, from (see pg 117): nat-c qqh
- **trifles**, at (see pg 117)
- **urinating**; before (see pg 117)
- **wakens**:
  - **noise**; in a fright from least (see pg 117): lach frc,qqh lyc qqh
- **waking**, on (see pg 117)

GESTURES, makes:
- **angry** (see pg 118)
- **arms** or legs; involuntary motions of:
  - **sleep**; during:
- **automatic** (see pg 118)
- **awkward** in (see pg 118)
- **convulsive** (see pg 118)
- **frightful** (see pg 118)
- **hands**; involuntary motions of the:
  - **strong** motions:
    - **sleep**; during: sulph brm
- **light** (see pg 119)
- **repeating** the same actions:
  - **box** walking: cann-i hnb

Gestures, makes – **repeating** the same actions: ...
- **crib** biting:
- **playing** with a ball; obsessed by:
- **tongue** moving to and fro:
- **weaving**:
- **wind**-sucking:
- **ridiculous** or foolish (see pg 120)
- **strange** attitudes and positions (see pg 120): med frc
- **tics**; nervous (see pg 120)
- **violent** (see pg 120)

GOING OUT; aversion to (see pg 120)

GOURMAND (see pg 120)

GREED, cupidity (see pg 120)

GRIEF:
- **castration**; after:
- **condition**; about his (see pg 121): ign frc nat-m frc sep frc
- **offenses**; from long past (see pg 121)
- **ovariectomy**; after:
- **past** events, about (see pg 121)
- **prolonged** (see pg 121)
- **silent** (see pg 121): *Ph-ac* brm
- **trifles**, over (see pg 121)
- **waking**, on (see pg 121)

GRIMACES:
- **strange** faces; makes (see pg 121)

GROWLING:
- **children**; at: phos brm
- **dog**; at any male: nat-m brm
- **sleep**; when disturbed in: nux-v brm sep brm
- **strangers**; at (see pg 121): puls brm
  - **commanded** by them; if: caust brm

GRUMBLING (see pg 121)
- **night** (see pg 121)

GRUNTING:
- **angry**, when (see pg 121)
- **sleep**, during (see pg 121)

HARD for inferiors and kind for superiors (see pg 121): lyc elg,ffd,hnb

HARDHEARTED (see pg 121)

HATRED (see pg 122): staph dyc1
- **persons**:
  - **offended** him; hatred of persons who (see pg 122)
  - **owner** offended him; after the:
- **revengeful**; hatred and (see pg 122)

HAUGHTY (see pg 122)
- **pregnancy**, during (see pg 122)

HEEDLESS (see pg 122): ign fmx sil fmx

HELD:
- **amel.** being held (see pg 122)
- **desire** to be held (see pg 122)

HELPLESSNESS; feeling of (see pg 122)
- **cats**; towards other: puls brm

HIDING:
- **bones** and other eatable items: sep$_{brm}$
- **children**; her:
- **food**; desire to hide: ars$_{frc}$ calc$_{frc}$ sep$_{frc}$ sulph$_{frc}$
- **himself** (see pg 123): acon$_{klp}$ **Bell**$_{fmx}$ calc$_{klp}$ mag-c$_{brm}$ op$_{brm}$ *Puls*$_{fmx}$ *Stram*$_{klp}$ ter$_{fmx}$
  - **bed**; under the: ign$_{brm}$ sulph$_{brm}$
  - **dark** places; in: chin$_{brm}$
  - **fear**, on account of (see pg 123): med$_{brm}$
    : **owner**; behind the:
    : **dogs**; from fear of: sil$_{brm}$
    : **vet**; from fear of: lyc$_{hnb}$
  - **flatus** has been noticed: ashamed that: nat-m$_{hnb}$

HIGH PLACES:
- **desire**: merc$_{frc}$

HIGH-SPIRITED (see pg 123)

HISSING [cats, etc.; of]
- **neighbors**; at:
  - **feeding** him; when they are: sep$_{brm}$

HOME:
- **desires** to go (see pg 123)
- **leave** home:
  - **aversion** to:
    : **alone**; when: sep$_{brm}$
  - **desire** to (see pg 123): nat-m$_{brm}$ puls$_{brm}$ ther$_{brm}$
    : **night**; at (see pg 123): phos$_{brm}$

HOMESICKNESS (see pg 123): *Calc* $_{ffd}$
- **silent** ill humor, with (see pg 123)

HOMOSEXUALITY:

HOUSE:
- **in** the house; being:
  - **aversion** being kept in the house (see pg 124): puls$_{brm}$
    : **night**: phos$_{brm}$

HOWLING (see pg 124)
- **night** (see pg 124): stram$_{lkk}$

HUMANS:
- **animal** only loves humans:

HUNTING:
- **excessively**: med$_{brm}$

HURRY:
- **always** in a (see pg 124): arg-n$_{frc}$
- **awkward** from hurry (see pg 124)
- **drinking**, on (see pg 124): cham$_{brm}$
- **eating**; while (see pg 124): arg-n$_{qqh}$ calc$_{frc}$ phos$_{frc}$ sulph$_{frc}$
- **menses**:
  - **before**:
  - **during** (see pg 124)
- **movements**, in (see pg 124)
- **trifles**; about (see pg 124)
- **walking**, while (see pg 125)
- **work**, in (see pg 125): sulph$_{brm}$

HYDROPHOBIA (see pg 125)

HYSTERIA:
- **changing** symptoms (see pg 126)
- **discharges**; after suppression of (see pg 126)
- **fainting**, hysterical (see pg 126)
- **fright**:
  - **after** (see pg 126)
- **grief**, from (see pg 126)
- **hemorrhage**:
  - **after** (see pg 126)
  - **with** (see pg 126)
- **injure** herself; desire to:
- **looked** at; when (see pg 126)
- **loss** of:
  - **blood**; after (see pg 126)
  - **fluids**; after:
- **menopause**; at (see pg 126)
- **menses**:
  - **after** (see pg 126)
  - **before** (see pg 126)
  - **during** (see pg 126)
- **moon**:
  - **increasing** agg.:
- **music** amel. (see pg 126)
- **pregnancy** and delivery; during (see pg 126)
- **puberty**, at (see pg 126)
- **sexual**:
  - **excesses**, after (see pg 126)
  - **excitement**; from suppression of sexual (see pg 126)
- **veterinarian**; when being at the: nux-v$_{brm}$ tarent$_{wha}$

IDIOCY:
- **bite**; desire to (see pg 127)
- **idiotic** actions (see pg 127)
- **masturbation**; after (see pg 127)
- **shrill** shrieking, with (see pg 127)

IMBECILITY:
- **epilepsy**; before (see pg 127)
- **sexual** excitement, with (see pg 127)
- **shrieks** when occupying with him (see pg 127)

IMITATION, mimicry (see pg 127)

IMPATIENCE (see pg 127)
- **always**:
- **children**; about his (see pg 128)
- **contradiction**; at slightest (see pg 128)
- **convulsions**:
  - **before**:
- **coryza**, with (see pg 128)
- **heat**, with (see pg 128)
- **itching**, from (see pg 128)
- **pain**, from (see pg 128)
- **perspiration**, during (see pg 128)
- **room**, in a warm crowded (see pg 128)
- **tossing** about (see pg 128)
- **trifles**, about (see pg 128)
- **urinating**; before (see pg 128)

- **waking**, on:
- **walking**, while (see pg 128)
- **IMPETUOUS** (see pg 128)
- **heat**, with (see pg 128)
- **perspiration**, with (see pg 128)
- **urination**; before (see pg 128)
- **IMPRESSIONABLE** (see pg 128)
- **unpleasantly** impressed by everything:
- **IMPULSE;** morbid (see pg 128)
- **rash** (see pg 128)
- **run**; to (see pg 129)
- **sexual** (see pg 129)
- **violence**, to do (see pg 129)
- **IMPULSIVE** (see pg 129)
- **INCONSOLABLE**:
- **alone**; agg. when (see pg 129)
- **suicide**, even to:
- **INDEPENDENT** (see pg 129)
- **INDIFFERENCE** (see pg 129): *Calc*$_{elg}$
- **adverse** circumstances; to (see pg 130)
- **air**, in open (see pg 130)
- **anxiety**, after (see pg 130)
- **caresses**, to (see pg 130)
- **children**; towards:
  - **mother** towards her children; indifference of (see pg 130): **SEP**$_{hnb}$
- **coition**:
  - **after** (see pg 130)
  - **during** (see pg 130)
- **company**, society:
  - **to** (see pg 130)
  - **while** in (see pg 130)
- **concussion** of brain, after:
- **desire**, nor action of the will; has no (see pg 130)
- **ennui**, with (see pg 130)
- **epilepsy**, in:
- **everything**, to (see pg 130)
- **excitement**, after (see pg 130)
- **exertion**:
  - **after** (see pg 130)
  - **during**:
- **external** things; to (see pg 131)
  - **false** pregnancy; during: sulph$_{brm}$
- **family**, to his (see pg 131)
- **fever**, during (see pg 131): *Apis*$_{qqh}$ *Arn*$_{qqh}$
- **irritability**, with: sep$_{frc}$
- **joy** of others; to (see pg 131)
- **joyless** (see pg 131): sil$_{brm}$
- **lies** with eyes closed (see pg 131)
- **life**, to (see pg 131)
- **loved** ones, to (see pg 131)
- **masturbation**, after (see pg 131)
- **menopause**; in: lach$_{frc}$

- **Indifference**: ...
- **menses**:
  - **before** (see pg 131) ·
  - **during** (see pg 131)
- **mental** exertion:
  - **after** (see pg 131)
  - **during** (see pg 0)
- **morose** (see pg 131)
- **others**, toward (see pg 131)
  - **partner**; except towards the: caust$_{brm}$
- **owners**; to (see pg 131): phos$_{brm}$
  - **coming** home; when owners are: syph$_{brm}$
- **pain**:
  - **to** pain (see pg 131)
- **playing**; to: calc-p$_{brm}$ sulph$_{brm}$
- **pleasure**, to (see pg 131)
- **puberty**, in (see pg 131)
- **relations**, to (see pg 131)
- **reprimands**, to all (see pg 131)
- **sadness**; with (see pg 131): sep$_{bnfl.es}$
- **sex**; to opposite (see pg 131)
- **sleepiness**, with (see pg 131)
- **stool**, after (see pg 131)
- **surroundings**, to the (see pg 131)
- **taciturn** (see pg 131)
- **vexation** with distress in stomach; after least:
- **weather**:
  - **stormy** (see pg 131)
- **INDIGNATION**:
- **alternating** with:
  - **mirth** (see pg 132)
- **pregnant**, while (see pg 132)
- **INITIATIVE**, lack of (see pg 132)
- **INJUSTICE**, cannot support (see pg 132)
- **INSANITY**:
- **amenorrhea**, from:
- **anger**, from (see pg 133)
- **anxiety**, with (see pg 133)
- **apoplexy**:
  - **after** (see pg 133)
- **brutal** (see pg 133)
- **bulimia**; with (see pg 133)
- **cheerful**, gay (see pg 133)
- **chilliness**, with (see pg 133)
- **company**; with desire for:
  - **light**; and:
- **convulsions**, with (see pg 133)
- **crazy** person; behaves like a (see pg 133)
- **despair**; with:
- **dictatorial** (see pg 133)
- **eating**:
  - **dirt** (see pg 133)
  - **dung** (see pg 133)
  - **refuses** to eat:
- **envy**, with:
- **erotic**:
  - **menses**:

- **erotic** – **menses**: ...
  - after:
    - before (see pg 133)
- **eruptions**; after suppressed (see pg 133)
- **escape**, desire to (see pg 133)
- **foolish**, ridiculous (see pg 133)
- **fright**, from (see pg 133)
- **grief**, from (see pg 133)
- **heat**; with (see pg 133)
- **hemorrhage**, after (see pg 133)
- **hysterical** (see pg 133)
- **injuries** to the head, from (see pg 133)
- **jealousy**; from:
- **ketosis**; in:
- **lascivious** (see pg 133)
- **loquacious** (see pg 133)
- **love**; from disappointed (see pg 133)
- **malicious** (see pg 133)
- **masturbation**, from (see pg 133)
- **melancholy** (see pg 134)
- **menopause**, during (see pg 134)
- **menses**:
  - before (see pg 134)
  - during (see pg 134)
  - suppressed, with (see pg 134)
- **mental** exertion; from (see pg 134)
- **mild**:
- **mortification**:
  - fear of; from:
  - from (see pg 134)
- **neuralgia**:
  - disappearance of; with (see pg 134)
  - face; with neuralgia of:
- **noisy**:
- **old** people; in (see pg 134)
- **pain**; from intolerable (see pg 134)
- **paralysis**, with (see pg 134)
- **paroxysmal** (see pg 134)
- **periodical** (see pg 134)
- **perspiration**:
  - fits of insanity followed by perspiration (see pg 134)
- **pregnancy**, in (see pg 134)
- **puerperal** (see pg 134)
- **quarrelsome** (see pg 134)
- **restlessness**, with (see pg 134)
- **sexual** excesses, from (see pg 134)
- **silent** (see pg 134)
- **sleeplessness**, with (see pg 134)
- **staring** of eyes (see pg 134)
- **strength**; with increased (see pg 134)
- **suicidal** disposition, with (see pg 134)
- **threatening** destruction and death (see pg 134)
- **touched**, will not be (see pg 134)
- **travel**, with desire to (see pg 134)
- **urinating** on the floor (see pg 134)
- **wantonness**, with (see pg 135)

INSECURITY; mental:
- **working**; while: plb$_{brm}$

INTERRUPTION:
- **agg.** (see pg 135)
- **aversion** to (see pg 135)
- **intolerance** (see pg 135)

INTROSPECTION (see pg 135)

IRRESOLUTION:
- **acts**, in (see pg 136): sil$_{frc}$
- **anxious**:
- **bathing**; if he should go: puls$_{brm}$
- **changeable** (see pg 136)
- **laziness**; with (see pg 136)
- **trifles**, about (see pg 136): sil$_{frc}$
- **waking**, on (see pg 136)

IRRITABILITY (see pg 136)
- **day** and night (see pg 136)
- **daytime** (see pg 136)
- **morning** (see pg 137)
- **forenoon** (see pg 137)
- **noon** (see pg 137)
- **afternoon** (see pg 137)
- **evening** (see pg 137)
- **night** (see pg 137)
  - waking, on:
    - walk; having to go for the last: phos$_{brm}$
  - walking agg.:
- **abortion**:
  - in:
  - threatened, in:
- **air**, in open (see pg 137)
- **alone**:
  - when (see pg 137)
  - wishes to be alone (see pg 137)
- **anxiety**, with (see pg 137)
- **aroused**, when (see pg 137)
- **cardiac** symptoms, with (see pg 138)
- **castration**; after:
- **cats**; towards:
  - other cats in the same household: puls$_{brm}$
- **causeless** (see pg 138)
- **children**, in (see pg 138)
- **chill**, during (see pg 138)
- **coition**:
  - after (see pg 138)
  - amel. (see pg 138)
- **cold**; after taking (see pg 138)
- **consolation**:
  - agg. (see pg 138)
- **contradiction**; from (see pg 138)
- **convulsions**:
  - before (see pg 138)
    - epileptic (see pg 138)
  - between (see pg 138)
- **cough**, from (see pg 138)
- **delivery**, during (see pg 138)
- **dentition**, during (see pg 138)
- **diabetes**, in (see pg 138)
- **diarrhea**:
  - after (see pg 138)

- **disturbed**, when (see pg 138): nux-v$_{frc}$ sulph$_{frc}$
- **dogs**; towards (see pg 138): tarent$_{brm}$
  - **dark** dogs; towards: lyc$_{brm}$
  - **male** dogs; towards: caust$_{brm}$ lyc$_{brm}$ phos$_{brm}$ stram$_{brm}$
  - **puppies**; towards: **Staph**$_{brm}$
  - **sniffing**; who are:
    - **front**; from the: nat-m$_{brm}$
- **dominant** animals; in:
- **easily** (see pg 138)
- **estrus**:
  - **after**:
  - **before**:
  - **during**:
- **excited**, when (see pg 138)
- **exertion**; from (see pg 138)
- **family**, to her (see pg 138)
- **females**; in:
  - **females** of another species; towards:
  - **females** of the same species; towards:
- **fever**; during: nux-v$_{qqh}$
- **grief**, from (see pg 138)
- **handled**; being:
- **heat**:
  - **after** (see pg 139)
  - **during** (see pg 139)
- **impotence**, with (see pg 139)
- **itching**, from (see pg 139)
- leukorrhea ceases; as soon as:
- liver trouble, in:
- **looked** at (see pg 139)
- **loved** ones, to (see pg 139)
- **masturbation**, after (see pg 139)
- **medical** examination; during: cham$_{hnb}$ nux-v$_{hnb}$
- **menopause**; during (see pg 139)
- **menses**:
  - **after** (see pg 139)
  - **before** (see pg 139)
  - **during** (see pg 139)
- **mental** exertion; from (see pg 139)
- **noise**, from (see pg 139)
- **ovariectomy**; after:
- **ovariohysterectomy**; after:
- **pain**, during (see pg 139)
  - **colic**; from (see pg 139): cham$_{hnb}$ op$_{brm}$
- **people**; with (see pg 139): lyc$_{brm}$
- **perspiration**, during (see pg 139)
- **pregnancy**, during (see pg 139)
- **prolapsus** uteri, in (see pg 139)
- **puberty**, in (see pg 139)
- **quarreling**; when owners are: phos$_{brm}$
- **remorse**; with easy and quick (see pg 139)
- **sadness**, with (see pg 139)
- **sexual** desire; from loss of (see pg 139)
- **sexual** excesses; from (see pg 139)
- **sexual** excitement; from:
- **sexual** weakness; with:
- **sleep**; when aroused by noise during (see pg 140)
- **spoken** to, when (see pg 140)

Irritability: ...
- **sudden** (see pg 140)
- **suspicious** (see pg 140)
- **taciturn** (see pg 140)
- **thunderstorm**:
  - **before** (see pg 140)
  - **touch**, by (see pg 140)
    - **Feet**; of the: phos$_{brm}$
- **trifles**, from (see pg 140)
- **waking**, on (see pg 140): tarent$_{wha}$
  - **alone**; when: tarent$_{wha}$
- **warm** room, in (see pg 140)
- **water**; on hearing or seeing (see pg 140)
- **weather**; in rainy or cloudy (see pg 140)
- **worm** affections; in (see pg 140)

JEALOUSY (see pg 140): calc$_{ffd}$ canth$_{dyc}$ **HYOS**$_{dyc}$ **LACH**$_{dyc,hnb}$ lyc$_{ffd}$ murx$_{pkj1}$ orig$_{pkj1}$ plat$_{pkj1}$
- **animal** or an inanimate object; for (see pg 140)
- **children**:
  - **between** (see pg 140)
  - **in** (see pg 140)
- **crime**, to a (see pg 140)
- **irrational** (see pg 140)
- **irresistible** as foolish as it is (see pg 140)
- **kill**, driving to (see pg 140): lach$_{frc,itm}$
- **loquacity**, with (see pg 140)
- **love**; from disappointed (see pg 140)
- **people** around, of (see pg 140)
- **quarrelling**, reproaches and scolding; with (see pg 140)
- **rage**, with (see pg 140)
- **sadness**, with (see pg 140)
- **sexual** excitement, with:
- **toys**; about: stram$_{brm}$
- **vindictive**: lach$_{frc}$ lyc$_{frc}$ nux-v$_{frc}$
- **women**:
  - **between** (see pg 141)
  - **in**:

JOY (see pg 141)

JUMPING:
- **aversion** to jump into the car: sep$_{brm}$
- **children**; in (see pg 141)
- **convulsions**:
  - **after**:
- **impulse** to jump (see pg 141)
- **suddenly**, as from pain (see pg 142)

KICKING:
- **children**; in (see pg 142)
  - **carried**; child becomes stiff and kicks when (see pg 142)
- **legs**; with:
  - **convulsions**; during (see pg 142)
- **sleep**, in (see pg 142)
- **veterinarian** or the owner; the:
  - **anger**; from:
  - **fear**; from:
    - **medical** examination; during:

- **veterinarian** or the owner; the
  - **medical** examination; during: nux-v$_{hnb}$
  - **pain**; from:
    - medical examination; during:
  - **reason**; without:
  - **warning**; without: nat-m$_{hnb}$
- **wall**; the:
  - **food** first; if other animals get their: aur$_{hnb}$
- **worm**-complaints; during (see pg 142)

KILL; desire to:
- **anger**; from:
- **beloved** ones (see pg 142)
- **child**, the own:
  - **delivery**; during:
- **children**; in:
  - **parents**; to kill the (see pg 142)
- **contradicts** her; the person that (see pg 142)
- **everyone** he sees (see pg 142)
- **fear**; desire to kill from:
- **herself**; sudden impulse to (see pg 142)
- **menses**:
  - **before** (see pg 142)
  - **during** (see pg 142)
- **offense**; sudden impulse to kill for a slight (see pg 142)
- **sudden** impulse to kill (see pg 142)

KLEPTOMANIA (see pg 142)
- **food**; stealing: calc$_{frc}$ phos$_{frc}$ sulph$_{frc}$
  - **neighbor**; from:

KNIFE; cannot look at a (see pg 142)

LAMENTING (see pg 143): *Calc*$_{ffd}$ **Lyc**$_{ffd}$

LASCIVIOUS (see pg 143)
- **erections**:
  - **with**:
- **followed** by:
  - **epilepsy**:
- **impotence**, with (see pg 143)
- **prostate**; with enlarged (see pg 143)

LAZINESS:
- **air**, in open (see pg 146)
  - **amel.** (see pg 146)
- **amenorrhea**, in:
- **anger**, after:
- **children**, in (see pg 146)
- **chill**, during (see pg 146)
- **coition**, after (see pg 146)
- **eating**, after (see pg 146)
- **masturbation**, after:
- **nervous** exhaustion, in:
- **paddock** or riding hall; in: nat-m$_{brm}$
- **physical** (see pg 146)
- **sadness**, from (see pg 146)
- **sleep**, after (see pg 146)
- **sleepiness**, with (see pg 146): sulph$_{frc}$
- **sudden** (see pg 147)
- **waking**, on (see pg 147)

Laziness: ...
- **walking**:
  - **while** (see pg 147)
- **weather**; in damp (see pg 147)

LEAD TYPE BEHAVIOR:
- **alpha** type:
- **beta** type:
- **omega** type:

LIE on bare floor; wants to (see pg 147)

LIGHT:
- **aversion** to (see pg 147)
- **desire** for (see pg 147)

LOATHING:
- **general** loathing (see pg 147)

LOOKED AT; to be:
- **cannot** bear to be looked at (see pg 148): lyc$_{ffd}$ nux-v$_{ffd}$
- **evading** the look of other persons:
  - **spoken** to; when (see pg 148): plb$_{hnb}$

LOOKING:
- **not** looking:
  - **owner**; at the:
    - absent; when he has been:
      - **days**; for some: nat-m$_{dyc}$ staph$_{dyc}$
      - **hours**; for some: ign$_{hnb}$
- **wall**; is looking at the: aur$_{brm}$

LOQUACITY (see pg 148)
- **daytime** (see pg 148)
- **afternoon** (see pg 148)
- **evening** (see pg 148)
- **night** (see pg 148)
- **alternating** with:
  - **sadness** (see pg 148)
  - **taciturnity** (see pg 148)
- **chill**, during (see pg 149)
- **coughing**:
  - **after** (see pg 149)
- **excited** (see pg 149)
- **fever**; during (see pg 149)
- **insane** (see pg 149)
- **menopause**; during (see pg 149)
- **menses**:
  - **during** (see pg 149)
- **mental** exertion, after (see pg 149)
- **perspiration**, during (see pg 149)
- **pregnancy**, during (see pg 149)
- **rapid** (see pg 149)
- **sleep**, during (see pg 149)
- **vivacious** (see pg 149)

MAGNETIZED:
- **amel.** (see pg 150)
- **easily** magnetized (see pg 150)

MALICIOUS (see pg 150): *Lach*$_{hnb}$

- **anger**, with (see pg 150)
- **loved** ones, to (see pg 150)
- **sadness**, in (see pg 150)

MANIA:
- **alternating** with:
  - **depression** (see pg 150)
- **coldness**, with (see pg 150)
- **demonic** (see pg 150)
- **eruptions**; after suppressed (see pg 150)
- **fever**, during (see pg 150)
- **heat:**
  - **during** (see pg 150)
- **lascivious** (see pg 151)
- **lochia**, from suppressed (see pg 151)
- **menses:**
  - **before** (see pg 151)
  - **during** (see pg 151)
  - **suppressed**, after (see pg 151)
- **mental** exertion, after (see pg 151)
- **paroxysmal** (see pg 151)
- **periodical** (see pg 151)
- **perspiration**; with cold (see pg 151)
- **puerperal** (see pg 151)
- **scratching** themselves (see pg 151)
- **sexual** mania:
  - **increased** sexual desire; from (see pg 151)
  - **men**; in (see pg 151)
  - **women**, in (see pg 151)
- **shrieking** in (see pg 151)
- **spit** and bite at those around him, would (see pg 151)
- **trembling**, with (see pg 151)
- **violence**, with deeds of (see pg 151)

MANNISH:
- **behavior:**
  - **women**; in (see pg 151): aur$_{dyc,hnb}$ calc$_{dyc}$
    - **cover**; desire to:
      - **jumping** and clinging:
      - **marking** often with urine, like a male animal does: sep$_{hnb}$
      - **urination**; lifts leg during: lyc$_{brm}$ sep$_{hnb}$
- **women:**
  - **ovaries**; with cysts in:

MARKING WITH FECES: calc$_{klp}$ puls$_{klp}$

MEMORY:
- **active:**
  - **alternating** with:
    - **dullness** (see pg 152)
    - **lassitude** (see pg 152)
    - **weakness** of memory (see pg 152)
- **confused** (see pg 152)
- **loss** of memory:
  - **apoplexy**, after:
  - **coma**, after (see pg 152)
  - **concussion** of the brain; after (see pg 152)
  - **epileptic** fits, after (see pg 152)
  - **fear**, from:

Memory – loss of memory: ...
- **injuries**; after (see pg 153)
- **insanity**, in:
- **mental** exertion, from:
- **sunstroke**, after (see pg 153)
- **weakness** of memory:
  - **done**; for what he just has (see pg 153)
  - **everyday** things, for (see pg 153)
  - **faces**; for (see pg 153)
  - **facts**, for (see pg 153)
    - **past** facts; for (see pg 153)
  - **fright**; from:
  - **grief**, after (see pg 153)
  - **pain**; from (see pg 154)
  - **periodical** (see pg 154)
  - **persons**, for (see pg 154)
  - **sexual** excesses; from (see pg 154)
  - **sudden** and periodical (see pg 154)
  - **vexation** agg. (see pg 154)

MENOPAUSE agg. (see pg 154)

MENSES:
- **after** (see pg 154)
- **before** (see pg 154)
- **during** (see pg 154)
- **suppressed** menses; after (see pg 154)

MENTAL EXERTION:
- **agg.** (see pg 155)
- **amel.** (see pg 155)
- **aversion** to (see pg 155): Sil$_{brm}$
  - **estrus**; during: sep$_{brm}$
  - **menses**; during:
- **desire** for (see pg 155)

MENTAL SYMPTOMS:
- **abortion**; after: ign$_{dyc}$ puls-vg$_{dyc}$ sep$_{dyc}$
- **accompanied** by:
  - **Lyme** disease: tarent$_{brm}$
- **acute** mental symptoms (see pg 156)
- **alternating** with:
  - **physical** symptoms (see pg 156)

MILDNESS (see pg 156): Calc$_{ffd}$ **Nat-m**$_{ffd}$ **Puls**$_{ffd}$
- **epileptic** convulsions; after (see pg 156)

MIRTH:
- **air**; in open (see pg 157)
- **foolish** (see pg 157)
- **heat**; during (see pg 157)

MISANTHROPY (see pg 157)

MISCHIEVOUS (see pg 157)

MISTAKES; making:
- **localities**, in (see pg 157): sep$_{brm}$
- **space**; in:
  - **time**; and in (see pg 158)
- **time**, in (see pg 158)

MOANING:
- **daytime** (see pg 159)
- **morning** (see pg 159)
- **afternoon** (see pg 159)

- **evening** (see pg 159)
- **night** (see pg 159)
- **anxious** (see pg 159)
- **breath**; with every (see pg 159)
- **children**, in (see pg 159)
- **chill**, during (see pg 159)
- **constant** moaning and gasping for air (see pg 159)
- **contradicted**, when (see pg 159)
- **convulsions**, in (see pg 159)
- **cough**, during (see pg 159)
- **dentition**, in (see pg 159)
- **heat**, during (see pg 159): *Mur-ac* $_{qqh}$
- **honor**, from wounded (see pg 159)
- **ill** humor, from (see pg 159)
- **involuntary** (see pg 159)
- **lifted**, when (see pg 159)
- **menses**:
  · **after** (see pg 159)
  · **during** (see pg 159)
- **offense**, happened long ago; for trifling (see pg 159)
- **old** age, in (see pg 159)
- **pain**, from (see pg 159)
- **perspiration**, during (see pg 159)
- **pollutions**, after (see pg 159)
- **restlessness**, with (see pg 159)
- **sleep**, during (see pg 159)
- **stool**; before (see pg 159)
- **touch**, on (see pg 160)
- **trifle**, about every (see pg 160)
- **waking**, on (see pg 160)

MOOD:
- **agreeable** (see pg 160): phos$_{frc}$ puls$_{frc}$ verat$_{frc}$
- **alternating** (see pg 160)
- **changeable** (see pg 160)
- **insupportable** (see pg 160)
- **repulsive** (see pg 160)

MOONLIGHT agg. (see pg 160)

MOROSE:
- **daytime** (see pg 161)
- **morning** (see pg 161)
- **forenoon** (see pg 161)
- **noon** (see pg 161)
- **afternoon** (see pg 161)
- **evening** (see pg 161)
- **night** (see pg 161)
- **air**, in open (see pg 161)
- **alternating** with:
  · **affectionate** (see pg 161)
  · **cheerfulness** (see pg 161)
- **caressing** agg.:
- **causeless** (see pg 161)
- **children**, in (see pg 161)
- **chill**, during (see pg 161)
- **coition**, after (see pg 161)
- **contradiction**, by (see pg 162)

Morose: ...
- **convulsions**:
  · **before** (see pg 162)
- **cough**:
  · **before** fits of (see pg 162)
- **dentition**, in (see pg 162)
- **eating**, after (see pg 162)
- **epistaxis** amel. (see pg 162)
- **fever**:
  · **after** (see pg 162)
  · **during** (see pg 162)
- **hurry**, with (see pg 162)
- **interruption**, from (see pg 162)
- **menopause**; at (see pg 162)
- **menses**:
  · **after** (see pg 162)
  · **before** (see pg 162)
  · **during** (see pg 162)
  · **suppressed**, in (see pg 162)
- **pain**, after (see pg 162)
- **perspiration**, during (see pg 162)
- **puberty**, in (see pg 162)
- **taciturn** (see pg 162)
- **thunderstorm**, from (see pg 162)
- **trifles**, about (see pg 162)
- **waking**, on (see pg 162): Lyc$_{frc,qqh}$
- **walking** in open air; after (see pg 162)
- **weather**:
  · **bad**; from:
  · **cloudy**; from (see pg 162)
  · **rainy**; from (see pg 162)
- **worm** affection, in:

MUSIC:
- **agg.** (see pg 162)
- **amel.** (see pg 162)
- **aversion** to (see pg 162)
- **desire** for (see pg 163)
  · **didgeridoo**; listening to: aur$_{brm}$

MUTILATING his body (see pg 163): merc$_{frc}$ nux-v$_{frc}$ phos$_{frc}$ stram$_{brm}$ tub$_{frc}$

MUTTERING:
- **apoplexy**, in (see pg 163)

NAIVE:
- **intelligent**, but very (see pg 163)

NEGLECTING:
- **children**, her (see pg 163): lyc$_{frc}$ sep$_{frc}$

NIBBLE; desire to (see pg 164)

NOISE:
- **amel.** (see pg 164)
- **aversion** to (see pg 164)
- **inclination** to make noise (see pg 164)

NYMPHOMANIA (see pg 164): *Canth*$_{dyc1}$ *Ferul*$_{dyc1}$ gels$_{dyc1}$ **Hyos**$_{dyc1}$ hyper$_{gsd4}$ **ORIG**$_{dyc1}$ *Phos*$_{dyc1}$ pic-ac$_{dyc1}$ *Tarent*$_{dyc1}$

- **chorea**, with:
- **coition** agg. (see pg 164)
- **loquacity**, with (see pg 164)
- **menopause**; at (see pg 164)
- **menses**:
  - **after** (see pg 164)
  - **before** (see pg 164)
  - **during** (see pg 164)
  - **suppressed**, after (see pg 164)
- **metrorrhagia**, during (see pg 164)
- **pregnancy**, during (see pg 164)
- **puerperal** (see pg 164)
- **urination**; with frequent: plat$_{qqh}$ staph$_{qqh}$
- **worms**, from (see pg 164)
- **young** girl, in a (see pg 164)

OBSTINATE (see pg 164): Calc$_{ffd,gl3}$ *Crot-h*$_{ffd}$
nat-m$_{brm}$ **Nux-v**$_{gl3}$
- **alternating** with:
  - **mildness** (see pg 165)
- **children** (see pg 165)
- **eruption**, during (see pg 165)
- **fever**, during (see pg 165)
- **menorrhagia**, in (see pg 165)
- **menses**:
  - **during**:
    : **beginning** of menses (see pg 165)
  - **resists** wishes of others (see pg 165)
- **simpleton**, as a (see pg 165)

OCCUPATION:
- **amel.** (see pg 165)
- **desire** to (see pg 165)

OFFENDED, easily:
- **castration**; after:
- **ovariectomy**; after:

OPTIMISTIC:
- **weakness**; in spite of the (see pg 165): sulph$_{frc}$

OUTDOORS; staying:
- **desire** to stay outdoors:
  - **two** hours; staying outdoors exactly: sulph$_{brm}$

PATIENCE (see pg 166)

PERFIDIOUS (see pg 166)

PERSEVERANCE (see pg 166)

PERT (see pg 166)

PESSIMIST (see pg 166)

PICKING with the beak:
- **feathers**:
  - **others**; of:
  - **own**; his:

PLAYFUL (see pg 167)
- **alternating** with:
  - **sadness** (see pg 167)

PLAYING:
- **aversion** to play (see pg 167): lyc$_{brm}$

Playing – aversion to play: ...
  - **adults**; in (see pg 167): calc-p$_{brm}$ ign$_{brm}$ lyc$_{brm}$
    nat-m$_{brm}$ phos$_{brm}$ tab$_{brm}$
    : **cats**; with other: sil$_{brm}$
  - **children**; in (see pg 167): calc$_{brm}$ *Lyc*$_{ffd}$ nat-m$_{ffd}$
  - **observing**; only: calc-p$_{brm}$
  - **sticks**; with: sep$_{brm}$
- **desire** to play:
  - **breed**; only wants to play with dogs of the same:
    lyc$_{brm}$
  - **rude** way, in a: lyc$_{brm}$
  - **smaller** animals; only with: puls$_{brm}$
  - **toys**; with:
    : **animals**: phos$_{brm}$
    : **one** particular toy only; playing with: bell$_{brm}$
    sulph$_{brm}$

PLEASING:
- **desire** to please others (see pg 167): sulph$_{frc}$

PRECOCITY of children (see pg 168)

PREGNANCY:
- **during** pregnancy (see pg 168)

PRESUMPTUOUS (see pg 168)

PROSTRATION of mind (see pg 169): *Puls*$_{frc}$
- **abortion**, after (see pg 169)
- **anxiety**, after (see pg 169)
- **coition**, after (see pg 169)
- **convulsions**, from (see pg 169)
- **diarrhea**:
  - **suppression** of; prostration of mind from (see pg 169)
- **eating**, after (see pg 169)
- **epilepsy**, in (see pg 169)
- **excitement**, after (see pg 169)
- **eye** strain, from (see pg 169)
- **fever**:
  - **after**, prolonged (see pg 169)
  - **during** (see pg 169)
- **grief**; from (see pg 169)
- **heart** failure, with (see pg 169)
- **injuries**, from (see pg 169)
- **menses**:
  - **after** (see pg 169)
  - **before** (see pg 169)
  - **during**:
- **nursing**, after (see pg 169)
- **old** age, in (see pg 169)
- **pollutions**, after (see pg 169)
- **prostatic** complaints; in (see pg 169)
- **sexual** excesses; after (see pg 169)
- **trembling**, with (see pg 170)
- **trifles**, from (see pg 170)
- **vexation**, from (see pg 170)
- **waking**, on (see pg 170)

PUBERTY; in (see pg 170)

PULLING:
- **hair** (see pg 170): staph$_{brm}$

- **hair**: ...
  - **desire** to pull:
    - **her** own hair:
      - **alone**; when: staph$_{brm}$

QUARRELLING:
- **aversion** to (see pg 170)

QUARRELSOME:
- **anger**, without (see pg 170)
- **causeless** (see pg 170)
- **delivery**, during:
- **disturbed**, if (see pg 170)
- **dominant** animals; in:
- **family**, with her (see pg 170)
- **jealousy**; from (see pg 170): Lach$_{hnb}$
- **menses**:
  - **beginning** of; at:
  - **during** (see pg 171)
- **pains**:
  - **before** (see pg 171)
  - **during** (see pg 171)
- **pugnacious** (see pg 171)
- **recriminations** about trifles (see pg 171)
- **sleep**, in (see pg 171)
- **waking**, on (see pg 171)

QUEER:
- **gait**, in (see pg 171)
- **gestures**; in:
  - **Arms**; of (see pg 171)
  - **Head**; of (see pg 171)

QUICK to act (see pg 171)

QUIET disposition (see pg 171): Calc$_{brm}$ op$_{elg}$
- **delivery**, after:
- **heat**, during (see pg 171)
- **menses**, during (see pg 171)
- **noise**, intolerable to (see pg 171)
- **sleep**, after (see pg 171)

QUIET; wants to be:
- **pain**; during (see pg 171): phos$_{brm}$ ruta$_{brm}$
  - **colic**: nux-v$_{brm}$
- **repose** and tranquillity; desires (see pg 171)

QUIETED, cannot be:
- **carried**; only by being (see pg 171)

RAGE:
- **day** and night (see pg 171)
- **morning**:
  - **bed**; in (see pg 171)
- **evening** (see pg 171)
- **night** (see pg 171)
- **alone**, while (see pg 171)
- **alternating** with:
  - **anxiety** (see pg 171)
  - **cheerfulness** (see pg 171)
  - **convulsions** (see pg 171)
  - **fear** (see pg 172)
  - **loquacity** (see pg 172)

Rage – alternating with: ...
- **quiet**; desire to be (see pg 172)
- **sleep**:
- **unconsciousness**:
- **weeping** (see pg 172)
- **aroused**, when (see pg 172)
- **biting**, with (see pg 172)
- **chill**, during (see pg 172)
- **cold** applications to head amel. (see pg 172)
- **consolation**, from:
- **constant** (see pg 172)
- **contradiction**, from (see pg 172)
- **convulsions**; rage with (see pg 172)
- **delivery**, during:
- **delusion** puts him into rage (see pg 172)
- **drinking**, while (see pg 172)
- **epilepsy**:
  - **after** epilepsy; rage (see pg 172)
  - **with** epilepsy; rage (see pg 172)
- **flies**; from: lyc$_{elg}$
- **foaming** mouth, with (see pg 172)
- **followed** by:
  - **repentance** (see pg 172)
- **kill** people, tries to (see pg 172)
- **love**; from disappointed:
- **malicious** (see pg 172)
- **medicine**, from forcible administration of (see pg 172)
- **menses**:
  - **beginning** of; at (see pg 172)
  - **during** (see pg 172)
- **pain**, from (see pg 172)
- **paroxysms**, in (see pg 172)
- **shining** objects, from (see pg 172)
- **sleep**:
  - **followed** by continuous deep:
  - **in** (see pg 172)
- **staring** looks, with (see pg 172)
- **strength** increased (see pg 172)
- **suffering**, from (see pg 172)
- **suicidal** disposition, with (see pg 172)
- **taken** up, child on being:
- **tearing** clothes:
- **touch**, renewed by (see pg 172)
- **trifles**, at (see pg 172)
- **violent** (see pg 172)
- **water**, at sight of (see pg 172)
- **weeping**, with (see pg 172)
- **worm** affections; in (see pg 172)

RANKING:
- **alpha** type: aur$_{hnb,klp}$ lyc$_{hnb,klp}$ plat$_{klp}$ sep$_{hnb}$ sulph$_{klp}$
- **beta** type:
- **omega** type: calc$_{klp}$ carc$_{klp}$ puls$_{klp}$

RASH (see pg 172): hep$_{frc}$ merc$_{frc}$ nux-v$_{frc}$

RECOGNIZING:
- **not** recognize; does:
  - anyone (see pg 173)
  - relatives; his (see pg 173)

REFUSING:
- **everything** offered to him (see pg 173)
- **help** (see pg 173): sil_ffc
- **medicine**; to take the (see pg 173)
- **treatment**; every (see pg 173)

REMORSE:
- **menses**, after (see pg 174)
- **quickly**, repents (see pg 174)
- **trifles**, about (see pg 174)

RESERVED (see pg 174): lyc_ffd **Nat-m**_ffd nux-v_brm
- **menses**, during (see pg 175)

RESIGNATION (see pg 175): sulph_brm

RESPONSIVE (see pg 175)

REST:
- **cannot** rest when things are not in the proper place (see pg 175)
- **desire** for (see pg 175)

RESTLESSNESS (see pg 175): **Tarent**_brm
- **day** and night (see pg 176)
- **daytime** (see pg 176)
- **morning** (see pg 176)
- **forenoon** (see pg 176)
- **noon** (see pg 176)
- **afternoon** (see pg 176)
- **evening** (see pg 176)
- **night**:
  - midnight:
    - before (see pg 176)
    - at (see pg 176)
    - after (see pg 176)
  - heart; from uneasiness about (see pg 176)
  - mewing the whole night; cat is: nat-m_brm phos_brm
  - waking; on (see pg 176)
- **air**; in open:
  - amel. (see pg 176)
- **alone**, when (see pg 176)
- **anger**; restlessness from (see pg 177)
- **anxious** (see pg 177)
- **barking**; with: phos_brm
- **cardiac** symptoms, with (see pg 177)
- **children**, in (see pg 177)
- **chill**:
  - beginning of; at (see pg 177)
  - during (see pg 177)
- **coition**:
  - after (see pg 177)
  - during (see pg 177)
- **company**, in (see pg 177)
- **convulsions**:
  - after (see pg 177)
  - before (see pg 178)

Restelessness: ...
- **coughing**, with (see pg 178)
- **delivery**, during (see pg 178)
- **drives** him from place to place (see pg 178)
- **driving** about (see pg 178)
- **eating** (see pg 178)
  - after (see pg 178)
- **eructation**, from insufficient (see pg 178)
- **eruptions**:
- **exertion**, after (see pg 178)
- **false** pregnancy; during: lyc_brm
- **fear**; from (see pg 178)
- **feverish** (see pg 178): acon_qqh
- **followed** by:
  - faintness (see pg 178)
  - sadness:
- **heat**:
  - after (see pg 178)
  - during (see pg 178)
- **hemorrhages**; after (see pg 178)
- **hysterical** (see pg 178)
- **internal** (see pg 178)
- **lying**, while (see pg 178)
  - cannot lie down: lyc_brm
- **medical** examination; during: tarent_brm
- **menopause**; at (see pg 178)
- **menses**:
  - after (see pg 178)
  - before (see pg 178)
  - during (see pg 178)
  - suppressed, during (see pg 178)
- **mental** exertion:
  - amel. (see pg 178)
  - during (see pg 178)
- **metrorrhagia**, during (see pg 178)
- **moon**:
  - full moon; during:
    - hurting oneself because of restlessness: calc_hnb
- **motion**:
  - agg. (see pg 179)
  - amel. (see pg 179)
- **move**:
  - must constantly (see pg 179)
  - weak to; but too:
- **nausea**:
  - from (see pg 179)
  - with (see pg 179)
- **noise**; from: tab_brm
  - stable; in the:
- **pain**, from (see pg 179)
- **paroxysms**:
  - after (see pg 179)
  - during (see pg 179)
- **periodical** (see pg 179)
- **perspiration**:
  - amel. (see pg 179)
  - during (see pg 179)

- **pregnancy**, during (see pg 179)
- **room**, in (see pg 179)
- **sadness**:
  - **with** (see pg 179)
- **sexual** excitement, in (see pg 179)
- **sitting**, while (see pg 179)
- **sleep**:
  - **before** (see pg 179)
  - **loss** of sleep; from (see pg 179)
  - **starting** from; on (see pg 179)
- **sleepiness**, with (see pg 179)
- **stable**; in the:
- **strangers**:
  - **presence** of strangers agg. (see pg 179)
- **thunderstorm**:
  - **before** (see pg 179): rhod_{brm}
  - **during** (see pg 179)
- **travelling** by car; while:
- **tremulous** (see pg 179)
- **urinary** complaints; during:
- **urination**:
  - **before** (see pg 179)
- **waking**, on (see pg 179)
- **walking**, while (see pg 179)
- **warm**:
  - **bed** (see pg 179)
  - **room** (see pg 179)
- **weaning**; after: acon_{elg} ign_{elg}
- **working**, while (see pg 180): phos_{brm}

RETIRING:

RIDING:
- **car**, in a:
  - **agg.**:
  - **aversion** to:
- **carriage**; in a:
  - **aversion** to (see pg 180): caps_{brm}
  - **desire** to (see pg 180): cham_{frc} lyc_{frc} tub_{hnb}

ROCKING:
- **agg.** (see pg 180)
- **amel.** (see pg 180)
- **desire** for being rocked (see pg 180)

ROLLING:
- **dirt**; in his own (see pg 180)
- **feces** or cow-dung; in: carc_{brm} sep_{brm}
  - **never**: lyc_{brm}
- **floor**; on the (see pg 180)
- **side** to side (see pg 180)

RUDENESS (see pg 180): sulph_{brm}

RUNS about:
- **dangerous** places, in most (see pg 181)
- **fright**, as if in (see pg 181)
- **menses**:
  - **before** (see pg 181)
- **paroxysms**, agg. evening; runs in (see pg 181)
- **room**, in (see pg 181)
- **streets**; in:

Runs about – **streets**; in: ...
  - **night**:
- **unsteady** (see pg 0)

SADNESS:
- **day** and night (see pg 181)
- **daytime** (see pg 181)
- **morning** (see pg 181)
- **noon** (see pg 181)
- **afternoon** (see pg 182)
- **evening** (see pg 182)
- **night** (see pg 182)
- **air**, in open (see pg 182)
- **alone**:
  - **when** (see pg 182)
- **amenorrhea**, in:
- **anger**:
  - **after** (see pg 182)
  - **from** (see pg 182)
- **anxious** (see pg 183)
- **canine** hunger, with (see pg 183)
- **causeless** (see pg 183)
- **cheerfulness**, after (see pg 183)
- **children**, in (see pg 183)
- **coition**, after (see pg 183)
- **cold**, from becoming (see pg 183)
- **company**:
  - **agg.** (see pg 183)
  - **amel.** (see pg 183)
  - **aversion** to company, desire for solitude (see pg 183)
  - **desire** for company (see pg 183)
- **continence**, from (see pg 183)
- **coughing**:
  - **after** (see pg 183)
  - **during**:
- **darkness**, in (see pg 183)
- **delivery**:
  - **after** (see pg 183)
  - **during** (see pg 183)
- **diarrhea**:
  - **during** (see pg 183)
  - **suppressed**; from (see pg 183)
- **disappointment**, from (see pg 183)
- **disease**, about (see pg 183)
- **eating**:
  - **after** (see pg 183)
  - **before** (see pg 183)
  - **while** (see pg 183)
- **epilepsy**:
- **epistaxis**, after (see pg 183)
- **errors** of diet, from (see pg 183)
- **eruptions**:
  - **suppressed** eruptions; with (see pg 183)
- **estrus**:
  - **after**:
  - **before**:
  - **during**:

- excitement:
  - after (see pg 183)
- exertion, after (see pg 183)
- fear:
  - from (see pg 184)
- flowers; from smell of (see pg 184)
- friends, as if having lost affection of (see pg 184)
- grief, after (see pg 184)
- heart; from:
  - affections (see pg 184)
- heat:
  - after (see pg 184)
  - during (see pg 184)
- house:
  - in (see pg 184): nux-v$_{frc}$
- idleness, while (see pg 184)
- impotence, with (see pg 184)
- injuries:
  - from (see pg 184)
  - head, of the (see pg 184)
- itching, from (see pg 184)
- leukorrhea amel.:
- light:
  - soft or colored; from (see pg 184)
- love; from disappointed (see pg 184)
- masturbation, from (see pg 184)
- menopause, during (see pg 184)
- menses:
  - after (see pg 184)
  - before (see pg 184)
  - during (see pg 185)
- mental exertion, after (see pg 185)
- mercury, after abuse of (see pg 185)
- milk; after disappearance of (see pg 185)
- misfortune; as if from (see pg 185)
- mortification, after (see pg 185)
- music:
  - agg. (see pg 185)
- noise, from (see pg 185)
- old age; in (see pg 185)
- pain, from (see pg 185)
- past events; about (see pg 185)
- periodical (see pg 185): puls$_{brm}$
- pollutions, from (see pg 185)
- pregnancy, in (see pg 185)
- puberty, in (see pg 185)
- puerperal (see pg 185)
- sexual excesses; from (see pg 185)
- sexual excitement:
  - with sexual excitement (see pg 185)
- shock, from (see pg 185)
- sighing, with (see pg 185)
- slight, from an undeserved (see pg 185)
- stomach complaints; with (see pg 185)
- suicidal disposition, with (see pg 185)
- summer (see pg 185)
- sunshine, in (see pg 185)
- taciturn (see pg 185)
- thunderstorm amel. (see pg 186)

Sadness: ...
- trifles, about (see pg 186)
- urination:
  - amel. (see pg 186)
- urine; with copious flow of: calc$_{qqh}$ nat-m$_{qqh}$ ph-ac$_{qqh}$
- vexation, after (see pg 186)
- waking:
  - when (see pg 186)
- walking:
  - air, in open (see pg 186)
  - amel. (see pg 186)
  - during and after (see pg 186)
- warm room, in (see pg 186)
- weather:
  - clear (see pg 186)
  - cloudy (see pg 186)
  - sultry (see pg 186)
  - wet (see pg 186)

SATYRIASIS (see pg 186): bufo$_{bnfl.es}$ calc$_{qqh}$ Canth$_{dyc,pkj,plr1}$ ferul$_{dyc1}$ Gels$_{dyc1}$ hyos$_{dyc,pkj1}$ hyper$_{gsd4}$ orig$_{bnfl.es,dyc1}$ Phos$_{dyc1}$ Pic-ac$_{dyc,qqh}$ Plat$_{plr1}$ staph$_{pkj1}$ Stram$_{pkj1}$ tarent$_{bnfl.es,dyc1}$

SCENERY; loves to look at: nux-v$_{brm}$

SCRATCHING with hands:
- head; on waking child scratches (see pg 186)
- walls; lime off the (see pg 186)

SEARCHING:
- floor, on (see pg 186)

SEASIDE:
- amel.: carc$_{qqh}$ med$_{qqh}$ nat-m$_{qqh}$

SELF-CONTROL:
- increased (see pg 187)
- loss of self-control (see pg 187)

SELFISHNESS (see pg 187)

SENSES:
- acute (see pg 187)
- confused (see pg 187)
- dull (see pg 187)

SENSITIVE (see pg 187)
- alternating with:
  - indifference (see pg 188)
- certain persons, to (see pg 188)
- children (see pg 188)
- chill, during (see pg 188)
- combing; to: apis$_{brm}$
- complaints; to the most trifling (see pg 188)
- everything; to (see pg 188)
- excitement (see pg 188)
- external impressions, to all (see pg 188)
- heat, during (see pg 188)
- light, during (see pg 188)
- menses:
  - before (see pg 188)
  - during (see pg 188)

- **mental** impressions; to (see pg 188)
- **motion** in the room (see pg 188)
- **music**, to (see pg 189)
  - menses; before:
  - **piano**, to (see pg 189)
  - **violin**, to (see pg 189)
- **noise**, to (see pg 189): Calc$_{ffd}$ Lyc$_{ffd}$
  - **car** passing on the street (see pg 189)
  - **chill**, during (see pg 189)
  - **clocks**, ringing of bells; striking of (see pg 189): sep$_{brm}$
  - **cracking** of wood; to: sep$_{brm}$
  - **crackling** of paper, to (see pg 189): acon$_{klp}$ calc$_{klp}$ lyc$_{klp}$ nat-m$_{brm}$
  - **fever**; during: nux-v$_{qqh}$
  - **labor**, during (see pg 189)
  - **menses**, during (see pg 189)
  - **music** amel. (see pg 189)
  - **painful** sensitiveness to (see pg 189)
  - **scratching** on linen, silk or strings, to (see pg 189)
  - **shrill** sounds, to (see pg 189)
  - **sleep**, on going to (see pg 189)
  - **slightest** noise; to the (see pg 189)
  - **stepping**, of (see pg 189)
  - **sudden** (see pg 189)
  - **talking**, of (see pg 189)
  - **television**; of the: phos$_{brm}$
  - **voices**, to (see pg 189)
  - **water** splashing, to (see pg 189)
- **odors**, to (see pg 189)
- **pain**, to:
  - **beside** oneself from pain; being (see pg 190)
- **puberty**, in (see pg 190)
- **quarrels**; to (see pg 190): phos$_{frc}$
- **reprimands**, to (see pg 190): lyc$_{frc}$
- **reproaches** (see pg 190)
- **rudeness**, to (see pg 190)
- **steel** points directed toward her (see pg 190)
- **surroundings** (see pg 190)
- **touch**, to (see pg 190)
  - **fever**; during: arn$_{qqh}$ lach$_{qqh}$ nux-v$_{qqh}$
- **want** of sensitiveness (see pg 190)

SENTIMENTAL:
- **menses**:
  - **before** (see pg 190)
- **moonlight**, in (see pg 190)
- **twilight** (see pg 190)
- **young** persons; in (see pg 190)

SERVILE (see pg 191)

SHINING objects:
- **agg.** (see pg 191)
- **amel.**:
- **aversion** to (see pg 191)
- **surface** of water agg. (see pg 191)

SHRIEKING:
- **night** (see pg 191): nat-m$_{brm}$

Shrieking: ...
- **alternating** with:
  - **unconsciousness** (see pg 191)
- **anxiety**, from (see pg 191)
- **approached**; when being:
  - **cat**; by a: merc$_{brm}$
  - **dog**; by a: arn$_{brm}$
- **brain** cry (see pg 191)
- **children**, in (see pg 191)
- **chorea**, in (see pg 192)
- **convulsions**:
  - **after** (see pg 192)
  - **before** (see pg 192)
  - **between** (see pg 192)
  - **during** (see pg 192)
- **cough**:
  - **after**:
  - **agg.** (see pg 192)
- **dentition**, during (see pg 192)
- **fever**, during (see pg 192)
- **hydrocephalus**, in (see pg 192)
- **menses**:
  - **after** (see pg 192)
  - **before** (see pg 192)
  - **during** (see pg 192)
- **mirrors**; when looking at his image in: syph$_{brm}$
- **obstinate** (see pg 192)
- **pain**, with the (see pg 192): calc$_{brm}$ phos$_{brm}$
  - **Heart**: lat-m$_{brm}$
- **paroxysmal** (see pg 192)
- **rage**; during (see pg 192)
- **sleep**, during (see pg 192): chin$_{brm}$
  - **falling** asleep; when: chin$_{brm}$
  - **loudly**: stram$_{brm}$
- **stool**:
  - **before** (see pg 192): sulph$_{brm}$
  - **during** (see pg 193)
- **stupor** in (see pg 193)
- **sudden** (see pg 193)
- **thunderstorm**, during (see pg 193)
- **touched**, when (see pg 193)
  - **pain**; when having: ars$_{brl}$ thuj$_{brl}$
- **trifles**, at (see pg 193)
- **urination**:
  - **before** (see pg 193)
- **waking**:
  - **on** (see pg 193): apis$_{qqh}$ lach$_{frc,qqh}$ Lyc$_{qqh}$ thuj$_{qqh}$

SIGHING:
- **causeless** (see pg 193)
- **epileptic** convulsions:
  - **before** (see pg 193)
- **heat**, during (see pg 193)
- **honor**, from wounded (see pg 193)
- **hysteria**, in (see pg 193)
- **involuntary** (see pg 193)
- **shock** from injuries, in (see pg 193)

- **sleep**, in (see pg 193)

SITTING:
- **aversion** to sit (see pg 194)
- **inclination** to sit (see pg 194)
  - **stiff**, quite (see pg 194)
  - **still** (see pg 194)
- **suddenly** sits up:

SLOWNESS (see pg 195)
- **behindhand**; always (see pg 195)
- **eating**, while (see pg 195)
- **motion**, in (see pg 195): $Calc_{ffd}$ $crot\text{-}h_{ffd}$
- **old** people, of (see pg 195)
- **work**, in (see pg 195)

SNAPPISH (see pg 195): $plat_{qqh}$

SNIFFING AROUND for a long time to find a decent spot; must: $calc\text{-}p_{brm}$

SOCIABILITY (see pg 195)

SPITTING (see pg 197)
- **cud**; not chewed:
  - **morning**: $lach_{hnb}$
- **neighbors**; at:
  - **feeding** him; when they are: sep_{brm}

SPOKEN TO; being:
- **agg.** (see pg 197)
- **aversion** (see pg 197)

SPYING everything (see pg 198)

STARING, thoughtless (see pg 198)
- **corner** of a room; into: $syph_{brm}$

STARTING (see pg 198)
- **daytime** (see pg 198)
- **morning**:
  - **sleep**; starting from (see pg 198)
- **noon** (see pg 198)
- **afternoon** (see pg 198)
- **evening** (see pg 198)
- **night** (see pg 198)
  - **midnight** in sleep:
    : **about** (see pg 198)
    : **after** (see pg 198)
    : **before** (see pg 198)
- **anxious** (see pg 198)
- **called** by name, when (see pg 198)
- **coition**, after (see pg 198)
- **consciousness**; on recovering (see pg 198)
- **convulsive** (see pg 198)
- **crackling** of paper, from (see pg 198): $caust_{klp}$ $ther_{brm}$
- **dentition**, during (see pg 198)
- **door**:
  - **opened**; when a door is (see pg 198)
  - **slammed**; when a door is (see pg 198)
- **easily** (see pg 198): $\textbf{KALI-C}_{fmx}$
- **eating**, after (see pg 199)
- **excitement** (see pg 199)
- **feet**, as if coming from the (see pg 199): $nat\text{-}m_{brm}$

Starting: ...
- **frequently** (see pg 199)
- **fright**; from and as from (see pg 199)
- **heat**, during (see pg 199)
- **itching** and biting, from (see pg 199)
- **lying**, while (see pg 199)
- **menses**:
  - **before** (see pg 199)
  - **during** (see pg 199)
- **noise**, from (see pg 199): $Calc_{ffd}$ $calc\text{-}p_{brm}$ Lyc_{ffd} $tarax_{brm}$
  - **pregnancy**; during: $nat\text{-}m_{fmx}$
- **pain**:
  - **from** (see pg 199)
- **palpitation**, from (see pg 199)
- **paroxysmal** (see pg 199)
- **prick** of a needle, at the (see pg 199)
- **sleep**:
  - **before** (see pg 199)
  - **during** (see pg 199): $Nat\text{-}m_{qqh}$ $Phos_{qqh}$
  - **from** (see pg 199)
  - **going** to sleep; on (see pg 199)
- **sneezing** of others, at (see pg 200)
- **spoken** to, when (see pg 200)
- **touched**, when (see pg 200): $mag\text{-}c_{brm}$
- **trifles**, at (see pg 200)
- **uneasiness**, from (see pg 200)
- **urinate**, on beginning to (see pg 200)
- **violent** (see pg 200)
- **waking**, on (see pg 200)

STRANGER:
- **presence** of strangers:
  - **agg.** (see pg 200): $Lyc_{brm,ffd}$ $nat\text{-}m_{brm,ffd}$
  - **amel.** (see pg 200)

STRIKING:
- **anger**, from (see pg 200)
- **bystanders**, at (see pg 200)
- **children**; in (see pg 200)
- **children**; striking one's own (see pg 200)
- **convulsions**, after (see pg 200)
- **himself**:
  - **abdomen**, his (see pg 200)
  - **chest**, his (see pg 200)
  - **face**, his (see pg 200)
  - **head**:
    : **his** (see pg 201)
    - **knocking** his head against wall and things (see pg 201)
- **imaginary** objects; about him at (see pg 201)
- **rage**; with (see pg 201)
- **strangers**: $nux\text{-}v_{brm}$ sep_{brm}
- **wall**, the (see pg 201)
  - **food** first; if other horse has received: $nux\text{-}v_{brm}$

- **worm** affections, in (see pg 201)

STUPEFACTION:
- **convulsions**:
  - **between** (see pg 201)
- **diarrhea**; with (see pg 201)
- **epistaxis**, after (see pg 201)
- **eruptions**; from suppressed (see pg 201)
- **heat**; during (see pg 202)
- **injury** to head, after (see pg 202)
- **menses**, during (see pg 202)
- **mental** exertion; after (see pg 202)
- **restlessness**, with (see pg 202)
- **sun**, agg. in (see pg 202)
- **urine** amel.; copious (see pg 202)
- **vertigo**:
  - **after** (see pg 202)
  - **during** (see pg 202)
- **vomiting**; after:
  - **children**; in (see pg 202)
- **weather**, hot (see pg 202)

STUPOR (see pg 202): crot-h$_{ffd}$
- **concussion** of brain, from (see pg 202)
- **convulsions**, after (see pg 202)
- **diarrhea**:
  - **after** (see pg 202)
  - **during** (see pg 202)
- **fever**, during (see pg 202): *Apis*$_{qqh}$ **Arn**$_{qqh}$ merc$_{qqh}$
- **hydrocephalus**, in (see pg 203)
- **jaundice**, in:
- **jaw** dropping; with:
- **meningitis**, in (see pg 203)
- **murmuring**, muttering (see pg 203)
- **old** age, in:
- **pain**, after (see pg 203)
- **pneumonia**, in:
- **restlessness**, with:
- **sexual** excitement, with (see pg 203)
- **sudden** (see pg 203)
- **uremia**, in:
- **vomiting**:
  - **after** (see pg 203)
  - **during** (see pg 203)

SUCKING:
- **cloth** or clothes:
- **fingers**:
  - **owners** fingers; sucking the: ign$_{brm}$
- **milk**; her own:
- **objects** into the mouth; sucking: lyc$_{ffd}$
  - **adults**; in: lac-c$_{elg}$ lac-e$_{elg}$ lac-f$_{elg}$

SUICIDAL disposition:
- **anger** driving to suicide (see pg 203)
- **anguish**; during (see pg 203)
- **anxiety**, from (see pg 203)
- **car**; throwing himself under a (see pg 203)
- **courage**, but lacks (see pg 203)
- **drowning**, by (see pg 203)
  - **love**, from disappointed (see pg 203)

Suicidal disposition: ...
- **fire**, to set oneself on (see pg 203)
- **fright**, after (see pg 203)
- **heat**, during (see pg 203)
- **homesickness**, from (see pg 203)
- **intermittent** fever, during (see pg 203)
- **love**; from disappointed (see pg 203)
- **menses**:
  - **before** (see pg 203)
  - **during** (see pg 203)
- **pains**, from (see pg 203)
- **pregnancy**, during:
- **sadness**, from (see pg 204)
- **starving**, by (see pg 204): nat-m$_{frc}$
- **throwing**:
  - **height**; himself from a (see pg 204)
  - **river**; himself into the (see pg 204)
  - **windows**, from (see pg 204)
- **walking** in open air, while (see pg 204)

SULKY (see pg 204)

SUSCEPTIBLE: lyc$_{frc}$

SWIMMING:
- **aversion**: sep$_{brm}$ **Sulph**$_{brm}$

SYMPATHETIC (see pg 205)

SYMPATHY from others:
- **aversion** to (see pg 205)
- **desire** for (see pg 205)

TACITURN:
- **air**, in open (see pg 205)
- **company**, in (see pg 205)
- **eating**, after (see pg 205)
- **fright**, after:
- **heat**, during (see pg 205)
- **menses**, during (see pg 205)
- **mortification**, after:
- **obstinacy**, from (see pg 205)
- **pregnancy**, during:
- **sadness**, in (see pg 205)
- **sickness** or injuries, about:
- **walking** in open air, after (see pg 205)

TEARING:
- **himself** (see pg 207)
- **things** in general (see pg 207)

TENSION, mental (see pg 207)

THOUGHTS:
- **compelling** (see pg 208): *Ars*$_{dyc}$ *Lach*$_{dyc}$ *Staph*$_{dyc}$

THREATENING (see pg 210)

THROWING OFF THE RIDER (see pg 210): nat-m$_{brm}$
- **anger**; from:
- **contradiction**; from: aur$_{hnb}$ lyc$_{hnb}$
- **fear**; from:

TIDY (see pg 211)
- **branches** in the fur coat are extremely disturbing when walking: sulph$_{brm}$

TIMIDITY (see pg 211): bar-ar$_{sxj,vkw}$
- **alone**, when (see pg 211)
- **bashful** (see pg 211)
- **children**; in (see pg 211)
- **company**, in (see pg 211)
- **fright**, after (see pg 211)
- **public**; about appearing in (see pg 211)

TORMENTING:
- **others** (see pg 212)

TORPOR (see pg 212)

TOUCHED:
- **aversion** to be (see pg 212): Ant-c$_{dyc}$ Arn$_{dyc}$
  · **children**; by her own: arn$_{hnb}$
  · **owner**; by the:
  · **sleep**; during: lyc$_{ffd}$ nux-v$_{brm}$ sep$_{brm}$ stram$_{brm}$ tab$_{brm}$ tarent$_{wha}$
  · **strangers**; by:
  · **ticklishness** (see pg 212): sep$_{brm}$
    : **Chest**: sep$_{brm}$
  · **veterinarian**; by the:

TRANQUILLITY:
- **anger**, after (see pg 212)
- **hemoptysis**, hemorrhages, in (see pg 212)
- **stool**, after (see pg 212)

TRAVELLING:
- **desire** for (see pg 212): cham$_{frc}$ lyc$_{frc}$
  · **jumping** to and fro when travelling by car: tub$_{hnb}$

TRIFLES:
- **important**; seem (see pg 213)

TWILIGHT agg. (see pg 213)

UNCONSCIOUSNESS:
- **air**, in open (see pg 213)
- **alone**, when (see pg 213)
- **apoplexy**, in (see pg 213)
- **asphyxia**, with (see pg 213)
- **awareness** of surroundings, with (see pg 213)
- **brain** diseases, in (see pg 213)
- **burning**, in:
- **coition**, after (see pg 213)
- **cold**:
  · **taking** a cold; after (see pg 213)
- **coma** vigil:
- **concussion** of brain, from (see pg 213)
- **convulsions**:
  · **after** (see pg 214)
  : **epileptic** (see pg 214)
- **cough**:
  · **during** (see pg 214)
  · **from** cough (see pg 214)
- **crowded** room, in a (see pg 214)
- **delirium**:
- **delivery**, during (see pg 214)
- **diarrhea**, after:
  · **vomiting**; and (see pg 214)
- **dream**, as in a (see pg 214)
- **emotion**, after (see pg 214)

Unconsciousness: ...
- **eruptions**:
  · **suppression** of eruptions; after (see pg 214)
- **excitement**, after (see pg 214)
- **exertion**, after (see pg 214)
- **eyes**:
  · **cannot** open (see pg 214)
  · **fixed**; with (see pg 214)
  · **open**, with:
- **fever**, during (see pg 214): Arn$_{qqh}$
- **frequent** spells of unconsciousness (see pg 214)
- **head**:
  · **bending** forward, on (see pg 214)
  · **moving**; on (see pg 214)
- **hydrocephalus**, in (see pg 214)
- **incomplete** (see pg 214)
- **jaundice**, in (see pg 214)
- **jaw** dropping (see pg 214)
- **lies** as if dead (see pg 214)
- **looking**:
  · **downward**, on (see pg 214)
  · **upwards** (see pg 214)
- **lying**, while (see pg 214)
- **meningitis**, in (see pg 214)
- **menses**:
  · **after** (see pg 214)
  · **before** (see pg 214)
  · **during** (see pg 214)
  · **suppression** of (see pg 214)
- **mental** insensibility (see pg 214)
- **noise** arouses; every (see pg 214)
- **odors**, from (see pg 214)
- **old** age, in (see pg 214)
- **pain**, from (see pg 214)
- **periodical** (see pg 214)
- **pneumonia**, in (see pg 215)
- **pregnancy**, during (see pg 215)
- **raising** arms above head, on (see pg 215)
- **remains** fixed in one spot (see pg 215)
- **restlessness**, with (see pg 215)
- **riding**, while (see pg 215)
- **semi**-consciousness (see pg 215)
- **sexual** excitement, with:
- **shock** from injury, in (see pg 215)
- **shrieking**:
  · **with** (see pg 215)
- **sighing**, with (see pg 215)
- **sudden** (see pg 215)
- **sunstroke**, in (see pg 215)
- **trance**, as in a (see pg 215)
- **transient** (see pg 215)
- **trifles**, at (see pg 215)
- **turning** in a circle, during (see pg 215)
- **uremic** coma (see pg 215)
- **urine**:
  · **suppression** of; with (see pg 215)
- **vertigo**, during (see pg 215)

- **vomiting**:
  - **amel.** (see pg 215)
  - **with** (see pg 215)
- **wakes** often, but only for a short time (see pg 215)
- **waking**:
  - **after** (see pg 215)
  - **on** (see pg 215)
- **walking**, while (see pg 215)
- **warm** room, in (see pg 215)

UNFRIENDLY humor (see pg 216)

UNGRATEFUL (see pg 216)

UNOBSERVING [=inattentive] (see pg 216)

UNSYMPATHETIC (see pg 216)

UNTIDY (see pg 216): calc$_{frc}$ nat-m$_{frc}$
- **branches** in the fur coat do not disturb at all when walking: sulph$_{brm}$

URINATING:
- **male** does not lift his leg (see pg 216): calc$_{ffd}$
  - **does** lift his leg when at home; but: lyc$_{ffd}$
- **ride**; horses urinating during a short:

VANITY (see pg 216): nat-m$_{brm}$

VIOLENCE:
- **aversion** to (see pg 216)

VIOLENT:
- **activity**, with bodily (see pg 216)
- **alternating** with:
  - **affection**: aur$_{brm}$
  - **cheerfulness** (see pg 216)
  - **sadness** (see pg 217)
  - **taciturnity** (see pg 217)
  - **tranquillity** (see pg 217)
  - **unconsciousness** (see pg 217)
- **animals**; towards certain (see pg 217): nat-m$_{klp}$ staph$_{klp}$
  - **different** species; of:
  - **same** species; of the: lach$_{hnb}$
- **contradiction**; from (see pg 217)
- **deeds** of violence; rage leading to (see pg 217)
- **dominant** animals; in:
- **exhaustion**; until:
- **friends**; towards his (see pg 217)
- **pain**, from (see pg 217): nux-v$_{frc}$
- **persons**; towards certain:
- **reproached**, when hearing another (see pg 217)
- **sick**, when (see pg 217)
- **sleep**:
  - **before** (see pg 217)
- **touch**, from (see pg 217)
- **trifles**, at (see pg 217)

VIVACIOUS (see pg 217): agar$_{brm}$
- **alternating** with:
  - **dullness** (see pg 217)
  - **grief** (see pg 217)
  - **sadness** (see pg 217)
- **rising**, after (see pg 217)

WAKING:
- **owners**; the:
  - **morning**:
    - **7 h**: caust$_{brm}$
- **when** (see pg 217)

WALKING:
- **air**; in the open:
  - **amel.** (see pg 217): lyc$_{frc,qqh}$ plat$_{frc,qqh}$
- **amel.** (see pg 217)
- **aversion** to (see pg 217)
- **circle**, walks in a (see pg 217)
- **hither** and thither, walks (see pg 217)
- **owner**; only close to the: lyc$_{brm}$ phos$_{brm}$ puls$_{brm}$
- **rapidly**:
- **street**:
  - **middle** of the street and not on the sidewalk; walking in the: calc$_{brl}$

WANDERING:
- **desire** to wander (see pg 217)
  - **night** (see pg 217)
  - **house**; desires to wander about the:
  - **pregnancy**, during:
  - **restlessly**, wanders about (see pg 218)

WANTS:
- **nothing** (see pg 218)

WASHING:
- **aversion** to wash (see pg 218)

WATER:
- **loves** (see pg 218)

WEATHER:
- **cloudy**:
  - **agg.** (see pg 218): sep$_{frc}$
- **rain**:
  - **trickling** of the rain amel. (see pg 218)
- **thunderstorm**:
  - **before** (see pg 218)
  - **during** (see pg 218)
- **wind**:
  - **intolerance** to (see pg 219)

WEEPING:
- **dominant** dog; if meeting a: staph$_{brm}$
- **pains**:
  - **with** the (see pg 221): plb$_{brm}$ sil$_{brm}$
- **sleep**, in (see pg 222): tarent$_{brm}$
  - **first** sleep; in: chin$_{brm}$
- **telephone** is ringing; when: arn$_{brm}$
- **trifles**, at (see pg 222): calc$_{brm}$

WICKED disposition (see pg 223)

WILDNESS:
- **children**, in (see pg 223)
- **convulsions**; before (see pg 223)
- **trifles**, at (see pg 223)

- **vexation**, from (see pg 223)

WILL:
- **loss** of will power (see pg 223)
- **weakness** of (see pg 223)

YIELDING disposition (see pg 224): Lyc_{brm} nat-m$_{brm,klp}$
- **animals** of the same species; towards other: lyc$_{brm}$

Vertigo

FEVER:
- **during**:

HIGH:
- **places** (see pg 231)

INJURIES of head; after (see pg 231)

MÉNIÈRE'S DISEASE (see pg 232): acon$_{dyc1}$ borx$_{dyc1}$ bry$_{dyc1}$ caust$_{dyc1}$ cocc$_{dyc1}$ con$_{dyc1}$ gels$_{dyc1}$ nat-m$_{dyc1}$ rhus-t$_{dyc1}$

OLD ANIMALS; IN:
- **vestibular** syndrome:

Head

ABSCESS (see pg 239)

ANEMIA:
- **Brain**; of (see pg 239)

APOPLEXY (see pg 239)

BALANCING:
- **difficult** to keep the head erect (see pg 239)

BENDING:
- **head**:
  • **backward**:
    : **must** bend head backward (see pg 240)
  • **forward**:
    : **must** bend head (see pg 240)

BLEEDING:
- **dehorning**; from:

BORES head in pillow (see pg 240): puls$_{brm}$

CEPHALHEMATOMA (see pg 240)

CEREBRAL HEMORRHAGE (see pg 240): **Acon**$_{pkj1}$ apis$_{pkj1}$ Arn_{pkj1} Aur_{pkj1} **Bry**$_{pkj1}$ crat$_{pkj1}$ hell$_{gsd4}$ kali-c$_{pkj1}$ **Lach**$_{gsd4}$ mill$_{gsd4}$ **Op**$_{gsd4}$

COLD:
- **air**:
  • **agg.** (see pg 240)

COLDNESS, chilliness, etc. (see pg 241)

CONCUSSION of brain (see pg 244)

CONGESTION (see pg 244)
- **Brain**:
  • **chill**; with: bell$_{qqh}$
  • **fever**; during: bapt$_{qqh}$ echi$_{qqh}$

HEAD: ...

DANDRUFF (see pg 249)

DROPSY (see pg 250)

EDEMA:
- **Brain**; of (see pg 250): apis$_{mld1}$ bell$_{mld1}$ cic$_{mld1}$ stry$_{mld1}$

ERUPTIONS (see pg 251)
- **Occiput**:
  • **Ear** to ear; from:

ERYSIPELAS (see pg 253)

EXOSTOSIS (see pg 253): hecla$_{dyc1}$

FONTANELLES:
- **open** (see pg 254)

FUNGUS (see pg 256)

HAIR (see pg 385)
- **baldness**:
  • **castration**; after:
  • **ovariectomy**; after:
- **gray**; becoming (see pg 386): **Lyc**$_{ffd}$
  • **prematurely** (see pg 387): Lyc_{klp} sil$_{klp}$
- **shaggy**:

HEADSHAKER: acon$_{dyc}$ aesc$_{dyc}$ agar$_{dyc}$ all-c$_{dyc}$ anac$_{dyc}$ apis$_{dyc}$ ars$_{dyc}$ arum-m$_{dyc}$ arund$_{dyc}$ bell$_{dyc}$ borx$_{dyc}$ caust$_{dyc}$ cedr$_{dyc}$ cham$_{dyc}$ chin$_{brm,dyc}$ cina$_{dyc}$ coff-t$_{dyc}$ colch$_{dyc}$ coloc$_{dyc}$ euphr$_{dyc}$ galph$_{dyc}$ hyper$_{dyc}$ kali-bi$_{hnb}$ lyc$_{brm}$ mag-c$_{dyc}$ mag-p$_{dyc}$ mez$_{dyc}$ nat-m$_{dyc}$ nux-v$_{brm,dyc}$ olnd$_{dyc}$ plan$_{dyc}$ plat$_{dyc}$ puls$_{ggp}$ sabad$_{dyc}$ samb$_{dyc}$ sep$_{brm}$ spig$_{dyc}$ thuj$_{dyc}$ tub$_{dyc}$ verb$_{dyc}$ wye$_{dyc}$ zinc$_{dyc}$
- **strangles**; after: puls$_{ggp}$

HEAT (see pg 256)
- **coldness**:
  • **Extremities**; with coldness of (see pg 258): **Bell**$_{qqh}$ gels$_{qqh}$
- **fever**:
  • **during**:
    : **agg.**: verat-v$_{qqh}$
- **nose**; except:
  • **fever**; during: arn$_{qqh}$

HYDROCEPHALUS (see pg 264)

INFLAMMATION:
- **purulent**:
  • **dehorning**; from:
- **Brain** (see pg 264): aeth$_{mld}$ agar$_{mld}$ bufo$_{mld}$ cic$_{mld}$ cupr-act$_{mld}$ ferr-p$_{mld}$ mag-p$_{mld}$ sol-ni$_{mld}$ tarent$_{mld}$ zinc$_{mld}$
  • **dehorning**; from:
  • **purulent**:
- **Meninges** (see pg 264): agar$_{mld,mld4}$ $Apis_{dyc}$ **Bell**$_{dyc}$ calc-s$_{qqh}$ caust$_{bnf}$ cic$_{dyc,mld,mld4}$ con$_{bnf}$ $Cupr_{brm}$ cyt-l$_{mld}$ ferr-p$_{mld}$ hyper$_{bnf}$ lath$_{mld}$ nux-v$_{bnf}$ stry$_{bnf}$ symph$_{bnf}$

INJURIES of the head; after (see pg 265): acon$_{qqh}$ bar-c$_{dyc1}$ gels$_{gsd4}$ Op_{qqh}

ITCHING of scalp (see pg 265)

JERKING of the head (see pg 266)

KNOCKING head against things (see pg 267)

LARGE SIZE (see pg 267)

LEAN on something, desire to (see pg 267)

LICE (see pg 267)

LUPUS (see pg 267)

MOTIONS in head (see pg 268)

MOTIONS of head (see pg 269)
- **involuntary** (see pg 269): lyc$_{ffd}$
- **rolling** head (see pg 269)

NECROSIS:
- **Cerebral** cortex: agar$_{dyc,mld5}$ cic$_{dyc,mld5}$ hell$_{dyc,mld5}$ stram$_{mld5}$ stry$_{dyc}$ zinc$_{mld5}$
- **Skull**; of the (see pg 270): phos$_{dyc1}$

PERSPIRATION of scalp (see pg 370)
- **except** the head; general perspiration (see pg 370): Thuj$_{qqh}$
- **sleep**:
  - **during** (see pg 371): *Calc-p*$_{qqh}$ *Sil*$_{qqh}$
  - **sweetish** odor: calc$_{qqh}$ sil$_{qqh}$

RAISING:
- **head**:
  - **difficult**:
    : **night** (see pg 376)
  - **frequently** from pillow (see pg 376)
  - **impossible** (see pg 376)

RESTLESSNESS (see pg 377)

RUBBING:
- **agg.** (see pg 377)

SCLEROSIS; cerebral (see pg 377): bar-c$_{qqh}$ kali-p$_{qqh}$ plb$_{qqh}$ sec$_{qqh}$

SENSITIVENESS (see pg 377)

SHAPE:
- **brachycephalic**:
- **broad**:
- **domed** forehead:
- **trochocephalus**:

SUNSTROKE (see pg 380): chin$_{bnf1.es}$ cupr$_{gsd4}$ kali-c$_{bnf1.es}$

TREMBLING (see pg 382)
- **fear**; from: cic$_{brm}$

TUMORS:
- **swellings**; tumorous (see pg 382)
- **Brain** (see pg 382)

TURNED:
- **left** in convulsions; to (see pg 382)

TWISTING head (see pg 382)

ULCERS (see pg 383)

WARM:
- **coverings** on head:
  - **agg.** (see pg 383)

HEAD: ...

WARTS: sep$_{brm}$

WASHING:
- **head**:
  - **agg.** (see pg 383)

WENS (see pg 384)

Eye

AGGLUTINATED (see pg 389): *Sulph* $_{fmx}$

ANEMIA of:
- **Conjunctiva** (see pg 389)
- **Optic** nerve (see pg 389)
- **Retina** (see pg 389)

ATROPHY:
- **Lachrymal** glands: seneg$_{dyc1}$ verat$_{dyc1}$ zinc$_{dyc1}$
- **Optic** nerve (see pg 390)
- **Retina**: crot-h$_{mld3}$ ham$_{mld3}$ phos$_{mld3}$
  - **progressive**: phos$_{klp}$

BLEEDING from eyes (see pg 390): chin$_{frl1}$

BRILLIANT (see pg 390)

CANCER (see pg 390)
- **fungus** (see pg 390)

CATARACT (see pg 390): arg-n$_{mld3}$ naphtin$_{dyc,itm,mld,pkj1}$ *Santin* $_{mld3}$ thuj$_{mmj1}$

CATARRH:
- **fever**; during: merc$_{frc,qqh}$

CLOSED (see pg 391)

CLOSING THE EYES:

COLDNESS (see pg 392)

CONTRACTION:
- **Lids**; of (see pg 393)

CRACKS:
- **Canthi**; in (see pg 393)

DEGENERATION:
- **Cornea** (see pg 393)

DETACHMENT of retina (see pg 393)

DISCHARGES:
- **right** eye: nat-m$_{brm}$
- **thick** (see pg 394): sulph$_{fmx}$

DISCOLORATION:
- **blue** (see pg 394)
- **red** (see pg 395): Bell$_{hnb}$ *Lyc*$_{brm}$
  - **fever**; during (see pg 395): ail$_{qqh}$ bapt$_{qqh}$ lach$_{qqh}$
  - **Canthi** (see pg 395): ars$_{brm}$
- **yellow** (see pg 396)
- **Iris**:
  - **heterochromia**: calc$_{brm}$

DULLNESS (see pg 397)

ECCHYMOSIS (see pg 397)

EMBOLISM of arteria retina (see pg 397)

ENLARGED:
- **Lens** (see pg 397)

ERUPTIONS:
- **About** the eyes (see pg 397): ant-c$_{elg}$ *Ars*$_{elg}$
  - crusts (see pg 397): nux-v$_{brm}$
- **Cornea**:
  - blisters; small (see pg 397)
- **Lids**:
  - crusts:
    : Margins of lids (see pg 398)
  - pimples:
    : red: sulph$_{brm}$

EVERSION of lids (see pg 398): borx$_{mld3}$ caust$_{brm}$
Lyc$_{brm}$ petr$_{pkj}$
- injuries; after: caust$_{brm}$

EXCORIATION:
- **painful** (see pg 398)
- **Canthi** (see pg 398)
- **Lids** (see pg 398)

EYE GUM (see pg 398)

FALLING:
- **Lids**; of (see pg 399)

FILMY (see pg 399)

FIRE agg.; looking into (see pg 399)

GLASSY appearance (see pg 399)

GLAUCOMA (see pg 399): apis$_{mld3}$ bar-c$_{itm}$
cocain$_{itm,pkj1}$
- **sclerosis**; from: calc-f$_{itm}$ plb$_{itm}$ sec$_{itm}$

GRANULAR:
- **Canthi**; outer (see pg 399)
- **Lids** (see pg 399)

HARDNESS (see pg 399)

HEAT in (see pg 400)

HERPES CORNEA:

HYPERESTHESIA:
- **Retina** (see pg 401)

INFLAMMATION (see pg 401)
- **air** agg.; draft of: lyc$_{brm}$
- **children**; in:
  - infants (see pg 401)
- **cold**:
  - agg. (see pg 402): puls$_{brm}$
- **wind**: puls$_{brm}$
- **Conjunctiva** (see pg 402): aesc$_{mld3}$ arn$_{mld3}$
  borx$_{dyc,mld3}$ con$_{dyc1}$ croc$_{dyc1}$ hyper$_{pkj1}$ merc-c$_{itm}$
  nat-m$_{dyc1}$ sabad$_{dyc1}$ sanic$_{dyc1}$ symph$_{mld3}$
  - accompanied by:
    : coryza (see pg 403): sil$_{spk1}$
  - chronic (see pg 403): nat-m$_{brm}$
  - granular (see pg 403): sep$_{brm}$

Inflammation – Conjunctiva: ...
  - herpetic: phos$_{brm}$ sep$_{brm}$
- **Cornea** (see pg 403): arg-n$_{itm}$ *Kali-bi*$_{bnfl.es,dyc,mld3}$
  led$_{mld3}$ *Merc-c*$_{dyc,mld3}$ phos$_{dyc1}$ sang$_{mld3}$ sil$_{mmj1}$
  symph$_{mld3}$
  - herpetic (see pg 403): lyc$_{brm}$ sep$_{brm}$
  - superficialis chronica:
  - superficialis punctata:
  - ulcerative:
- **Iridochoroiditis**:
  - recurrent: alum$_{dyc}$ bell$_{dyc}$ cinnb$_{dyc}$ con$_{dyc}$ euphr$_{dyc}$
    kali-i$_{dyc}$ merc$_{dyc}$ phos$_{dyc}$ puls-vg$_{dyc}$ rhus-t$_{dyc}$ seneg$_{dyc}$
    spig$_{dyc}$
- **Iris** (see pg 403): acon$_{mld3}$ led$_{bnfl.es,mld3}$ phos$_{mld3}$
  Puls$_{fmx}$ symph$_{mld3}$
- **Keratoconjunctivitis**:
  - epidemic:
  - herpetic:
  - phlyctenular (see pg 403): con$_{dyc}$ kali-bi$_{dyc}$
    kali-i$_{dyc}$ led$_{dyc}$ merc$_{dyc}$ merc-c$_{dyc}$ tub$_{dyc}$
  - sicca:
- **Lachrymal** ducts (see pg 404): arg-n$_{mld3}$
- **Lachrymal** sacs (see pg 404): borx$_{pkj1}$ iod$_{mld3}$
  merc-c$_{mjs1}$
- **Lids** (see pg 404): agar$_{mld3}$ alum$_{mld,pkj1}$ borx$_{pkj1}$
  urt-u$_{mld3}$
  - purulent: hep$_{mld3}$ merc-c$_{mld3}$ puls$_{mld3}$ staphycoc$_{mld3}$
  - Lower (see pg 404): cham$_{frc}$
  - Upper (see pg 404): ign$_{frc}$
- **Meibomian** glands (see pg 404): aeth$_{dyc1}$ rhus-t$_{dyc1}$
- **Membrana** nictitans:
  - granular (see pg 404): arg-n$_{klp}$ phos$_{klp}$ puls$_{klp}$ syph$_{klp}$
    : right: sulph$_{brm}$
- **Uvea** (see pg 404): puls$_{fmx}$

INJECTED (see pg 404)
- **fever**; during: verat-v$_{qqh}$

INJURIES; after (see pg 405)

INSENSIBILITY (see pg 405)

INVERSION of lids (see pg 405): agar$_{pkj1}$ hyos$_{pkj1}$

IRRITATION (see pg 405)

ITCHING:
- **morning** (see pg 405): calc$_{brm}$

LACHRYMATION (see pg 406): canth$_{frc}$
- **right** (see pg 406): coloc$_{brm}$
- **left** (see pg 406): calc$_{brm}$ *Ign*$_{hnb}$
- **morning** (see pg 406): *Sep*$_{brm}$
- **cold**:
  - air agg. (see pg 407)
- **excitement** agg. : coloc$_{brm}$
- **profuse** (see pg 407): acon$_{dyc,pkj1}$ all-c$_{bnfl.es,dyc,itm}$
  cob$_{bnfl.es,dyc,itm}$ **Euphr**$_{bnfl.es,itm}$ merc$_{dyc,pkj1}$ nat-s$_{itm}$

LIGHT; from:
- **moonlight**:
  - amel. (see pg 408)

LUPUS:
- **Lids** (see pg 408)

MELANOSIS (see pg 408)

MOVEMENT:
- **convulsive** (see pg 408)
- **involuntary** (see pg 409): nat-m$_{brm}$
- **pendulum** like, from side to side (see pg 409): cocc$_{fmx}$ con$_{fmx}$

NARROWING of intervals between lids (see pg 409)

NEAR the eyes; bringing objects:
- **aversion** to (see pg 409)

OPACITY:
- **Cornea**:
  - **arcus** senilis (see pg 409)

OPEN lids (see pg 409)
- **sleep**; during (see pg 410): *Bell*$_{brm}$ *Lyc*$_{brm}$ thuj$_{brm}$
- **spasmodic** (see pg 410)

OPENING the lids:

PAIN (see pg 410)

PARALYSIS:
- **Eyeballs**:
  - **Muscles**:
    - **External** recti (see pg 428)
    - **Internal** recti (see pg 428)
    - **Superior** oblique (see pg 428)
- **Optic** nerve (see pg 428)

PERSPIRATION on eyebrows and lids (see pg 429)

PHOTOMANIA (see pg 429)

PHOTOPHOBIA (see pg 429)
- **fever**; during (see pg 429): nat-m$_{brm}$

PROTRUSION:
- **exophthalmos** (see pg 430)

PUPILS:
- **contracted**:
  - **left** (see pg 440): sulph$_{brm}$
  - **fever**; during: acon$_{qqh}$
- **dilated**:
  - **fever**; during (see pg 441): ail$_{qqh}$ bell$_{qqh}$ verat-v$_{qqh}$
- **insensible** to light (see pg 441): puls$_{brm}$
- **unequal** (see pg 441): sulph$_{brm}$

RESTLESS eyes (see pg 431)

ROUGH cornea (see pg 431)

RUBBING the eyes:
- **desire** to (see pg 431)

SCLEROSIS:
- **Lens**; crystalline:
  - **Center** of: bar-c$_{mld3}$

SCROFULOUS affections (see pg 431)

SICKLY look around the eyes (see pg 431)

SPASMS:
- **Eyes** (see pg 432): agar$_{f111}$
- **Lids** (see pg 432): cic$_{f111}$ phys$_{f111}$ rheum$_{f111}$ sulph$_{f111}$

EYE: ...

SPOTS, specks, etc. :
- **Cornea**; on (see pg 432)

STAPHYLOMA (see pg 432)

STARING (see pg 432)

STRABISMUS (see pg 433)

STRICTURE of lachrymal duct (see pg 433)

STYES (see pg 433)

SUNKEN (see pg 434)

SWELLING (see pg 434)
- **Lids** (see pg 434)
- **Membrana** nictitans:

THICKENING:
- **Lids**:
  - **Margins** of:
    - **tyloma**:

TINGLING (see pg 436)

TIRED EXPRESSION (see pg 436)

TUMORS:
- **Lids**:
  - **nodules** in the lids (see pg 436)

TWITCHING (see pg 437)

ULCERATION:
- **Cornea** (see pg 437): calen$_{fmx}$ *Puls*$_{fmx}$
- **Lids** (see pg 438): ant-c$_{mld3}$ kali-bi$_{mld3}$ nit-ac$_{mld3}$ ran-b$_{mld3}$ vario$_{mld}$

UNSTEADY look (see pg 438)

WARM:
- **agg.**:
  - **heat** (see pg 438)

WARTS (see pg 438)

WEAK (see pg 438)

WINKING (see pg 439)

WRINKLED conjunctiva (see pg 439)

Vision

ACUTE (see pg 443)

BLURRED (see pg 443)

DIM (see pg 447)

EXERTION:
- **amel.** (see pg 450)

EXERTION OF THE EYES agg. (see pg 450)

LOSS OF VISION (see pg 454)
- **night** (see pg 454)

WEAK (see pg 458)

Ear

ABSCESS:
- **Behind** the ears (see pg 461): lyc$_{qqh1}$

ADHESIONS in middle ear (see pg 461)

BALD spot above (see pg 461)

CALCAREOUS deposit on tympanum (see pg 461)

CANCEROUS affections: ars$_{pkj1}$ graph$_{pkj1}$ hep$_{pkj1}$ hydr$_{pkj1}$ mez$_{pkj1}$ thuj$_{pkj1}$
- **melanoma**:

CARIES, threatened (see pg 461)

CATARRH:
- **Eustachian** tubes (see pg 461)
- **Middle** ear (see pg 461)

CHILDREN; in (see pg 461)

CICATRICES:
- **retraction** of cicatrices: calc-f$_{bnf1.es}$ graph$_{bnf1.es}$ sil$_{bnf1.es}$

COLDNESS (see pg 462)

CONTRACTION (see pg 463)

DISCHARGES (see pg 463)
- **blood**:
  · **hematoma** (see pg 463): arn$_{brm}$ lach$_{brm}$
- **mites**; caused by:
- **odor**:
  · **urine**; like: urea$_{hnb}$
- **purulent** (see pg 464): sulph$_{brm}$

DISCOLORATION:
- **blue**:
  · blue eared pig syndrome: lach$_{dyc}$ sec$_{dyc}$
- **redness** (see pg 464)
  · **Lobes** (see pg 465): nat-m$_{brm}$

DRYNESS (see pg 465)

ERECT; concha becoming:
- **late**; too: calc$_{qqh}$ calc-s$_{qqh}$

ERUPTIONS (see pg 465)
- **eczema** (see pg 465): ars$_{mld3}$ calc$_{bnf1.es,itm}$ graph$_{bnf1.es}$ hep$_{mld3}$ merc$_{mjs1}$ petr$_{bnf1.es}$ puls$_{bnf1.es,itm}$ rhus-t$_{mld3}$ sil$_{bnf1.es,itm}$ sulph$_{spk1}$
- **scabies**: ars-i$_{mld3}$ con$_{dyc1}$ graph$_{bnf1.es,itm}$ mez$_{brm}$ psor$_{bnf1.es,dyc,itm,pkj1}$ puls$_{bnf1.es,itm}$ sulph$_{dyc,pkj,spk1}$
- **Behind** the ears:
  · **cracks** (see pg 466)
- **Lobes**, on:
  · **scurfs** (see pg 467): ars$_{mjs1}$ sulph$_{mjs1}$
- **Tip**:

EXCORIATION:
- **Behind** (see pg 467)

EXOSTOSIS (see pg 467)

FULLNESS, sensation of (see pg 467)

FUNGOUS excrescences (see pg 467)

HANGING DOWN: lyc$_{brm}$

Hanging down: ...
- **right**: lyc$_{ffd}$

HEAT (see pg 467): caust$_{qqh1}$
- **cold**:
  · **feet**; with coldness of:

HEMATOMA (see pg 468): arn$_{dyc,qqh}$ ham$_{dyc1}$ mill$_{pkj1}$
- **right** ear: phos$_{qqh}$
- **left** ear: lach$_{pkj,qqh}$

INFLAMMATION (see pg 468): aur$_{pkj1}$ con$_{pkj1}$ kali-br$_{itm}$ sil$_{fmx}$
- **right**: sulph$_{brm}$
- **left** (see pg 468): sil$_{brm}$
  · **recurrent**: nat-m$_{brm}$
- **accompanied** by:
  · **black** pigmentation: graph$_{klp}$ thuj$_{klp}$
  · **bulge** of cartilage:
  · **Skin**; eruptions of:
- **parasitica**; otitis: bac$_{klp}$ sulph$_{klp}$ tub$_{klp}$
- **External** ears:
  · **accompanied** by:
    ⁞ **black** pigmentation:
  · **parasitic**:
  · **sensitive** to touch:
- **Meatus** (see pg 469): Calc$_{ffd}$ Lyc$_{ffd}$ pyrog$_{bnf1.es,itm,qqh1}$ Sil$_{fmx}$
  · **chronic**: lyc$_{brm}$ nat-m$_{brm}$
- **Media** (see pg 469): ars$_{frc}$ kali-s$_{pkj1}$ maland$_{mld3}$ Sil$_{fmx}$

ITCHING (see pg 469): puls$_{brm}$

LUMPS; hard:
- **Behind** ear (see pg 470)

LUPUS on the lobe (see pg 470)

MOISTURE (see pg 470)

NECROSIS: sec$_{dyc}$

NODES:
- **Auricle**, on (see pg 470)
- **Behind** the ears (see pg 470)
- **External** ears; on:
  · **copper**-colored nodes (see pg 470)

ODORS (see pg 480)

PAIN (see pg 480)
- **cold**:
  · **air**:
    ⁞ **agg.** (see pg 484)
- **music**:
  · **from** (see pg 486)

PERFORATION:
- **Tympanum** (see pg 494)

PERSPIRATION (see pg 494)

POLYPUS (see pg 494)

RUSH of blood to right ear (see pg 495)

SENSIBILITY:
- **External** ear:

SENSITIVE:

- **touch**; to: arn$_{hnb}$ hep$_{klp}$
- **Lobes** (see pg 495)

STOPPED sensation (see pg 495)

STROKES, blows in ears (see pg 496): hyper$_{gsd4}$

SUPPURATION (see pg 496): ars$_{bnfl.es,qqh1}$ kali-m$_{pkj1}$ lach$_{bnfl.es,qqh1}$ pyrog$_{bnfl.es,pkj1}$ sep$_{qqh1}$

SWELLING (see pg 496)
- **Lobes**:
  · **hematoma**: *Arn*$_{brm}$
  ⋮ **bluish**: lach$_{brm}$

TENSION (see pg 496)

TUBERCLE, hard:
- **Behind** the ear:
- **Lobe**; on the (see pg 497)

TUMORS:
- **steatoma** (see pg 497)
- **wens**:
  · **Behind** the ears (see pg 497)
  · **Lobe**; on (see pg 497)

ULCERATION:
- **Lobes**:
  · **Edges**: ars$_{pkj1}$ nit-ac$_{pkj1}$
  · **Hole** for earrings; in (see pg 497)
- **Margins**:

VESTIBULAR SYNDROME:
- **old** people; in: *Carb-an*$_{brm}$ hell$_{klp}$

WART-LIKE growth, inflamed and ulcerated:
- **Behind** the ears (see pg 497)
- **External** ears; on (see pg 497)

WAX:
- **increased** (see pg 498): *Lyc*$_{fmx}$ sulph$_{brm,fmx}$

Hearing

IMPAIRED (see pg 501)
- **direction** of sound, cannot tell (see pg 502)

LOST (see pg 504)

Nose

ALTERNATING SIDES:

ABSCESS (see pg 505)

ADENOIDS (see pg 505)

AGGLUTINATION of nostrils (see pg 505)

AIR:
- **inspired** air; sensitive to (see pg 505)

ATROPHY:
- **Inside** (see pg 505)

BROAD and flat (see pg 505)

CANCER (see pg 505): *Phos*$_{fmx}$
- **bleeding**: phos$_{fmx}$

NOSE: ...

CARIES (see pg 505)

CATARRH (see pg 505): *Squil*$_{qqh}$
- **extending** to:
  · **Antrum**:
  · **Chest**:
  · **Frontal** sinuses:

CERE; complaints of:

CHAPPED (see pg 506)

COLD:
- **air**:
  · **agg.** (see pg 507)

COLDNESS (see pg 507)

CONGESTION (see pg 507): stict$_{qqh}$

CONSTRICTION (see pg 508)

CONTRACTION (see pg 508)

CORYZA (see pg 508): ail$_{mld5}$ *Ars-i*$_{brm}$ naphtin$_{qqh}$ samb-c$_{qqh}$ sul-i$_{mld5}$
- **chronic** (see pg 509): *Lyc*$_{brm}$ puls$_{brm}$ *Sil*$_{brm}$
- **cough**:
  · **with** (see pg 510): sil$_{brm}$ stict$_{brm}$
- **cutting** the hair, from (see pg 510)
- **fever**:
  · **with** (see pg 511): **Bry**$_{qqh}$ nux-v$_{qqh}$
- **vaccination**; after:

CRACKLING noise in (see pg 513)

CRACKS (see pg 513)

CRAMPS of nose (see pg 513)

DEPIGMENTATION: cob$_{dyc1}$ cupr$_{dyc1}$ ferr$_{dyc1}$ lyc$_{brm}$ mang$_{dyc1}$ puls$_{hnb}$ zinc$_{dyc1}$
- **white**:
  · **spots**: puls$_{hnb}$ syph$_{klp}$

DESQUAMATION (see pg 513)

DILATED nostrils (see pg 513)

DIPHTHERIA in (see pg 513)

DISCHARGE (see pg 513)
- **crusts**, scabs, inside (see pg 514)
- **dripping** (see pg 515): lyc$_{brm}$
- **greenish** (see pg 516): *Phos*$_{fmx}$
- **offensive**:
  · **fetid** (see pg 516)
- **purulent**:
  · **dehorning**; from:
- **viscid**, tough (see pg 517): *Phos*$_{fmx}$
- **white** (see pg 518): ars-i$_{brm}$
  · **right**: phos$_{fmx}$
  · **thick**: ars-i$_{brm}$
- **yellowish** green (see pg 518): agar$_{brm}$

DISCOLORATION:
- **copper**-colored spots (see pg 518)
- **pigmentation**:
  · **black**: thuj$_{klp}$

- **pigmentation**: ...
  - **brown**:
  - **pink**:
- **redness** (see pg 518)
- **spots** (see pg 519)
- **yellow**:
  - **saddle** (see pg 519)

DISTENSION (see pg 519)

DRYNESS:
- **Inside** (see pg 519)

EDEMA (see pg 520)

EPISTAXIS (see pg 520): eup-per$_{dyc1}$ fic-r$_{mld,mld5}$ tril-c$_{qqh}$

EXCORIATION (see pg 524)

EXOSTOSIS (see pg 524)

FRECKLES (see pg 524)

FROSTBITTEN (see pg 524)

GANGRENE (see pg 524)

HAIR:
- **falling**:
  - **Nostrils** (see pg 543)

HARDNESS (see pg 524)

HAY FEVER (see pg 524)

HEAT in (see pg 525)

HORNY skin: graph$_{klp}$ thuj$_{klp}$

INFLAMMATION (see pg 525): all-c$_{bnfl.es}$ hydr$_{bnfl.es}$ merc-c$_{bnfl.es}$
- **atrophic**: ars$_{dyc}$ kali-i$_{dyc}$ lem-m$_{dyc}$ nat-m$_{dyc}$ stict$_{dyc}$

ITCHING (see pg 525)
- **rubs** (see pg 526)

JERKING at root of nose; sudden (see pg 526)

KNOBBY:
- **Tip** (see pg 526)

LACERATION (see pg 526)

LIPOMA (see pg 526)

LIQUIDS:
- **come** out through the nose on attempting to swallow (see pg 526)

LUMP:
- **Posterior** nares (see pg 526)

LUPUS (see pg 526)

LYING:
- **agg.** (see pg 526)

MEMBRANE, mucous (see pg 526)

MOIST after eating (see pg 526)

MOTION:
- **Wings**; of:
  - **constant** (see pg 526)
  - **fan**-like (see pg 526)
    - **pneumonia**, in (see pg 526): Lyc$_{fmx}$

NECROSIS (see pg 526)

NODOSITIES (see pg 527)

NOSTRILS drawn in (see pg 527)

NUMBNESS (see pg 527)

OBSTRUCTION (see pg 527)

ODORS; imaginary and real (see pg 529)

OILY (see pg 530)

OPERATION; after (see pg 530)

OZENA (see pg 530): Puls$_{brm}$ sec$_{frc}$ squil$_{frc}$

PAIN (see pg 530)
- **sore** (see pg 532)

PERFORATED:
- **Septum** (see pg 537)

PERSPIRATION on (see pg 537)
- **Tip**: calc$_{frc}$

PICKING:
- **affected** parts; the (see pg 537)
- **Nose** (see pg 537)

PINCHED (see pg 537)

POINTED (see pg 537)

POLYPUS (see pg 537)

PROTUBERANCES (see pg 537)

PUFFINESS (see pg 537)

PULSATION (see pg 537)

QUIVERING (see pg 537)

RATTLING (see pg 537)

ROUGHNESS inside (see pg 537)

SCURFY:
- **Nostrils** (see pg 537)

SENSITIVE (see pg 537)

SHINY (see pg 537)

SINUSES; complaints of (see pg 543): ars$_{mld4}$ fl-ac$_{mld3}$ hecla$_{mld3}$ hep$_{bnfl.es,mld,mld,mld5}$ hippoz$_{mld3}$ *Hydr*$_{mld,mld4}$ merc-c$_{mld,mld4}$ sil$_{bnfl.es,mld,mld,mld4}$ thuj$_{qqh}$

SMELL:
- **acute** (see pg 538)
- **diminished** (see pg 538): sulph$_{brm}$
- **wanting** (see pg 538)

SNEEZING (see pg 538)
- **coryza**:
  - **without** (see pg 539): calc-p$_{brm}$ nat-m$_{brm}$
- **occupation** amel.: nat-m$_{brm}$
- **paroxysmal** (see pg 540)

SNUFFLING (see pg 541)

SOOTY nostrils (see pg 541)

SPASMS in muscles (see pg 541)

STIFFNESS (see pg 541)

SWELLING (see pg 541)

TENSION (see pg 542)

THICK (see pg 542)

TUMOR:
- **Nostrils**:
  - left: graph$_{hnb}$
  - lardaceous: graph$_{hnb}$

TWITCHING (see pg 542)

ULCERS (see pg 542)

VEINS, varicose (see pg 543)

WARTS (see pg 543)

WEATHER agg.; changing (see pg 543)

WET; too:
- **sensation** in nose (see pg 543)

WINTER agg. :

WRINKLED skin (see pg 543)

Face

ABSCESS (see pg 545)

ACTINOMYCOSIS:
- **Jaw**:
  - **Lower**: calc-f$_{dyc}$ fl-ac$_{dyc}$ hecla$_{dyc}$ kali-i$_{dyc}$

ADHESION of skin to forehead (see pg 545)

ANGIOMA (see pg 545)

APHTHAE (see pg 545)

ATROPHY:
- **Masseter** muscles; painful atrophy of: bell$_{brm}$

BEAK; complaints of:
- **crumbly**:
- **distorted**:

BLEEDING of lips (see pg 545)

BLOATED (see pg 545)

CANCER (see pg 545)
- **lupus** (see pg 545)
  - **exedens**; lupus:
    : **Maxilla**:
      : left:
  - **Eyebrows** (see pg 545)
- **Lips** (see pg 545)
  - **Lower**:
    : **Middle** of: hydr$_{pkj1}$ nat-m$_{pkj1}$
  - **Mouth**; corners of: ars$_{pkj1}$

CARIES of bone (see pg 546)

CHAPPED (see pg 546)

CHEWING motion of the jaw (see pg 546)

CHILLINESS (see pg 546)

CLENCHED jaw (see pg 546)

COLDNESS (see pg 546)

CONGESTION (see pg 548)

FACE: ...

CONTRACTION (see pg 549)

CONVULSIONS, spasms (see pg 549)

CRACKED:
- **Lips** (see pg 549)
- **Mouth**; corners of (see pg 550)

CRACKING in articulation of jaw (see pg 550)

CRAMP (see pg 550)

DISCOLORATION:
- **pale** (see pg 552)
- **red** (see pg 554)
  - **excitement** (see pg 556)
- **yellow** (see pg 558)

DISLOCATION of jaws:
- **easy** (see pg 559)

DISTORTION (see pg 559)

DRAWN (see pg 559)

DROPPING:
- **Jaws** (see pg 559)

DRYNESS (see pg 559)

EMACIATION (see pg 560)
- **Temporal** muscles:

EMPYEMA:
- **Sinuses**:
  - **Maxillary** (see pg 560)

ERUPTIONS (see pg 560)
- **accompanied** by:
  - **Lips**:
    : **swelling**: thuj$_{brm}$
- **acne** (see pg 560): **Sulph**$_{elg}$
  - **Chin** (see pg 561): calc-p$_{brm}$ lach$_{brm}$ ph-ac$_{brm}$
- **boils**:
  - **Nose** (see pg 562)
- **carbuncles**:
  - **Chin**; on (see pg 562)
- **comedones** (see pg 562)
- **crusty**, scabby (see pg 562)
- **desquamating** (see pg 562)
- **ecthyma**; contagious: ant-t$_{itm}$ kali-bi$_{itm}$ merc$_{itm}$ nit-ac$_{itm}$ vario$_{itm}$
- **eczema** (see pg 563)
  - **Lips** (see pg 563): graph$_{klp}$ hep$_{klp}$ nit-ac$_{klp}$
  - **Mouth**:
    : **Corners** of (see pg 563): caps$_{pkj1}$ mez$_{pkj1}$ nit-ac$_{pkj1}$
  - **Nose**:
    : moist:
    : ulcers; with:
    : **Margin** of skin and crossing of mucous membrane:
- **herpes**:
  - **circinatus** (see pg 563): *Nat-m*$_{ffd}$
- **Lips**:
  - **Lower** (see pg 569): puls$_{brm}$

- **Nose** (see pg 569)
ERYSIPELAS (see pg 569)
EVERTED lips (see pg 570)
EXCORIATION:
- **Lips**:
  • **Upper**:
    : **Above**: sulph_{brm}
- **Mouth**; corners of (see pg 570): *Cund*_{dyc}
EXOSTOSIS (see pg 570)
EXPRESSION:
- **anxious** (see pg 570)
- **besotted** (see pg 570): nat-m_{brm}
- **cadaverous** (see pg 570): ars_{hnb}
- **cold**, distant (see pg 570)
- **foolish** (see pg 571)
- **frightened** (see pg 571)
- **insane**: aur_{brm}
- **intoxicated** (see pg 571)
- **old** looking (see pg 571)
  • **prematurely** (see pg 571): ars_{hnb} lyc_{hnb}
- **sickly** (see pg 571)
- **sleepy** (see pg 571)
- **suffering** (see pg 571): sep_{brm}
FORMICATION (see pg 572)
FRECKLES (see pg 572)
FULLNESS (see pg 572)
FUNGUS growth:
- **Jaws**:
  • **Lower** (see pg 572)
GANGRENE (see pg 572)
GREASY (see pg 572): lyc_{brm} stram_{brm}
HAIR:
- **brittle**:
  • **Whiskers**:
HEAT (see pg 572)
- **fever**:
  • **during**:
    : **agg.** (see pg 574): calc_{qqh}
HIPPOCRATIC (see pg 575)
INDURATIONS (see pg 575)
- **red**, hard lumps (see pg 575)
- **Parotid** glands (see pg 575)
INFLAMMATION:
- **Muscles**:
  • **eosinophilic**: cedr_{dyc} phos_{dyc} phyt_{dyc} puls-vg_{dyc}
- **Parotid** glands:
  • **mumps** (see pg 576)
- **Temporal** muscle: acon_{dyc1} arn_{dyc1} cedr_{dyc1} gels_{dyc1} hyper_{dyc1} kali-i_{dyc1} merc_{dyc1}
INVOLUNTARILY, mouth opens (see pg 576)
ITCHING (see pg 576)
- **Chin** (see pg 577): carc_{brm}

LICKING:
- **lips**:
  • **heat**; during (see pg 577)
LOCKJAW (see pg 577)
NECROSIS of:
- **Jaws**:
  • **Lower** (see pg 578)
  • **Upper** (see pg 578)
NODOSITIES (see pg 578)
NUMBNESS (see pg 578)
OVERSHOT JAW (see pg 578): syph_{brm}
PAIN (see pg 578)
- **corrosive** (see pg 581)
- **Jaws**:
  • **Joints**:
    : **chewing** agg. (see pg 587): puls_{brm}
  • **Nerves**:
    • **Trigeminal** neuralgia (see pg 592): chin_{brm} sep_{brm}
PARALYSIS (see pg 593): *Am-p*_{mld4} **Caust**_{mld4} *Gels*_{mld4} plb_{mld4}
- **right** (see pg 593): *Caust*_{ffd}
- **cold**; from (see pg 594): acon_{pkj1}
- **injuries**; after (see pg 594): arn_{pkj1} hyper_{pkj1}
- **Lips** (see pg 594): am-p_{mld4} arn_{mld4} caust_{mld4} gels_{mld4} plb_{mld4}
PEELING off of lips (see pg 594)
PERSPIRATION (see pg 594)
PICKING (see pg 595)
POINTED (see pg 595)
PULSATION (see pg 595)
QUIVERING (see pg 595)
RISUS sardonicus (see pg 595)
ROUGH skin (see pg 595)
SADDLE across the nose (see pg 596)
SENSITIVE (see pg 596)
SHINY (see pg 596)
- **oily**; as if (see pg 596)
SHORTENED, lower jaw seems (see pg 596)
SHRIVELLED (see pg 596)
SLIMY lips (see pg 596)
SMUTTY (see pg 596)
SORDES on the lips (see pg 596)
SPOTS:
- **colored** (see pg 596)
- **ulcerating** (see pg 596)
STICKING:
- **Lips**:
  • **together** (see pg 596)
STIFFNESS (see pg 596)
SUNBURN (see pg 596)

SUNKEN (see pg 596)

SUPPURATION:
- **Chin**:
  - **old** boils (see pg 597)
- **Jaws**:
  - **Lower** (see pg 597)
- **Mouth** closed by ulceration; corner of (see pg 597)

SWELLING (see pg 597)
- **bee** stings; from (see pg 597): apis$_{fmx}$ *Lach*$_{fmx}$
- **Lips** (see pg 598): borx$_{mld3}$ calc-s$_{mld3}$ staphycoc$_{mld3}$

TENSION of skin (see pg 599)

TIC (see pg 600)

TINGLING (see pg 600)

TREMBLING (see pg 600)

TUMOR:
- **cystic** tumor:
  - **Cheek**; on (see pg 600)
  - **Lips**; on (see pg 600)
  - **Parotid** gland:
    - **right** (see pg 600)

TWITCHING (see pg 601)

ULCERS (see pg 601)
- **Lips**:
  - **eosinophilic** ulcers: fl-ac$_{klp}$ nit-ac$_{klp}$

UNDERSHOT JAW:

VEINS distended (see pg 602)

WARTS (see pg 602)
- **papillomatosis**:
- **Mouth**:
  - **Corner**:

WEAKNESS:

WRINKLED (see pg 602)
- **Forehead** (see pg 602): **LYC**$_{dyc}$

Mouth

ABSCESS:
- **Gums**; of (see pg 605)
- **Tongue** (see pg 605)

ADHERES to roof of mouth; tongue (see pg 605)

APHTHAE (see pg 605): ph-ac$_{plrl}$

ATROPHY:
- **Gums** (see pg 606)
- **Tongue** (see pg 606)

BLEEDING (see pg 606)
- **Gums** (see pg 606)
  - **cleaning** them, when (see pg 606)

BOILS at gums (see pg 607)

MOUTH: ...

BURNS:
- **Tongue**:
  - **And** lips (see pg 607)

CANCER:
- **Gums** (see pg 607): hydr$_{mjs1}$
- **Tongue** (see pg 607): rad-br$_{pkj1}$ semp$_{pkj1}$

CARIES:
- **Gums** (see pg 607)
- **Palate** (see pg 607)

CHOREA, tongue (see pg 607)

CLAMMY (see pg 608)

CLOSED (see pg 608)

COLDNESS:
- **Tongue** (see pg 608)
  - **Tip**: carb-v$_{sxj}$

CONDYLOMATA:
- **Palate** (see pg 609)
- **Tongue** (see pg 609)

CONGESTION of gums (see pg 609)

CONSTRICTION (see pg 609)

CONTRACTION (see pg 609)

CRACKED (see pg 609)

CRACKLING of gums on pressure (see pg 610)

DENUDED spots:
- **Tongue**; on (see pg 610)

DESQUAMATION:
- **Cheek**; inside (see pg 610)
- **Palate**:
  - **sensation** of (see pg 610)

DETACHED from teeth; gums (see pg 610)

DISCHARGE:
- **brown** ichor on making incision near second molar; stinking (see pg 610)
- **offensive**:
- **putrid** (see pg 610)

DISCOLORATION:
- **Tongue**:
  - **blue** (see pg 612)
  - **dirty** (see pg 613): podo$_{qqh}$
  - **red**:
    - **fever**; during: lach$_{qqh}$
    - **Tip**:
      - **triangular**:
        - **fever**; during: rhus-t$_{qqh}$
  - **white** (see pg 615)
  - **yellow**:
    - **white**:
      - **Root** (see pg 619): nux-v$_{qqh}$

DROPPING:
- **food**: calc$_{brm}$

DRYNESS (see pg 619)
- **Tongue:**
  - **fever;** during (see pg 621): lach$_{qqh}$ mur-ac$_{qqh}$ verat-v$_{qqh}$

ECCHYMOSES:
- **dark** red, bloody (see pg 622)

EPULIS (see pg 622): ars$_{brm}$ calc-f$_{bnfl.es,dyc,mld,qqh}$ hecla$_{bnfl.es,mld,qqh}$ lyc$_{brm}$ *Nat-m*$_{brm}$ plb$_{brm}$ *Sil*$_{mld,qqh}$ symph$_{bnfl.es}$ *Thuj*$_{elg}$
- **soft** and painless (see pg 622): calc$_{hnb}$

ERUPTIONS:
- **herpes:**
  - **Tongue;** on (see pg 622)
- **pimples** (see pg 622)
- **vesicles** (see pg 622)

EXCRESCENCES (see pg 623)

EXOSTOSIS at roof of mouth (see pg 623)

FISTULA:
- **Gums** (see pg 623)

FLABBY tongue (see pg 623)

FOLDED tongue, like little bags on sides (see pg 623)

FOOD:
- **escapes** from mouth when chewing (see pg 623)

FROTH, foam from mouth (see pg 623)

FURRY:
- **Gums** (see pg 624)
- **Tongue** (see pg 624)

GANGRENOUS (see pg 624)
- **Gums:**
  - **scabs** (see pg 624)

GLAZED:
- **Palate** (see pg 624)

HARD:
- **spot** (see pg 624)
- **Palate** (see pg 624)
- **Tongue** (see pg 624)

HEAT (see pg 624)

INDENTED:
- **Gums** (see pg 625)
- **Tongue** (see pg 625)

INDURATION:
- **Tongue** (see pg 625): Sil$_{plr1}$

INFLAMMATION (see pg 625)
- **Gums** (see pg 625): lyc$_{brm}$ staph$_{pkj,qqh}$
  - **chronic** (see pg 625): lyc$_{klp}$
  - **thin** border nearest teeth: merc$_{elg}$ plb$_{elg}$
  - **ulcerative:** lyc$_{brm}$ staph$_{brm}$
- **Tongue** (see pg 625): kreos$_{qqh}$
  - **actinomycosis:** cist$_{dyc}$ iod$_{dyc}$ kali-i$_{dyc}$ lap-a$_{dyc}$

INJURIES:
- **Gums:** arn$_{plr1}$ con$_{plr1}$ ph-ac$_{plr1}$ symph$_{plr1}$
- **Tongue** (see pg 626): arn$_{plr1}$ carb-an$_{plr1}$ merc$_{plr1}$

ITCHING (see pg 626)

LACERATED Tongue (see pg 626)

MAPPED tongue (see pg 626)

MERCURIAL affections of gums:

MERCURY; after abuse of:

MUCOUS MEMBRANE:
- **blood** oozes from (see pg 627)
- **excoriation** (see pg 627)
  - **scaling** off (see pg 627)
  - **Tongue** (see pg 627)
    - **Tip** (see pg 627): ant-c$_{plr1}$ arn$_{plr1}$

MUCUS (see pg 627)
- **ropy** (see pg 628)
- **Tongue;** collection of mucus on (see pg 628)

NODOSITIES (see pg 628)

NUMBNESS (see pg 629)

ODOR:
- **offensive** (see pg 629): *Lyc*$_{brm}$ symph$_{qqh}$
- **putrid:**
  - **fever;** during: ail$_{qqh}$

OPEN (see pg 630): mag-c$_{brm}$
- **sleep** agg.; during (see pg 630): ars$_{brm}$ *Lyc*$_{brm}$ nat-m$_{brm}$ puls$_{brm}$

PAIN (see pg 630)

PARALYSIS:
- **Palate** (see pg 638)
- **Tongue** (see pg 638)

PASTY (see pg 638)

PATCHES, syphilitic (see pg 638)

POINTED Tongue (see pg 638)

PRICKLING (see pg 638)

PROTRUDING:
- **Tongue** (see pg 638): mag-c$_{brm}$
  - **oscillating** (see pg 639)
  - **rapidly,** darting in and out like a snake's (see pg 639)

PROUD flesh on gums (see pg 639)

PURPURA (see pg 639)

PUSTULES (see pg 639)

PUTRID gums (see pg 639)

RANULA (see pg 639): apis$_{dyc1}$

RATTLING (see pg 639)

RINGWORM (see pg 639)

ROUGHNESS (see pg 639)

SALIVA:
- **gluey** (see pg 640)
- **scanty** (see pg 640): apis$_{dyc1}$ *Lyc*$_{dyc1}$
- **thick** (see pg 641): *Ars*$_{fmx}$ merc$_{fmx}$
- **viscid** (see pg 641): anac$_{brm}$

SALIVATION (see pg 641): esin$_{mld5}$ jab$_{pkj1}$ *Merc* $_{fmx}$
Pilo$_{dyc,mld5}$ tril-p$_{mld5}$
- **excitement** agg. : lyc$_{brm}$ phos$_{ffd}$ puls$_{brm}$
- **fear**; from: cham$_{brm}$ cic$_{brm}$
- **fever**; during (see pg 643): merc$_{qqh}$
- **food**:
  • **looking** at; on: med$_{brm}$ phos$_{brm}$ sulph$_{brm}$
  • **smell** of: med$_{brm}$
- **purring**; on: bar-c$_{brm}$ hep$_{brm}$ merc$_{fmx}$ nat-m$_{brm}$
  sulph$_{brm}$
- **riding** in a car; on: caust$_{brm}$ lyc$_{brm}$
- **sleep**:
  • **during**:
    agg. (see pg 644): *Sulph* $_{brm}$
- **sniffing**; when: phos$_{brm}$ sulph$_{brm}$
- **vomiting**; before (see pg 644): lyc$_{brm}$
- **walking** agg. (see pg 644): sulph$_{brm}$

SCORBUTIC Gums (see pg 644)

SCRATCHING:
- **Gums** (see pg 644)
- **Palate** (see pg 644)
- **Tongue** (see pg 644)

SENSITIVE (see pg 644)

SHRIVELLED:
- **Gums** (see pg 644)
- **Palate** (see pg 644)
- **Tongue** (see pg 644)

SMACKING tongue (see pg 644)

SMOOTH tongue (see pg 644)
- **varnished**; tongue looks as if (see pg 644)

SOFT:
- **Tongue** (see pg 645)

SOFTENING of gums (see pg 645)

SORDES:
- **Gums** (see pg 645)
- **Lips** (see pg 645)
- **Tongue** (see pg 645)

SPASMS (see pg 645)
- **Tongue** (see pg 645)

SPONGY:
- **Gums** (see pg 646)
- **Tongue** (see pg 646)

STICKY, viscid (see pg 646)

STIFF:
- **Tongue** (see pg 646)

STOMATITIS, ulcerative (see pg 646): agar$_{brm}$
bell$_{mid,pkj1}$ chel$_{mld}$ cor-r$_{itm}$ fl-ac$_{mld}$ hydr$_{pkj}$ hyper$_{mld}$
kreos$_{itm,mld4}$ merc-cy$_{itm,mld3}$ rhus-t$_{mld}$
- **gangrenous** (see pg 647)

SUPPURATION:
- **Gums** (see pg 647)
- **Tongue** (see pg 647)

SWELLING (see pg 647)

MOUTH – Swelling: ...
- **Glands** (see pg 647)
- **Tongue** (see pg 648): Apis $_{fmx}$ *Lach* $_{fmx}$
  • **accompanied** by:
    : **hypocalcemia**:

THRUSH (see pg 656)

TREMBLING of tongue (see pg 656)
- **fever**; during: lach$_{qqh}$

TUBERCLES:
- **Gums**, painful (see pg 656)
- **Tongue** (see pg 656)

TUMORS (see pg 656)

TWITCHING:
- **Gums** (see pg 657)
- **Tongue** (see pg 657)

ULCERS (see pg 657): acet-ac$_{mld5}$ cist$_{plr1}$ con$_{plr1}$
nat-s$_{gsd4}$
- **Lips**; inner side of:
  • **Base** lardaceous: caps$_{hnb}$

VARICOSE veins:
- **Tongue** (see pg 658)

WARTS (see pg 658)
- **Tongue** (see pg 658)

WATERY, gums look (see pg 658)

WETTING lips constantly (see pg 658)

WITHERED Tongue (see pg 658)

WRINKLED (see pg 658)

Teeth

ABSCESS of roots (see pg 661): aur$_{brm}$ calc-s$_{qqh}$
Lyc $_{qqh}$ myris$_{pkj1}$ puls$_{brm}$

BLEEDING (see pg 661)

BREAKING off (see pg 661)

CARIES, decayed, hollow (see pg 661): merc-c$_{bnf1.es,pkj1}$
pyrog$_{bnf1.es}$
- **accompanied** by:
  • **urination**; involuntary: plan$_{qqh}$

CHATTERING (see pg 661)

CLENCHING teeth together:
- **desire** to clench teeth together; constant (see pg 662)
  • **clenched** firmly (see pg 662)

COLDNESS (see pg 662)

CRACKING when rubbing (see pg 663)

CRUMBLING (see pg 663)

CUPPED:
- **children**; in (see pg 663)

DENTITION:
- **difficult** (see pg 663): *Cina* $_{bnf1.es}$
  • **milk** tooth persists: calc$_{hnb}$ calc-f$_{hnb}$

DIRTY looking (see pg 664)

DISCHARGE from carious tooth (see pg 664)

DISCOLORATION:
- **black** (see pg 664): Staph$_{klp}$
- **yellow** (see pg 664)

DWARFED (see pg 664)

EDGES feel sharp and hurt gums (see pg 664)

ENAMEL deficient (see pg 664)

GRINDING (see pg 664): *Arn*$_{brm}$
- **pain**; during:
- **sleep** agg.; during (see pg 664): *Acon*$_{qqh}$

HEAT; sensation of (see pg 664)

INCRUSTATIONS (see pg 665)

INFLAMMATION:
- **Dentin** (see pg 665)

IRREGULAR (see pg 665)

ITCHING in (see pg 665)

LOOSENESS of (see pg 665): *Arg-n*$_{bnfl.es}$
- **falling** out (see pg 665)

MUCUS on teeth (see pg 665)
- **black**:
  · **crusts** (see pg 665)

NERVES, injuries to dental (see pg 682)

PAIN (see pg 666): calc-s$_{qqh}$
- **accompanied** by:
  · **Face**:
    : **spots**:
- **extraction** of teeth; after (see pg 672): hyper$_{dycl}$ myris$_{pkjl}$ pyrog$_{pkjl}$ ruta$_{dycl}$

PERIOSTITIS (see pg 680)

PROUD flesh, surrounded by (see pg 680)

SENSITIVE, tender (see pg 680)

SERRATED (see pg 680)

SHARP and hurt tongue; sides seem (see pg 681)

SORDES (see pg 681): frag$_{dyc,mld,qqh}$ lyc$_{qqh}$ nat-s$_{bnf}$ sil$_{bnfl.es,mld3}$ thuj$_{dyc}$ tub$_{bnf}$

STICK together, as if glued (see pg 681)

STICKY (see pg 681)

ULCERATION of roots (see pg 681)

WATER coming from; sour, fetid (see pg 681)

WEAKNESS in teeth (see pg 681)

WISDOM teeth, ailments from eruption of (see pg 681)

Throat

ANESTHESIA (see pg 683)

ANXIETY and apprehension in throat (see pg 683)

APHTHAE (see pg 683)

BLISTERED (see pg 683)

BLOOD:
- **hawks** up dark clotted blood (see pg 683)
- **oozing** (see pg 683)

CALCAREOUS deposit (see pg 683)

CANCER (see pg 683)

CASEOUS deposits in tonsils (see pg 683)

CATARRH (see pg 683)

CHEESY:
- **spots**; cheesy looking (see pg 683)

CHOKING (see pg 683)
- **drinking** agg. (see pg 684): phos$_{fmx}$ rhus-t$_{fmx}$

CLUCKING sound, esophagus (see pg 685)

COLD:
- **air**:
  · **agg.** (see pg 685)

CONDYLOMATA (see pg 685)

CONSTRICTION (see pg 685)

CRAMP (see pg 686)

DIPHTHERIA (see pg 686)

DRYNESS (see pg 688)

ELONGATED:
- **Uvula** (see pg 689)

ENLARGEMENT:
- **Esophagus**:

EROSION (see pg 689)

ERUPTIONS:
- **petechiae**:
  · **Pharynx**: lach$_{qqh}$
- **vesicles** (see pg 689)

EXCORIATION (see pg 689)

FISSURED:
- **Pharynx** (see pg 689)

FOOD:
- **lodges** in throat (see pg 689)
- **passes** into posterior nares (see pg 690)
- **Esophagus**:

GANGRENE (see pg 690)

GLUEY (see pg 690)

GURGLING; esophagus is (see pg 690)

HAWK; disposition to (see pg 691)

HAWKS up cheesy lumps (see pg 691)

HEAT (see pg 691)

INDURATION:
- **Tonsils**; of (see pg 691)

INFLAMMATION (see pg 692): calc-f$_{mld4}$ sal-ac$_{mld5}$ spong$_{ljy,plr1}$ vinc$_{mld5}$
- **Air** sacs:
- **Esophagus** (see pg 692): merc-c$_{mld3}$ sul-ac$_{mld3}$
- **Tonsils** (see pg 693): *Brom*$_{mld}$ calc$_{bnf1.es,klp}$ calc-p$_{bnf1.es}$ carc$_{klp}$ pyrog$_{qqh}$ tub-a$_{klp}$

INJURIES:

IRRITATION (see pg 693)

ITCHING (see pg 694)

LIQUIDS taken are forced into nose (see pg 694)

LUMP; sensation of a:
- **eating**:
  • **after**:
    ⁞ **agg.** (see pg 694): sil$_{dyc1}$

MAPPED:

MEMBRANE (see pg 695)

MUCOUS patches (see pg 695)

MUCUS (see pg 695)
- **transparent**: sulph$_{brm}$

NUMBNESS (see pg 697)

OBSTRUCTION (see pg 697)

PAIN (see pg 697)
- **swallowing**:
  • **food**:
    ⁞ **agg.** (see pg 704): bell$_{brm}$
  • **liquids**:
    ⁞ **agg.** (see pg 704)
- **warm**:
  • **drinks**:
    ⁞ **agg.** (see pg 704)
    ⁞ **amel.** (see pg 704)

PALENESS (see pg 708)

PARALYSIS (see pg 708)

PIMPLES:
- **Uvula** (see pg 708)

PULSATING (see pg 708)

PUSTULES (see pg 708)

REVERSED peristaltic action of esophagus (see pg 708)

RIGIDITY (see pg 708)

ROUGHNESS (see pg 708)

SCRAPING (see pg 709)

SCRATCHING (see pg 709)

SENSITIVE (see pg 709)

SHOCKS on waking (see pg 709)

SHRIVELLED uvula (see pg 709)

SPASMS (see pg 709)

THROAT: ...

SPOTS:
- **Pharynx**; in (see pg 710)

STIFFNESS (see pg 710)

STRICTURE of esophagus (see pg 710)

SUPPURATION:
- **Guttural** pouch: hep$_{mld4}$ hydr$_{mld4}$ kali-m$_{mld4}$ merc-c$_{mld4}$ sil$_{mld4}$
- **Tonsils** (see pg 710)

SWALLOW, constant disposition to (see pg 710)

SWELLING (see pg 712)
- **Tonsils** (see pg 712)

TENSION (see pg 713)

ULCERS:
- **Pharynx** (see pg 714): arg-n$_{qqh}$ lach$_{qqh}$ merc$_{qqh}$

VARICOSE (see pg 714)

External throat

ABSCESS (see pg 715): *Kali-i*$_{brm}$

CLOTHING agg. (see pg 715)

COLD AIR agg. :

COLDNESS (see pg 715)

CONGESTION (see pg 715)

CONSTRICTION (see pg 715): agar$_{trj}$ arn$_{trj}$ bell-p$_{trj}$ bry$_{trj}$ cimic$_{trj}$ hyper$_{trj}$

CRACKING in muscles (see pg 715)

CRAMP:
- **Sides** (see pg 715)

DISCOLORATION (see pg 715)

DISTENSION:
- **left** side (see pg 715)

DISTORTED (see pg 715)

ERUPTIONS (see pg 715)
- **flea-collars**; from:
- **pimples** (see pg 715): ruta$_{brm}$
- **urticaria** (see pg 716): carc$_{brm}$

EXCORIATION:
- **rubbing** of clothes; from (see pg 716)

FISTULAE (see pg 716)

FULLNESS:
- **Jugular**; in (see pg 716)
- **Throat**-pit (see pg 716)

GOITRE (see pg 716)
- **exophthalmic** (see pg 716)

HEAT (see pg 716)

INDURATION of glands (see pg 716)

INFLAMMATION: acon$_{plr1}$ arn$_{plr1}$ bry$_{plr1}$ hep$_{plr1}$

- **Thyroid** gland (see pg 716): flor-p$_{mld5}$ iod$_{mld5}$ kali-i$_{mld5}$ spong$_{mld5}$

ITCHING (see pg 717)
- **scratching**:
  - **hair**; with loss of: nat-m$_{hnb}$

JERKS:
- **left** (see pg 717)

LUMPS:
- **Throat**-pit (see pg 717)

NUMBNESS (see pg 717)

PAIN (see pg 717)

PARALYSIS (see pg 719)

PERSPIRATION (see pg 719)

PULSATION:
- **Carotids**:
  - **fever**; during (see pg 720): verat-v$_{qqh}$

SENSITIVE:
- **touch**; to slightest (see pg 720)

SPASMS:
- **Sides** of neck (see pg 720)

SPOTS (see pg 720)

STIFFNESS of sides (see pg 720)

STRAINING muscles (see pg 720)

STRETCHING OUT (see pg 720)

SWELLING (see pg 720)
- **Cervical** Glands:
  - **hard**:
    - **marbles**; like:
  - **soft**:

TENSION (see pg 720)

TIGHT around neck and waist; cannot bear anything (see pg 721)

TORTICOLLIS (see pg 721)

TOUCH agg. (see pg 721)

TREMBLING (see pg 721)

TWITCHING (see pg 721)

ULCERS (see pg 721)

UNCOVERING throat:
- **agg.** (see pg 721)

WARTS (see pg 721)

Stomach

ACIDITY (see pg 723)
- **Rumen**: nux-v$_{dyc}$

ACRIDITY (see pg 723)

AEROPHAGIA (see pg 723): arg-n$_{qqh}$

STOMACH: ...

APPETITE:
- **capricious** appetite (see pg 723): Chin$_{fmx}$ Cina$_{fmx}$ Ign$_{fmx}$ lyc$_{ffd,fmx}$ nux-v$_{fmx}$ *Phos*$_{brm,fmx}$ sil$_{fmx}$ sulph$_{brm,fmx}$
  - **accompanied** by:
    - **cancerous** affections: cina$_{fmx}$ phos$_{fmx}$ sulph$_{fmx}$
- **changeable** (see pg 723): ign$_{klp}$ nux-v$_{brm}$
- **diminished** (see pg 723): caps$_{brm}$ ign$_{klp}$ *Lyc*$_{klp}$
- **easy satiety** (see pg 724): calc-p$_{brm}$ *Sulph*$_{brm}$
- **increased** (see pg 724): Nat-m$_{klp}$
  - **eating**:
    - **after** (see pg 725): Lyc$_{fmx}$ sulph$_{fmx}$
      - **only** while eating; appetite returns (see pg 725): calc$_{fmx}$ lyc$_{fmx}$ *Sulph*$_{fmx}$
  - **fever**:
    - **during**:
      - **agg.** (see pg 725)
- **wanting** (see pg 727): apis$_{brm}$
  - **daytime**: nat-m$_{brm}$
  - **morning** (see pg 727): lyc$_{brm}$ phos$_{brm}$ stram$_{brm}$
  - **accompanied** by:
    - **diarrhea**:
    - **hypocalcemia**:
    - **ketosis**: ant-c$_{dyc}$ flor-p$_{dyc}$ lyc$_{dyc}$ senn$_{dyc}$
      - **cerebral** form: arg-n$_{dyc}$ cic$_{dyc}$ lyc$_{dyc}$ nux-v$_{dyc}$
  - **children**; in:
    - **weaned**; when being: ign$_{elg}$
  - **eating**:
    - **overeating**; after:
  - **food**:
    - **sight** of; at (see pg 728): chin$_{fmx}$ *Colch*$_{fmx}$
  - **owner** is absent; when: caust$_{brm}$
  - **perspiration**; during:
    - **pregnancy**; during: nat-m$_{fmx}$
  - **thirst**:
    - **with** (see pg 728)

CANCER (see pg 728)

CLOTHING:
- **disturbs** (see pg 729)
- **tight** clothes:
  - **amel.** (see pg 729)

CONSTRICTION:
- **Pylorus**, of (see pg 731): lyc$_{mld3}$ nux-v$_{mld3}$ sil$_{mld3}$ staph$_{dyc1}$

DISORDERED (see pg 732)

DISPLACEMENT:
- **Abomasum**:

DISTENSION (see pg 732)
- **accompanied** by:
  - **weakness**; extreme general: carb-v$_{brm}$
  - **old** dogs; in: carb-v$_{brm}$
- **tympanitic**:
  - **Rumen**:
    - **accompanied** by:
      - **motion** of rumen:

ERUCTATIONS (see pg 735): podo$_{qqh}$

- **eating**:
  - **after**:
    - **agg.** (see pg 737): tab$_{brm}$
- **farinaceous** food, after (see pg 737): puls$_{brm}$

FERMENTATION (see pg 744): kali-c$_{qqh}$

FLABBINESS (see pg 744)

FOREIGN body (see pg 744)

GAGGING (see pg 745)

GANGRENE (see pg 745)

GURGLING (see pg 745)

HEARTBURN (see pg 746)

HICCOUGH (see pg 748)

HYPERCHLORHYDRIA (see pg 751)

INDIGESTION (see pg 751): ant-c$_{pkj,plr,qqh}$ arg-n$_{qqh}$ bapt$_{pkj1}$ bry$_{gsd4}$ **Carb-v**$_{mld5}$ *Coff*$_{mld5}$ kali-bi$_{gsd4}$ **Lyc**$_{mld5}$ **Nux-v**$_{mld5}$ podo$_{pkj1}$ thuj$_{pkj1}$ verat$_{pkj1}$
- **hair**; of ball of: colch$_{dyc1}$ coloc$_{dyc1}$ grat$_{dyc1}$ nux-v$_{dyc1}$ raph$_{dyc1}$

INDURATION:
- **Pylorus** (see pg 752)
- **Walls**; of the (see pg 752)

INFLAMMATION (see pg 753): apom$_{mld3}$ calc$_{itm}$ calc-p$_{itm}$ carb-v$_{itm,plr1}$ iris$_{mld3}$ merc$_{itm,mjs,pkj1}$ petr$_{mld3}$
- **weather** agg.; cold wet: dulc$_{itm}$

LOATHING of food (see pg 753)

MOTION of rumen:
- **absent**: nux-v$_{dyc}$
- **often**; too:
- **seldom**; too:
- **strong**; too: nux-v$_{hnb}$
- **weak**; too:

NAUSEA (see pg 754): **Colch**$_{fmx}$ *Phos*$_{fmx}$ **Sulph**$_{fmx}$
- **breakfast**:
  - **during**:
    - **accompanied** by:
    - **diarrhea**; sudden:
- **riding**:
  - **carriage**; in a:
    - **agg.** (see pg 761): *Sil*$_{fmx}$
- **seasickness** (see pg 762): **Cocc**$_{bnfl.es}$ **Nux-v**$_{bnfl.es}$ **Petr**$_{bnfl.es}$

PAIN (see pg 764)
- **grass**; after eating: phos$_{brm}$

PERSPIRATION (see pg 781)

RETCHING (see pg 782): **Colch**$_{fmx}$ phos$_{fmx}$ *Sulph*$_{fmx}$

RUMINATION:
- **absent**:
- **short**; too:
- **slow**:
- **strong**; too:

SLOW digestion (see pg 784)

SUMMER (see pg 785)

THIRST (see pg 785)
- **chill**:
  - **during** (see pg 787): **Verat**$_{qqh}$
- **heat**:
  - **during** (see pg 787): *Puls*$_{fmx}$
- **large** quantities; for (see pg 788): carc$_{klp}$ **Phos**$_{fmx}$
  - **excitement** agg. : lyc$_{brm}$
  - **often**; and (see pg 788)
    - **pregnancy**; during: nat-m$_{fmx}$
  - **pregnancy**; during imaginary:
  - **walking** for a long time; after:
- **small** quantities, for:
  - **often**; and (see pg 788): calc$_{brm}$ calc-p$_{brm}$

THIRSTLESS (see pg 788): sil$_{fmx}$
- **pregnancy**; imaginary: puls$_{hnb}$

TORSION: acon$_{dyc1}$ colch$_{dyc1}$ coloc$_{dyc1}$

VOMITING (see pg 790): nat-s$_{spk1}$
- **morning**:
  - **empty** stomach; with:
- **night** (see pg 791): sep$_{brm}$
  - **midnight**:
    - **after** (see pg 791): puls$_{fmx}$
    - **towards** morning: lyc$_{brm}$
- **allergy**; from food: lyc$_{brm}$
  - **commercial** food: ph-ac$_{brm}$ phos$_{brm}$
- **bones**; after: caust$_{brm}$ nux-v$_{brm}$
- **cold**; on becoming (see pg 792): acon$_{qqh}$
- **diarrhea**:
  - **during** (see pg 792): phos$_{fmx}$
- **drinking**:
  - **after**:
    - **agg.** (see pg 793)
      - **large** quantities: nux-v$_{brm}$
    - **immediately** after (see pg 793): **Ars**$_{qqh}$
  - **large** quantities:
  - **warm** in stomach; as soon as water becomes (see pg 793): **Phos**$_{qqh}$
- **eating**:
  - **after**:
    - **agg.** (see pg 793): caust$_{klp}$ *Puls*$_{klp}$
      - **shortly** after eating: nat-m$_{brm}$
    - **grass**: carc$_{brm}$ lyc$_{brm}$ tritic$_{sxj}$
  - **fast** agg.: arg-n$_{qqh}$
- **excitement**; after (see pg 793): lyc$_{brm}$
- **fasting**; when: nat-m$_{brm}$
- **heat**:
  - **during** (see pg 793): puls$_{fmx}$
- **intoxication**; during (see pg 794): ars$_{qqh}$
- **leftovers**; after eating:
- **pregnancy** agg.; during:
  - **imaginary** pregnancy: sulph$_{brm}$
- **riding** in a carriage agg. (see pg 795): *Ars*$_{brm}$ med$_{brm}$ puls$_{brm}$ sep$_{brm,qqh}$
  - **after** (when the car stops): ars$_{elg}$
  - **while**: lyc$_{elg}$
- **warm**:
  - **room**:
    - **agg.** (see pg 796): acon$_{qqh}$

VOMITING; TYPE OF:
- **bile**:
  - **morning** (see pg 796): lyc$_{ffd}$
    - **empty** stomach; on: nat-m$_{brm}$
- **blood** (see pg 797)
- **food**:
  - **night** (see pg 798): lyc$_{brm}$
  - **eating**:
    - **after**:
      - **agg**. (see pg 798): mag-c$_{brm}$
      - **immediately** after (see pg 798): bar-c$_{brm}$ calc-p$_{brm}$ cham$_{brm}$ *Ferr-p*$_{hnb}$ phos$_{brm}$ puls$_{brm}$ sep$_{brm}$
        - **eating** again right away; then: med$_{brm}$ nat-m$_{brm}$ phos$_{brm}$
- **frothy** (see pg 799): ars$_{fmx}$ *Puls*$_{fmx}$
- **grass**: calc-p$_{brm}$ cic$_{brm}$ lyc$_{brm}$ nat-m$_{brm}$ sulph$_{brm}$ tritic$_{sxj}$
- **scraps**; eaten previously: phos$_{brm}$

Abdomen

ABSCESS: merc$_{mld5}$
- **Umbilicus**:
  - **painful**: hep$_{hnb}$ tarent$_{hnb}$
  - **painless**: sil$_{hnb}$

ATROPHY:
- **Liver** (see pg 803)
- **Spleen** (see pg 803)

BUBO (see pg 804)

CANCER:
- **accompanied** by:
  - **appetite**; wanting of: lyc$_{brm}$
  - **vomiting**: lyc$_{brm}$

CIRRHOSIS of liver (see pg 804): ars$_{qqh}$ berb$_{qqh}$ chel$_{qqh}$

CLOTHING; sensitive to (see pg 804): ign$_{brm}$

COLDNESS (see pg 805)

COMPLAINTS of abdomen:
- **Intestines**:
  - **accompanied** by:
    - **warmth**; desire for: tritic$_{sxj}$

CONGESTION:
- **Liver**; of (see pg 807): aloe$_{qqh}$ *Card-m*$_{bnfl.es,qqh}$ cean$_{qqh}$ chel$_{bnfl.es}$ chin$_{qqh}$ lept$_{qqh}$ puls$_{qqh}$ sep$_{qqh}$ **Sulph**$_{qqh}$
- **Spleen** (see pg 807): card-m$_{qqh}$ cean$_{qqh}$

CONTRACTION (see pg 807)

CRACKING and crackling (see pg 808)

CRACKS on surface of abdomen (see pg 808)

DISCHARGE from umbilicus (see pg 809): sil$_{hnb}$

ABDOMEN: ...

DISTENSION (see pg 809): alf$_{mld5}$ am-caust$_{mld5}$
- **painful** (see pg 811): absin$_{mld5}$ **Acon**$_{mld5}$ am-c$_{mld5}$ am-caust$_{mld,mld5}$ carb-v$_{bnfl.es,mld,mld5,qqh}$ chin$_{bnfl.es}$ colch$_{bnfl.es,mld,mld,mld5}$ euphr$_{mld5}$ hydr-ac$_{mld5}$ lyc$_{bnfl.es}$ raph$_{mld5}$
- **tympanitic** (see pg 811): **Lyc**$_{ffd}$
  - **calves**; in:
  - **cows**; in:
  - **Rumen**: ant-c$_{dyc}$ nux-v$_{dyc}$
    - **frothy** fermentation: colch$_{dyc}$

DROPSY:
- **ascites** (see pg 812): abrot$_{mld3}$ adon$_{mld3}$ aesc$_{mld3}$ ars-i$_{mld5}$ conv$_{mld3}$ crat$_{mld3}$ lycps-v$_{mld5}$ stroph-s$_{mld5}$
- **edema** (see pg 812)

DRYNESS:
- **Peritoneum**: bry$_{hnb}$
- **Skin**: lyc$_{brm}$

EMACIATION of muscles of abdomen (see pg 812)

ENLARGED (see pg 813): ars$_{fmx}$ kali-c$_{fmx}$ *Lyc*$_{fmx}$ nux-v$_{fmx}$ phos$_{fmx}$
- **young** animals; in:
- **Spleen**:
  - **children**; in (see pg 813): calc$_{hnb}$

EPILEPSY, begins in (see pg 813)

ERUPTIONS (see pg 813)

ERYSIPELAS (see pg 814)

EXCORIATIONS (see pg 814)

EXCRESCENCE at umbilicus; moist (see pg 814)

FATTY DEGENERATION of liver (see pg 814)

FERMENTATION (see pg 814)

FISTULAE:
- **Inguinal** glands; of (see pg 814)
- **Umbilicus**: sil$_{hnb}$

FLATULENCE (see pg 814)
- **obstructed** (see pg 815): tritic$_{sxj}$

FOREIGN BODY; ailments after swallowing a:

GOUTY metastasis (see pg 818)

GURGLING (see pg 818)

HAIR:
- **baldness**:
  - **licking**; from: ign$_{klp}$ nat-m$_{klp}$ puls$_{klp}$ staph$_{klp}$
- **falling** out:
  - **Sides**: tarent$_{brm}$

HARD (see pg 819)
- **Liver** (see pg 819): berb$_{bnfl.es}$ *Chel*$_{bnfl.es}$ *Lyc*$_{bnfl.es}$ *Nux-v*$_{bnfl.es}$ **Phos**$_{bnfl.es}$ solid$_{bnfl.es}$

- **Umbilicus** (see pg 819): sil$_{hnb}$

HERNIA; ABDOMINAL (see pg 821)

ILEUS (see pg 821)
- **operation**; after:
  - anesthesia; from:

IMPACTION (see pg 821)

INFLAMMATION (see pg 821): ant-c$_{qqh}$ calc-f$_{mld}$ chin$_{mld4}$ hep$_{mld}$ podo$_{mld,mld,mld5,qqh}$ rheum$_{plr,qqh}$
- **painful**: rhus-t$_{plr1}$
- **Liver** (see pg 822): aesc$_{dyc,mld3}$ aloe$_{mld4}$ berb$_{dyc,itm,mld,mld,mld5,pkj1}$ cean$_{dyc,mld5}$ crot-h$_{mld,mld5}$ dig$_{dyc,plr1}$ elaps$_{mld}$ hydr$_{mld4}$ iris$_{pkj1}$ kali-m$_{mld5}$ lept$_{dyc,mld5}$ *Ptel*$_{mld5}$ sol-v$_{dyc,pkj1}$ *Sulph*$_{mld,pkj1}$ tarax$_{dyc,pkj1}$
  - **chronic** (see pg 823): *Sulph*$_{fmx}$
- **Pancreas** (see pg 823): acon$_{dyc,mld3}$ *Atro*$_{dyc,mld3}$ cean$_{mld3}$ flor-p$_{bnf1.es}$ *Iris*$_{bnf}$ *Kali-i*$_{bnf}$ phos$_{mld,pkj1}$ puls$_{fmx}$
  - **acute** (see pg 823): bell$_{brm}$
- **Peritoneum**:
  - **accompanied** by:
    - Tongue:
      - dryness of tongue (see pg 823): bry$_{hnb}$
- **Small intestine** (see pg 823)
- **Spleen** (see pg 823): ferr-ar$_{pkj1}$ helia$_{pkj1}$
- **Umbilicus**:
  - **acute**: hep$_{dyc}$
  - **chronic**: calc-s$_{dyc}$ sil$_{dyc}$

ITCHING (see pg 823): carc$_{brm}$ *Sulph*$_{brm}$
- **Hypochondria** (see pg 824): sep$_{ffd}$

LIVER and region of liver; complaints of (see pg 894): *Sulph*$_{fmx}$

MOVEMENTS in (see pg 825)

NECROSIS:
- **Liver**: kali-c$_{mld}$ phos$_{mld}$ sil$_{mld}$

OBSTRUCTION:
- **Gall ducts**; of (see pg 825)

PAIN (see pg 826): am-caust$_{mjs,mld5}$
- **night** (see pg 828): phos$_{brm}$
- **cold**:
  - **drinks**:
    - after:
      - agg. (see pg 832)
  - **food**:
    - agg. (see pg 832)
- **constipation**:
  - **from** (see pg 832): *Alum*$_{itm}$ calc$_{bnf1.es}$ hydr$_{itm}$ mag-m$_{itm}$ *Nux-v*$_{itm,plr1}$ op$_{bnf1.es,itm,plr1}$ plb$_{bnf1.es,plr1}$ *Sulph*$_{itm}$
- **cramping** (see pg 832)
- **dentition**; during: cham$_{dyc1}$ podo$_{dyc1}$
- **diarrhea**:
  - **during**:
    - cramping (see pg 834): nux-v$_{brm}$

Pain: ...
- **hysterectomy**; after:
- **increasing**:
  - **gradually**:
    - decreasing:
      - gradually (see pg 837)
  - **quickly**:
    - decreasing:
      - quickly (see pg 837)
- **lying**:
  - **abdomen**; on:
    - amel. (see pg 838)
  - **side**; on:
    - left:
      - amel.:
        - cramping: con$_{brm}$ nux-v$_{brm}$
- **operation**; after:
  - **children**; in:
  - **ovariohysterectomy**; after:
  - **ovary** resection; after:
- **overloaded**; from being: ant-c$_{qqh}$ nux-v$_{dyc1}$ puls$_{plr1}$
- **owner** is stressed; if the:
  - **cramping**: nux-v$_{brm}$
- **periodical**:
  - **months**; every two: nux-v$_{brm}$
- **pressure**:
  - **agg.** (see pg 840): apis$_{dyc}$ arn$_{dyc}$ nat-m$_{dyc}$ staph$_{dyc}$
- **spasmodic** (see pg 842): acon$_{bnf1.es,itm,plr1}$ am-caust$_{itm}$ bell$_{qqh}$ cham$_{bnf1.es,plr1}$ cina$_{bnf1.es,itm}$ colch$_{bnf1.es,itm}$ coloc$_{bnf1.es,itm,mld5}$ cupr$_{bnf1.es}$ dulc$_{mld5}$ ign$_{qqh}$ nux-v$_{itm,mld5,qqh}$ staph$_{qqh}$
- **stool**:
  - **urging** to:
    - cramping (see pg 844): nux-v$_{brm}$
- **urination**:
  - **retention** of urine; from (see pg 845): ars$_{plr1}$ berb$_{plr,qqh}$ canth$_{plr,qqh}$ cham$_{plr1}$ hyos$_{plr1}$
- **walking**:
  - **amel.**:
    - cramping (see pg 846): op$_{brm}$
- **Liver**:
  - **lying**:
    - side; on:
      - right:
        - agg. (see pg 867): borx$_{hnb}$
    - **touch** agg. (see pg 868): borx$_{hnb}$

PANCREAS; complaints of (see pg 895): cean$_{dyc1}$ ph-ac$_{dyc1}$ puls$_{qqh}$ senec$_{dyc1}$

PARALYSIS of intestines (see pg 884): calc$_{qqh}$ *Kali-c*$_{qqh}$ raph$_{qqh}$
- **anesthesia**; from: op$_{hnb}$
- **discopathy**; from: nux-v$_{hnb}$
- **laparotomy**; after:
- **pain**; from:

PERISTALSIS:
- **increased** (see pg 884)
- **reversed** (see pg 884)

PERSPIRATION (see pg 884)

PORTAL congestion (see pg 884)
- **accompanied** by:
  - menses; painful (see pg 884)

PROTRUSION (see pg 885)
- **Umbilicus** (see pg 885)

RETRACTION (see pg 886)

RUMBLING (see pg 886): $Calc_{ffd}$
- **night:**
  - midnight:
    : after:
    : 4 h (see pg 887): lyc_{brm}
- **croaking** like frogs (see pg 887)
- **diarrhea:**
  - before (see pg 887): $phos_{fmx}$
  - during (see pg 887): $phos_{fmx}$

SENSITIVE:
- **Skin** (see pg 888)

SHOCKS (see pg 888)

SPLEEN; complaints of (see pg 896)

STIFFNESS (see pg 889)

SUPPURATION:
- **Glands;** inguinal (see pg 889)

SWASHING (see pg 889)

TABES mesenterica (see pg 890)

TENSION (see pg 890)

TREMBLING (see pg 892)

TUMORS (see pg 892)

TWITCHING and jerking (see pg 892)

ULCERS (see pg 892)

VEINS distended (see pg 893)

Rectum

ABSCESS:
- **Anal** sac: $apis_{pkj1}$ $bell_{pkj1}$ $calc-s_{mld5,qqh}$ $hep_{mld5,pkj1}$ $lach_{brm}$ lyc_{brm} $paeon_{pkj1}$ rat_{pkj1} $sil_{mld5,pkj,qqh}$
  - painful: hep_{brm}
- **Glands;** perianal (see pg 897): $syph_{brm}$

CANCER (see pg 897): $aesc_{bnfl.es}$ $hura_{bnfl.es}$ $stilboest_{mld5}$
- **Anal** sac: $aesc_{mld}$ $nit-ac_{mld}$ $stilboest_{mld}$

CATARRH of the rectum (see pg 897)

CAULIFLOWER excrescence (see pg 897)

CHOLERA (see pg 897)

CHRONIC complaints:
- **Anal** sac: sil_{hnb}

COLDNESS in anus (see pg 898)

CONDYLOMATA (see pg 898)

CONGESTION (see pg 898)

RECTUM: ...

CONSTIPATION (see pg 898)
- **accompanied** by:
  - uremia: $nat-m_{brm}$
- **anesthesia;** from: op_{hnb}
- **children;** in (see pg 899): Sep_{brm}
- **difficult** stool (see pg 900)
  - recedes; stool (see pg 900)
- **fever;** during (see pg 900): bry_{qqh}
- **home:**
  - stool at home not possible; passing: ars_{hnb}
- **ineffectual** urging and straining (see pg 900)
- **meconium;** of: $aloe_{qqh}$
- **old** animals; in:
- **sedentary** habits agg. (see pg 901): $nat-m_{brm}$ $Sulph_{brm}$ $thuj_{brm}$
- **walking:**
  - amel.: $thuj_{brm}$

CONSTRICTION (see pg 901)

DIARRHEA (see pg 902): $camph_{dyc1}$ $elat_{mld5}$ $senec_{dyc1}$
- **afternoon** (see pg 903): $phos_{brm}$
- **accompanied** by:
  - salivation (see pg 904): $merc_{fmx}$
- **allopathic** medicines; after:
- **canned** food; from: lyc_{brm}
- **children;** in:
  - leaving nest, house or stable; after:
- **chronic** (see pg 906): $Calc_{ffd}$ lyc_{klp} $nat-s_{klp}$ $Phos_{fmx}$ $puls_{klp}$ $Sulph_{klp}$ Tub_{klp}
- **drugs;** after:
  - antibiotics:
  - cortisone: $cortiso_{klp}$
- **eating:**
  - overeating agg.; after:
    : concentrated food:
- **excitement** agg. (see pg 907): $Arg-n_{dyc}$ $Calc-p_{dyc}$ $lyc_{brm,ffd}$
- **food:**
  - change of, after (see pg 908): lyc_{brm}
- **grass;** after eating: lyc_{brm}
- **grief;** from:
  - owners on holiday; when: $thuj_{brm}$
- **indiscretion** in eating, after the slightest (see pg 908): $lyc_{brm,fmx}$ $Phos_{fmx}$ $rhus-t_{fmx}$
- **leftovers;** after eating: $nat-m_{brm}$
- **meat:**
  - from (see pg 908): $nat-m_{brm}$
  - raw meat; from: tab_{brm}
- **nervous,** emotions agg. (see pg 909): tab_{brm}
- **nursing** the child agg.; after (see pg 909): $Chin_{brm}$
- **periodical** (see pg 909): $lyc_{brm,klp}$ tub_{klp}
- **salad;** from: $coloc_{brm}$
- **septic** conditions, from (see pg 910): $bapt_{bnfl.es,pkj1}$ $crot-t_{bnfl.es,pkj1}$ $cupr_{bnfl.es,pkj1}$ $merc_{bnfl.es,pkj1}$ $verat_{bnfl.es,pkj1}$
- **undigested:** $chin_{bnfl.es}$ $ferr_{bnfl.es}$ $graph_{bnfl.es}$ $hep_{bnfl.es}$
- **weakness,** without (see pg 910): ars_{brm} $Nux-v_{brm}$

- **weather**:
  - **warm**:
    - **agg.** (see pg 911): *Rhus-t*_{brm}

DISCOLORATION:
- **Anus**:
  - **red** (see pg 911): merc_{hnb}

DISTENSION (see pg 911)

DRAGGING, heaviness, weight (see pg 911)

DRYNESS (see pg 911)

DYSENTERY (see pg 911): Ars_{dyc} Canth_{gsd,pkjl} ph-ac_{mld4}

ERUPTIONS:
- **Anus**; about (see pg 912)
  - **boils** (see pg 912)
- **Perineum** (see pg 913)

EXCORIATION (see pg 913)

FISSURE (see pg 913)

FISTULA (see pg 913)
- **Anal sac**:
- **Glands**:
  - **Perianal**: lyc_{brm}

FLATUS (see pg 913)
- **evening** (see pg 914): **Sulph**_{fmx}
- **canned** food; from: lyc_{brm}
- **coughing**, on (see pg 914): tab_{brm}
- **diarrhea**, during (see pg 914): sep_{brm}
- **meat**; after: sulph_{brm}
- **observing** one's own flatus: nat-m_{brm,hnb}
- **onions** agg.:
- **rising**; when: lyc_{brm}
- **stool**:
  - **before** (see pg 915): sulph_{brm}

FULLNESS:
- **Anal sac**: ign_{brm} lyc_{brm} nat-m_{brm} nux-v_{brm} phos_{brm}

HEAT (see pg 915)

HEMORRHAGE from anus (see pg 915)
- **copious**:
  - **lovesickness**; from: phos_{hnb}

HERNIA; PERINEAL: phos_{brm}

INACTIVITY of rectum (see pg 919)

INFLAMMATION (see pg 919): coll_{mld3} podo_{mld3} ruta_{mld3}
- **Anal sac**: calc_{ffd} hep_{dyc} pyrog_{dyc} rhus-t_{brm} sanic_{dyc} sil_{dyc} sulph_{dyc}
  - **right**:
  - **left**: hep_{brm}
  - **greenish**: hep_{brm}
  - **purulent**:
- **Glands**; perianal: lyc_{brm} syph_{brm}

INSENSIBILITY (see pg 919)

INVOLUNTARY stool (see pg 919)
- **fever**; with (see pg 920): mur-ac_{qqh}

ITCHING (see pg 920)

MOISTURE (see pg 922)
- **corrosive**:
  - **Anal** glands:
- **offensive**:
  - **Anal** sac:
- **purulent**:
  - **Anal** sac: caust_{brm} lyc_{brm} phos_{brm}
- **putrid**:
  - **Anal** sac:
- **thick**:
  - **Anal** glands:
  - **Anal** sac:
- **thin**:
  - **Anal** glands:
  - **Anal** sac:
- **viscid**:
  - **Anal** glands:
  - **Anal** sac:
- **Anal** sac:

OPEN anus (see pg 922)

PAIN (see pg 922)
- **prostate** gland; from enlargement of:
  - **tenesmus**: phos_{brm} :
- **stool**:
  - **before**:
    - **tenesmus** (see pg 928): phos_{brm}
- **tenesmus** (see pg 929)
  - **enlarged** prostate; from: nux-v_{brm}
- **Anal** glands:
  - **touch** agg.:
- **Anal** sac:
  - **touch** agg.:
- **Perianal** glands:

PARALYSIS (see pg 932)

PARASITES:
- **coccidia**:
- **giardiasis**: sulph_{brm}
  - **accompanied** by:
    - **Pupil**; contraction of left: sulph_{brm}

PERSPIRATION about the anus and perineum (see pg 932)

POLYPI (see pg 933)

PROLAPSUS (see pg 933)

PULSATION (see pg 933)

RELAXED anus (see pg 934)

RETRACTION (see pg 934)

SENSITIVE (see pg 934)

SPASMS in (see pg 934)

STRICTURE (see pg 934)

SWELLING of anus (see pg 934)

TENSION (see pg 934)

TREMBLING in anus (see pg 934)

TUBERCLE on Perineum (see pg 934)

TUMORS:
- **Anal** sac:
- **Perianal** glands:

ULCERATION (see pg 934)

UNNOTICED stool (see pg 935)

URGING (see pg 935)
- **colic**, during (see pg 935): Nux-v$_{brm}$

WORMS:
- **complaints** of worms (see pg 937)
  - **tapeworm**:
    - **recurrent** infections with tapeworms: nat-m$_{brm}$ sulph$_{brm}$

Stool

BLOODY (see pg 939): cortiso$_{klp}$ **Phos**$_{hnb}$ *Rhus-t*$_{fmx}$

CHANGEABLE (see pg 940): *Sulph*$_{brm}$

FORCIBLE, sudden, gushing:
- **pulling** a wagon; when: sep$_{brm}$

GRANULAR (see pg 942): *Phos*$_{fmx}$

HARD:
- **followed** by:
  - **soft** stool (see pg 943): caust$_{klp}$ *Lyc*$_{fmx,klp}$ nux-v$_{brm}$

MUCOUS (see pg 944): lyc$_{klp}$ **Nat-s**$_{klp}$ **Puls**$_{klp}$
- **covered** with mucus (see pg 944): merc$_{klp}$ rhus-t$_{fmx}$ tab$_{brm}$ tub$_{klp}$
- **white** (see pg 945): **Nat-m**$_{brm}$

ODOR:

ODORLESS (see pg 946)

SHOOTING out (see pg 946): lyc$_{klp}$
- **exertion**; during physical:

UNDIGESTED (see pg 948): nux-v$_{brm}$

WATERY:
- **drops**:
  - **stool**; after the: lyc$_{brm}$

WHITE:
- **chalk**, like:
  - **curdy** (see pg 949): calc$_{hnb}$

Bladder

CANCER (see pg 951): crot-h$_{ffd}$

CATARRH, mucopus (see pg 951)

CONSTRICTION (see pg 951)

FUNGOID growths (see pg 952)

GANGRENE (see pg 952)

HEMORRHAGE (see pg 952)

HEMORRHOIDS of (see pg 952)

INACTIVITY of (see pg 952)

BLADDER: ...

INDURATION:
- **cartilaginous** (see pg 952)

INFLAMMATION (see pg 952): benz-ac$_{itm}$ form$_{bnfl.es}$ helon$_{mld5}$ staph$_{mld5}$ uva$_{mld,mld,mld4}$
- **catheterization**; after (see pg 952): arn$_{pkj1}$ staph$_{pkj,qqh}$
- **cold** agg.; becoming: rhus-t$_{spk1}$
- **hemorrhagic** (see pg 953): ign$_{brm}$
- **idiopathic**: ign$_{brm}$
- **old** people; in: carb-v$_{brm}$

INJURY, operations after (see pg 953)

INSENSIBILITY (see pg 953)

ITCHING (see pg 953)

MOTION in (see pg 953)

MOVEMENTS bring up urinary troubles (see pg 953)

PAIN (see pg 953)
- **urination**:
  - **after**:
    - **agg.** (see pg 955): equis-h$_{qqh}$ sars$_{qqh}$
  - **during**:
    - **agg.** (see pg 956): caps$_{qqh}$ *Clem*$_{qqh}$ pareir$_{qqh}$
- **Neck** of bladder:
  - **urination**:
    - **during**:
      - **end** of (see pg 957): equis-h$_{qqh}$

PARALYSIS (see pg 958): bry$_{qqh}$ con$_{mld4}$ kali-c$_{qqh}$
- **over-distension**, after (see pg 958): caps$_{brm}$

PARALYTIC weakness (see pg 958)

POLYPI (see pg 958)

RETENTION of urine (see pg 958): *Cann-i*$_{klp}$ *Chim*$_{klp}$ sabal$_{klp}$ ser-ang$_{qqh}$
- **daytime**: thuj$_{qqh}$
- **cold**:
  - **air** agg. (see pg 958): acon$_{qqh}$
- **company**; unable to pass urine in presence of (see pg 959): **Nat-m**$_{hnb}$
- **delivery**:
  - **after**; immediately (see pg 959): bry$_{qqh}$
- **discopathy**; from:
- **infection**; from:
- **long** time; for a: ars$_{qqh}$ caust$_{qqh}$ hyos$_{plr1}$

RHEUMATIC affections (see pg 959)

SPASM (see pg 959): acon$_{plr1}$ arn$_{plr,qqh}$ cann-i$_{plr1}$ coloc$_{pkj1}$ mag-m$_{qqh}$

SPASMODIC action of (see pg 959)

STONES in bladder (see pg 959): calc-p$_{dyc,itm}$ chim$_{bnfl.es,itm}$ equis-h$_{itm,pkj1}$ oxal-a$_{itm}$

SUPPURATION (see pg 960)

SWOLLEN (see pg 960)

TENESMUS (see pg 960)

TENSION (see pg 960)

THICKENING of walls of (see pg 960)

TUMORS (see pg 960)

ULCERATION (see pg 960)

URINATION:
- **dribbling** (see pg 960): $Canth_{klp}$ *Pareir*$_{klp}$ *Staph*$_{klp}$
  - **involuntary** (see pg 961): $caps_{brm}$ $Caust_{klp}$ cop_{klp} $nat-m_{brm}$
  - **retention**, with (see pg 961): $caps_{brm}$
- **dysuria** (see pg 961): *Apis*$_{qqh}$ **Bell**$_{qqh}$ *Berb*$_{qqh}$ *Caps*$_{pkj1}$ equis-h$_{pkj1}$ *Merc*$_{qqh}$ **Merc-c**$_{pkj,qqh}$ **Puls**$_{qqh}$ **Ter**$_{pkj,qqh}$
  - **painful** (see pg 962): *Tritic*$_{sxj}$
- **frequent**:
  - **night** (see pg 963): $apoc_{bnfl.es}$ $sabal_{qqh}$ *Sil*$_{qqh}$
  - **fever**:
    : **during**:
      : **agg.** (see pg 963)
  - **wet**; from becoming: $senec_{qqh}$
- **involuntary** (see pg 964): $calc-f_{dyc1}$ **Caust**$_{klp}$ $ferr-m_{qqh}$ **Phos**$_{klp}$ $phyt_{itm}$ *Thuj*$_{klp}$ tub_{itm}
  - **night** (see pg 964): $calc-p_{qqh}$
    : **adverse** circumstances; from: $staph_{pkj1}$
    : **jealousy**; from: $lach_{pkj1}$
    : **spasmodic** enuresis (see pg 965): $caps_{brm}$
  - **accompanied** by:
    : **Prostate** gland; swelling of (see pg 965): $sulph_{brm}$
  - **anxiety**; from: $calc-p_{brm}$ sep_{brm}
  - **atony**; from: $caust_{qqh}$
  - **castration**; after: $caust_{klp}$ $thuj_{klp}$
    : **men**; in:
    : **women**; in: $calc_{ffd}$ $cham_{lkk}$ $lach_{lkk}$ lyc_{ffd} med_{lkk} $phos_{brm,lkk}$ $plat_{lkk}$ $rhus-t_{brm}$ $sep_{brm,ffd,sxj}$ $stilboest_{sxj}$
  - **catheterization**, after (see pg 965): arn_{pkj1} $staph_{qqh}$
  - **children**; in (see pg 965): $phos_{hnb}$
  - **cough** agg.; during (see pg 965): $canth_{qqh}$
  - **dark**; in the: $mag-m_{qqh}$
  - **delivery**; after (see pg 965): bry_{qqh} equis-h$_{pkj1}$ $mag-m_{itm}$ $staph_{qqh}$
  - **demineralized** animal; in a: equis-h$_{qqh}$
  - **dentition**; during: $kreos_{qqh}$
  - **effort**; no urine flows during (see pg 965): $caps_{brm}$
  - **estrus**; during: $foll_{pkj1}$ med_{pkj1} $sars_{pkj1}$
  - **excitement** agg. (see pg 965): $arg-n_{pkj1}$ $caust_{brm,frc,pkj1}$ *Gels*$_{frc,pkj1}$ ign_{qqh} med_{brm} $phos_{frc}$ $puls_{frc,qqh}$
  - **fear**; from:
  - **fever**; during (see pg 965): $mur-ac_{qqh}$
  - **joy**; from: $phos_{hnb}$
  - **motion**:
    : **agg.** (see pg 965): $alet_{qqh}$ $arg-n_{qqh}$ $caust_{qqh}$ $nat-m_{qqh}$
  - **old** people; in (see pg 965): $caust_{dyc,pkj1}$ $ferr-p_{pkj1}$ $hyos_{pkj1}$ plb_{pkj1} $sars_{pkj1}$ $zinc_{pkj1}$
  - **ovariectomy**; after:
  - **rising**:
    : **sitting**; from:
      : **agg.** (see pg 966)

BLADDER – Urination – involuntary: ...
- **sexual** excitement agg. : $canth_{pkj1}$ $nat-m_{brm}$ $stram_{pkj1}$
- **sitting**:
  : **agg.** (see pg 966)
- **sleep**; during: $puls_{ffd}$
- **sneezing** agg. (see pg 966): $ferr-p_{qqh}$ *Kali-c*$_{qqh}$
- **surgical** operation; after a: $staph_{qqh}$
  : **genital** organs; in:
    : **female**; in: $lach_{pkj1}$
    : **male**; in: $caust_{pkj1}$
- **young** animals; in:
- **ride**; during the:
  - **doesn't** want to urinate: lyc_{brm}
- **seldom** (see pg 967): $sulph_{brm}$
- **unsatisfactory** (see pg 967): $acon_{pkj1}$ **Ars**$_{pkj1}$ $caps_{qqh}$ **Caust**$_{qqh}$ eup-per$_{pkj1}$ $hell_{pkj1}$ *Mag-m*$_{qqh}$ *Nux-v*$_{qqh}$
- **urging** to urinate (see pg 967):
  - **evening**:
    : **eating**; after: lyc_{brm}
  - **ineffectual** (see pg 969): $tritic_{sxj}$
- **walking** agg.:
  - **again** when not yet finished urinating: $phos_{brm}$

WEAKNESS:
- **atony**; from: $caust_{qqh}$ $kali-c_{qqh}$ $puls_{qqh}$

Kidneys

ABSCESS (see pg 973)

ADDISON'S disease (see pg 973)

CATARRH (see pg 973)

COMPLAINTS of kidneys:
- **followed** by:
  - **edema** of kidneys: $canth_{qqh}$

CONGESTION (see pg 973): $acon_{bnfl.es}$ $colch_{bnfl.es}$ $lyc_{bnfl.es}$ $phos_{bnfl.es}$ $ter_{bnfl.es}$
- **injuries**; after: $arn_{bnfl.es}$ $bell-p_{bnfl.es}$
- **intoxication**; from: $phos_{bnfl.es}$ $squil_{bnfl.es}$

EDEMA:
- **followed** by:
  - **complaints** of kidneys; other: $apis_{qqh}$

INFLAMMATION (see pg 974): $apoc_{bnfl.es,pkj1}$ $nat-m_{dyc,mld3}$ $ser-ang_{bnfl.es,itm,pkj1}$ $solid_{bnfl.es,ljy1}$ $uva_{ljy,mld1}$
- **parenchymatous**:
  - **acute** (see pg 974): $Apis_{brm}$
- **Glomeruli** (see pg 975): $Apis_{mld4}$ ars_{mld4} $bell_{mld4}$ $berb_{mld4}$ $kali-chl_{mld4}$ lyc_{mld4} $merc_{mld4}$ $nat-m_{mld4}$ $phos_{mld4}$ ter_{mld4}
- **Pelvis** (see pg 975): hep_{mld5} $kali-bi_{mld5}$ *Uva*$_{mld5}$
- **Pelvis** and kidneys (see pg 975): $benz-ac_{bnfl.es,itm,mld,mld4}$ $equis-h_{bnfl.es,itm}$ $form_{bnfl.es,itm}$ $hep_{bnfl.es,itm,mld,mld,mld4}$ $merc-c_{mld,mld,mld4}$ $sil_{itm,mld1}$ $ter_{bnfl.es,itm}$ $uva_{mld,mld4}$

IRREGULAR surface: ars_{klp}

LAMENESS, region of (see pg 975)

LARGE kidneys:

NEPHROSIS (see pg 975): acet-ac$_{mld4}$ ars$_{mld3}$ canth$_{mld4}$ con$_{mld4}$ nat-m$_{mld4}$ phos$_{mld3}$ plb$_{mld3}$ sil$_{mld3}$ solid$_{mld3}$ thuj$_{mld3}$ urt-u$_{mld3}$

NUMBNESS, region of (see pg 975)

PAIN:
- **right** (see pg 975): equis-h$_{qqh}$ helon$_{qqh}$ lyc$_{qqh}$ sars$_{qqh}$
- **left** (see pg 975): berb$_{qqh}$
- **cold**; exposure to: ser-ang$_{dyc,pkj1}$
- **cramping** (see pg 976): bell$_{pkj1}$ berb$_{pkj1}$ canth$_{pkj1}$ coloc$_{qqh}$ pareir$_{pkj1}$ sars$_{pkj1}$
- **injuries**; after: arn$_{qqh}$

POLYCYSTIC kidneys (see pg 979): sulph$_{brm}$

RENAL FAILURE:
- **chronic** (see pg 979): ars$_{elg,klp}$ mag-c$_{brm}$ med$_{brm}$ nat-m$_{brm}$ *Phos* $_{brm}$ plb$_{brm}$ staph$_{brm}$
  - **accompanied** by:
    - **thirstlessness**: ars$_{fmx}$ gels$_{fmx}$ puls$_{fmx}$

SMALL kidneys: ars$_{klp}$

STONES (see pg 980): **Benz-ac** $_{mld3}$ *Berb* $_{mld,mld,qqh}$ **Calc** $_{qqh}$ cann-i$_{mld,qqh}$ **Lith-c** $_{mld3}$ **Lyc** $_{mld,mld4}$ nux-v$_{qqh}$ **Pareir** $_{qqh}$ ph-ac$_{qqh}$ **Sars** $_{mld4}$ solid$_{mld4}$

SUPPRESSION of urine (see pg 980)

SWELLING (see pg 980)

Prostate gland

CANCER of prostate (see pg 981): bar-c$_{itm}$ calc$_{itm}$ Con $_{itm}$ *Iod* $_{itm}$ *Lyc* $_{itm}$ med$_{itm}$ *Sulph* $_{itm}$ **Thuj** $_{itm}$

EMISSION of prostatic fluid (see pg 981)

INDURATION (see pg 981)

INFLAMMATION (see pg 981)

IRRITATION in (see pg 982)

MASTURBATION, complaints after (see pg 982)

PAIN (see pg 982)
- **palpation**; on: ferr-pic$_{klp}$ sabal$_{klp}$

SUPPURATION (see pg 982)

SWELLING (see pg 982): caust$_{brm}$ chin$_{brm}$ *Med* $_{brm}$

Urethra

AGGLUTINATION of meatus (see pg 985)

AIR passes from the female urethra:
- **urination** agg.; during (see pg 985)

CARUNCLE (see pg 985)

CHORDEE (see pg 985)

CLOGGED by pieces of coagulated mucus (see pg 985)

COLDNESS (see pg 985)

CONSTRICTION (see pg 985)

CONTRACTION (see pg 985)

URETHRA: ...

CRACKS in meatus (see pg 985)

CRAMP (see pg 985)

CRAWLING (see pg 985)

DISCHARGE (see pg 985)
- **greenish** (see pg 986): Merc $_{qqh}$
- **purulent** (see pg 987): *Merc* $_{qqh}$ pareir$_{qqh}$

DROPPING from:
- **urination** agg.; after (see pg 987)

ERUPTIONS:
- **vesicles** (see pg 988)

EVERTED meatus (see pg 988)

EXCORIATION:
- **Meatus**; of (see pg 988)

EXCRESCENCES (see pg 988)

FUNGOID growth (see pg 988)

HARD:
- **node** (see pg 988)

HARDNESS (see pg 988)

HEAT (see pg 988)

HEMORRHAGE (see pg 988)

INDURATION (see pg 988)

INFLAMMATION (see pg 988): coc-c$_{mld5}$

IRRITATION (see pg 988)

ITCHING (see pg 988)

JERKING (see pg 989)

MOISTURE at meatus (see pg 989)

PAIN:
- **urination**:
  - **after**:
    - agg. (see pg 992): nat-m$_{qqh}$
  - **during**:
    - agg. (see pg 992): merc-c$_{qqh}$ pareir$_{qqh}$

PULSATION (see pg 996)

REDNESS:
- **spots** (see pg 996)
- **Meatus** (see pg 996)

SENSITIVE (see pg 997)

SPASM (see pg 997)

STRICTURE (see pg 997)

SWELLING (see pg 997)

TINGLING (see pg 997)

TUMOR (see pg 997)

TWITCHING (see pg 997)

ULCERATION (see pg 997)

URGING (see pg 997)

URINE:
- **stops** at fossa navicularis (see pg 997)

Urine

ACETONURIA (see pg 999)

ACRID (see pg 999)

ALBUMINOUS (see pg 999): *Ser-ang*$_{bnfl.es}$ *Uran-n*$_{mld5}$

ALKALINE (see pg 999)

BILE, containing (see pg 1000)

BLOODY (see pg 1000): **Arn**$_{bnfl.es}$ *Berb*$_{bnfl.es}$
Coc-c$_{bnfl.es,mld5}$ **Crot-h**$_{bnfl.es}$ **Ham**$_{bnfl.es,gsd,mld5}$
sarcol-ac$_{bnfl.es}$ *Sulph*$_{bnfl.es}$
- injuries; after: arn$_{bnfl.es}$ canth$_{bnfl.es}$ chin$_{bnfl.es}$
- prostate gland; from enlarged: med$_{brm}$

BURNING (see pg 1000)

CASTS, containing:
- **urate** (see pg 1001): solid$_{qqh}$

CLOUDY (see pg 1001)

COLD urine (see pg 1001)

COLOR:
- **coffee**, like (see pg 1002): benz-ac$_{qqh}$
- **yellow**:
  · **bright** (see pg 1003): caps$_{qqh}$

COLORLESS (see pg 1003)

COPIOUS (see pg 1003): *Equis-h*$_{pkjl}$ form$_{pkjl}$
Helon$_{qqh}$ *Lyc*$_{qqh}$ **Ph-ac**$_{qqh}$ **Puls**$_{pkjl}$

CUTICLE forming on the surface of the urine (see pg 1005)

FROTHY (see pg 1005)

GELATINOUS, lumpy:
- **left** standing for a while; when (see pg 1005)

INDICAN, containing:

MILKY (see pg 1005)

MUDDY (see pg 1006)

MYOGLOBINURIA: acon$_{mld4}$ arn$_{mld4}$ bell$_{mld4}$ bell-p$_{mld4}$
berb$_{mld,mld5}$ bry$_{mld4}$ cimic$_{mld4}$ cur$_{mld4}$ helon$_{mld4}$
rhus-t$_{mld4}$ thal$_{mld4}$

ODOR:
- **horrible**:
  · **left** standing for a while; when (see pg 1006):
    lyc$_{hnb}$
- **putrid** (see pg 1006): form$_{pkjl}$

ODORLESS (see pg 1006)

SCANTY (see pg 1007): *Acon*$_{qqh}$ **Apis**$_{qqh}$ **Ars**$_{qqh}$
Canth$_{qqh}$ *Kali-c*$_{qqh}$ par$_{qqh}$ **Puls**$_{qqh}$ solid$_{qqh}$ **Ter**$_{qqh}$
- **fever**; during (see pg 1007): **Apis**$_{qqh}$ gels$_{qqh}$

SEDIMENT (see pg 1007)
- **crystals** (see pg 1008): *Lyc*$_{klp}$
- **oxalate** of calcium, lime (see pg 1009)
- **phosphates** (see pg 1009): *Calc-p*$_{qqh}$ lyc$_{brm}$
- **purulent** (see pg 1009): calc-s$_{qqh}$ caps$_{qqh}$ *Merc*$_{pkjl}$
- **sand**:
  · **gravel** (see pg 1009): **Lyc**$_{brm}$ phos$_{brm}$ sulph$_{brm}$

URINE – Sediment: ...
- **thready** (see pg 1010): chim$_{pkj,qqh}$

SPECIFIC gravity:

SUGAR (see pg 1010)

THICK (see pg 1010)

VISCID (see pg 1011)

WHEY LIKE (see pg 1011)

Male genitalia/sex

ABSCESS (see pg 1013)

ADHERE to scrotum, testes (see pg 1013)

APHTHAE (see pg 1013)

ATROPHY (see pg 1013)

BLEEDING, from:
- **Penis**:
  · **Prepuce** (see pg 1013)
- **Scrotum** (see pg 1013)

CANCER:
- **Scrotum** (see pg 1013): merc$_{mjsl}$

COITION:
- **aversion** to (see pg 1013)

COLDNESS (see pg 1013)

CONDYLOMATA (see pg 1014)

CONGESTION (see pg 1014)
- **Scrotum** (see pg 1014)

CONSTRICTION:
- **Penis**:
  · **Glans**, behind (see pg 1014)
  · **Prepuce** (see pg 1014)

CONTRACTION (see pg 1014)

CRACKS (see pg 1014)

CRYPTORCHISM (see pg 1014)
- **puberty**; before:
- **Inguinal**:

DEVELOPMENT of genitalia:
- **delayed**: calc$_{brm}$ chin$_{brm}$

DISCOLORATION:
- **blue** (see pg 1015)
  · **spots**; blue (see pg 1015)
- **pale**: sil$_{brm}$

DRYNESS:
- **Penis**:
  · **Glans** (see pg 1015)

ELEPHANTIASIS scrotum (see pg 1016)

EMPYOCELE (see pg 1016)

ENLARGED:
- **Spermatic** cords (see pg 1016)
- **Testes** (see pg 1016)

In this chapter only remedies from veterinary authors are printed

ERECTIONS:
- **morning**:
  - **waking**; on:
    : **and** after (see pg 1016): sulph_{brm}
- **sleep**:
  - **during**:
    : **agg.** (see pg 1018)
- **stool**:
  - **during**:
    : **agg.** (see pg 1018): *Thuj* _{brm}

ERUPTIONS (see pg 1020): sil_{fmx}
- **Scrotum** (see pg 1021): sulph_{brm}
- **Testes**:

EXCITABILITY of genitals (see pg 1021)

EXCORIATION (see pg 1021)

EXCRESCENCES:
- **Testes** (see pg 1021)

FIRMNESS:
- **increased** testes (see pg 1021)

FISTULA:
- **Spermatic** cord:
  - **castration**; after: hyper_{hnb}

FISTULOUS openings at scrotum (see pg 1021)

FLACCIDITY (see pg 1021)

FORMICATION (see pg 1021)

GANGRENE (see pg 1022)

GURGLING in testes:
- **17 h**:
  - **sitting** agg. (see pg 1022)

HEAT (see pg 1022)

HEMATOCELE (see pg 1022)

HYDROCELE (see pg 1022)

INDURATION:
- **Penis** (see pg 1022)
- **Scrotum** (see pg 1023)
- **Spermatic** cords (see pg 1023)
- **Testes** (see pg 1023)

INFLAMMATION (see pg 1023): hep_{bnfl.es,pkj1}
- **Penis**: ,
  - **Glans** (see pg 1023): caps_{brm}
  - **Prepuce**:
    : **discharge**; with copious: caps_{brm} puls_{wha} tarent_{wha}
- **Testes** (see pg 1023): bry_{itm,mld3}

INJURIES (see pg 1023)

IRRITATION:
- **Penis**:
- **Scrotum** (see pg 1024)

ITCHING (see pg 1024)

MASTURBATION; disposition to (see pg 1025)
- **home**; when coming: lac-c_{brm} :

METASTASIS (see pg 1025)

MOISTURE (see pg 1025)

NODULES:
- **Scrotum**:
  - **hard** brown (see pg 1025)
- **Testes** (see pg 1025)

PAIN (see pg 1025)

PERSPIRATION (see pg 1033)
- **sweetish**; smells as if (see pg 1033): sulph_{qqh}
- **Scrotum** (see pg 1033): *Calc*_{frc}
  - **sweetish** odor (see pg 1033): calc_{qqh} sil_{qqh}

PHIMOSIS (see pg 1033)

PHTHISIS (see pg 1033)

POLLUTIONS (see pg 1033): **Chin**_{plr1} **Sep**_{plr1} **Sulph**_{plr1}
- **masturbation**; after (see pg 1035): lyc_{brm} phos_{brm}

PULSATION (see pg 1035)

RELAXED (see pg 1036)

RETRACTION (see pg 1036)
- **Testes**:
  - **painful** (see pg 1036): calc_{qqh}

SARCOCELE (see pg 1036)

SCURF:

SEMEN dribbling (see pg 1036)

SENSITIVENESS (see pg 1036)

SEXUAL DESIRE:
- **excessive** (see pg 1037)
- **increased** (see pg 1037): *Bufo*_{klp} *Hyos*_{klp} *Orig*_{klp} **Phos**_{klp}
  - **anorectic** when a bitch in estrus is nearby:
  - **blonde** bitches; loves: lyc_{brm}
  - **castrated** animals; in: med_{brm}
  - **whining**:
    : **day** and night:
    : **night**; the whole:
- **wanting** (see pg 1038)

SHINING Scrotum (see pg 1039)

SHRIVELLED (see pg 1039)

SPOTS (see pg 1039)

STERILITY (see pg 1039): agn_{bnfl.es} arn_{qqh} calad_{bnfl.es} *Con*_{pkj1} gels_{pkj1} lyc_{bnfl.es} ph-ac_{bnfl.es} sel_{bnfl.es} staph_{pkj1}

SUPPURATION:
- **Prepuce**, under the (see pg 1039)
- **Testes** (see pg 1039)

SWELLING (see pg 1039)

TENSION (see pg 1040)

THICKENING:
- **Penis**:
  - **Prepuce** (see pg 1040)
- **Scrotum** (see pg 1040)
- **Spermatic** cords (see pg 1040)

TICKLING:
- coition; during:
- **Penis:**
  - **Glans** (see pg 1040)
- **Scrotum** (see pg 1040)

TINGLING (see pg 1040)

TUBERCLES (see pg 1040)

TUMOR:
- **Testes** (see pg 1040)

ULCERS (see pg 1040)

VARICOCELE (see pg 1041)

WEAKNESS (see pg 1041)

Female genitalia/sex

ABORTION (see pg 1043): hydr$_{mld1}$

ABSCESS (see pg 1044)

ADHESIONS:
- **Ovaries:** calc-f$_{dyc}$ sil$_{dyc}$

ANESTRUS:

APHTHAE (see pg 1044)

ATONY of uterus (see pg 1044)
- palpation; upon:

ATROPHY:
- **Ovaries** (see pg 1044)
- **Uterus** (see pg 1044)

BLOTCHES (see pg 1044)

CANCER of:
- **Uterus** (see pg 1044): med$_{bnfl.es}$ *Puls*$_{bnfl.es}$

CASTRATION:
- ailments after: caust$_{klp}$ lach$_{klp}$ staph$_{klp}$ thuj$_{klp}$
  - **ovariohysterectomy;** after:
  - **Ovaries** resection; after:

CHEESY deposits (see pg 1044)

COITION:
- aversion to (see pg 1045)

CONDYLOMATA (see pg 1046): calc-s$_{qqh}$

CONGESTION:
- **Uterus** (see pg 1046): alet$_{qqh}$ helon$_{qqh}$ mag-m$_{qqh}$ mosch$_{qqh}$ plat$_{qqh}$
- **Vagina:** arg-n$_{qqh}$ bell$_{qqh}$:

CONTRACTIONS (see pg 1046)

CRACKS (see pg 1047)

CYSTS (see pg 1047)

DELIVERY:
- after; complaints:
  - **injuries** of parts (see pg 1047): arn$_{elg}$ bell-p$_{elg}$
    : **prevent** these injuries: caul$_{elg}$
    : **Muscles:** arn$_{elg}$ rhus-t$_{elg}$
    : **Nerves:** hyper$_{hnb}$

FEMALE GENITALIA/SEX – Delivery – after; complaints – **injuries** of parts: ...
  : Soft tissues; of the: arn$_{hnb}$ bell-p$_{hnb}$
  : **accompanied** by:
    . **swelling:** bell-p$_{hnb}$
  - **rise;** can't: arn$_{elg}$ bell-p$_{elg}$ hyper$_{elg}$ rhus-t$_{elg}$
    : **lying** for a few days; after: rhus-t$_{elg}$
  - **twins;** giving birth to:
- **during;** complaints (see pg 1047): *Cimic*$_{frc,itm,pkj1}$ nat-m$_{fmx}$
  - **slow** (see pg 1047): **Nat-m**$_{fmx}$

DEVELOPMENT of genitalia:
- **delayed** (see pg 1047)
  - **Ovaries:**

DIESTRUS:

DISCOLORATION:
- **red** (see pg 1047)
- **Uterus:**
  - **Cervix:**
    : **purple** (see pg 1047)

DISPLACEMENT of uterus (see pg 1047)
- **torsion:**

DISTENDED; sensation as if:
- **Uterus:**
  - **wind;** as if filled with (see pg 1047)

DRYNESS (see pg 1047): alum$_{qqh}$

ENDOMETRIOSIS (see pg 1047)

ENLARGED:
- **Ovaries** (see pg 1048)
- **Uterus** (see pg 1048)

EROSION of cervix (see pg 1048)

ERUPTIONS (see pg 1048)

ESTRUS:
- **absent:** calc-p$_{dyc}$ iod$_{dyc}$ phos$_{dyc}$ puls-vg$_{dyc}$ sep$_{dyc}$
  - **fat** animals; in:
  - **heifers;** in:
  - **old** animals; in:
  - **ovarian** cysts; from:
    : **follicular** cysts: apis$_{dyc}$ arist-cl$_{dyc}$ aur$_{dyc}$ bufo$_{dyc}$ lach$_{dyc}$ lil-t$_{dyc}$ murx$_{dyc}$
    : **right:** apis$_{dyc}$
    : **left:** lach$_{dyc}$
- **behavior;** with changes of:
  - **anger:**
  - **aversion** to male animals:
  - **passive:**
  - **quiet:**
- **bleeding:**
  - **long;** too:
    : **four** weeks:
  - **scanty:**
  - **short;** too:
- **discharge:**
  - **bright** colored:
  - **dark** colored:

- **discharge**: ...
  - **profuse**:
  - **red**:
  - **scanty**:
- **first estrus**:
  - **seventh** month; before:
  - **twelfth** month; after:
- **frequent**; too:
- **heifers**:
- **incessant**: murx$_{brm}$ sep$_{brm}$
- **irregular**:
- **long**; too:
- **periodical**:
  - **days**; every ten:
  - **week**; every:
  - **month**:
    : **every**:
    : **eight** months:
    : **nine** months:
    : **seven** months:
    : **three** months:
    : **two** months:
- **permanent**:

EXCITABILITY of genitals (see pg 1048)

EXCORIATION (see pg 1048)

EXCRESCENCES (see pg 1049)

FETUS:
- **dead**:
  - **mummification**:
  - **stillbirths**: caul$_{dyc}$

FISTULA at vagina (see pg 1049)

FLABBY:
- **Uterus**: alet$_{dyc}$ helon$_{dyc}$ sep$_{dyc}$

FLATUS from vagina (see pg 1049)

GANGRENE (see pg 1049)

GRANULATION:
- **Uterus**:
  - **Cervix** (see pg 1049)
- **Vagina** (see pg 1049)

HAIR falling out (see pg 1049)

HARDNESS (see pg 1049)
- **Ovaries** (see pg 1049): phyt$_{dyc}$ tub$_{dyc}$

INDURATION (see pg 1050)
- **Ovaries** (see pg 1050): calc-f$_{dyc}$ iod$_{dyc}$ lap-a$_{dyc}$

INFANTILISM; genital (see pg 1050)
- **Ovaries**: iod$_{dyc}$
- **Uterus**:

INFLAMMATION:
- **Uterus** (see pg 1051): bapt$_{bnfl.es,mld5}$ echi$_{mld4}$ helon$_{bnfl.es,mld,mld5}$ kali-bi$_{itm,pkj1}$ lil-t$_{mld,mld5}$ thuj$_{itm,pkj1}$
  - **accompanied** by:
    : **Mammae**; inflammation of: bry$_{dyc}$ caul$_{dyc}$ nux-v$_{dyc}$ phyt$_{dyc}$ puls-vg$_{dyc}$ sep$_{dyc}$ urt-u$_{dyc}$

Inflammation – Uterus: ...
  - **delivery**; after:
    : **prevent** this condition: lach$_{elg}$
  - **pyometra** (see pg 1051): apis$_{mld3}$ caul$_{mld,mld5}$ cimic$_{mld5}$ echi$_{mld5}$ helon$_{bnfl.es}$ hydr$_{bnfl.es,mld,mld5}$ kali-bi$_{bnfl.es,mld5}$ lach$_{brm}$ lil-t$_{mld5}$ ov$_{mld3}$ *Puls*$_{bnfl.es,brm,klp,mld5}$ pyrog$_{bnfl.es,mld5}$ sabad$_{mld5}$ sec$_{bnfl.es,brm,mld,mld5}$ *Sep*$_{bnfl.es,brm,mld5}$
- **Vagina** (see pg 1051): apis$_{itm,mld3}$ canth$_{bnfl.es,itm,mld,mld,mld4}$ helon$_{bnfl.es,mld3}$ hydr$_{bnfl.es,itm,mld,mld4}$ kali-bi$_{itm}$ kreos$_{itm,mld3}$ puls$_{itm,mld4}$

INJURIES (see pg 1051)
- **Nerves**:
  - **delivery**; after:

IRRITATION (see pg 1051)

ITCHING (see pg 1051)
- **Vulva**:
  - **estrus**; after: lyc$_{brm}$

LEUKORRHEA:
- **bright**:
  - **estrus**; during:
- **castration**; after: sulph$_{brm}$
- **children**; in:
  - **girls**; little (see pg 1054)
- **copious**:
  - **estrus**; during:
- **dark**:
  - **estrus**; during:
- **pregnancy** agg.; during (see pg 1056)
- **reddish**:
  - **estrus**; during:
- **scanty**:
  - **estrus**; during:
- **wanting**:
  - **estrus**; during:

LOCHIA (see pg 1058)
- **suppressed** (see pg 1058)
  - **fever**; with (see pg 1058): sabin$_{brm}$

LYING:
- **agg.**:
  - **Uterus** (see pg 1058)

MASTURBATION, disposition to (see pg 1059): *Sulph*$_{brm}$

MENOPAUSE (see pg 1059)

MENSES:
- **delayed** in girls, first menses (see pg 1062): *Lyc*$_{brm}$
- **return**:
  - **ceased**; after the regular menstrual cycle has (see pg 1066)

METESTRUS:

METRORRHAGIA (see pg 1068)
- **delivery**:
  - **after** (see pg 1069): *Arn*$_{elg}$ bell-p$_{elg}$

- **delivery – after:** ...
  : **bright** red:
  • **during** and after (see pg 1069)
- **paroxysms**; during (see pg 1070)

MOLES (see pg 1071)

NODULES (see pg 1071)

OVULATION:
- **during** (see pg 1071)

PAIN (see pg 1071)
- **labor** pains (see pg 1072)
  • **ceasing** (see pg 1072): Puls$_{brm}$
  • **painful**, too (see pg 1073): arn$_{frc}$ Cham$_{frc}$ Coff$_{frc}$
  • **spasmodic:**
    : **oxytocin**; abuse of: caul$_{hnb}$
  • **weak** (see pg 1073): Caul$_{elg}$
- **Vagina:**
  • **coition:**
    : **during** (see pg 1084)

PERSPIRATION (see pg 1086)
- **sweetish** odor: sulph$_{qqh}$

PLACENTA:
- **retained** (see pg 1086): alet$_{bnfl.es,mld5,qqh}$ Arn$_{elg}$ calc$_{elg}$
  caul$_{elg}$ cimic$_{itm,qqh}$ echi$_{bnfl.es}$ pyrog$_{bnfl.es,gsd,mld,mld5}$
  Sabin$_{elg}$ Sec$_{elg}$
  • **discharges**; with:
    : **odor:**
    : **fetid:**
    : **watery:**
  • **discharges**; without:
  • **fever**; with:
    : **milk** fever: calc$_{elg}$

POLYPUS (see pg 1086)

PREGNANCY:
- **during**; complaints:
  • **fetus:**
    : **little** fetus; too:
    : **many** fetuses; because of too: kali-c$_{dyc}$ ph-ac$_{dyc}$
- **imaginary:**
  • **adopting:**
    : **dolls**, toys:
    : **pups:**
  • **aggression**; with:
    : **defending** puppies:
  • **appetite**; wanting of:
  • **collecting** things:
  • **disobedience**; with:
  • **dullness**; with:
  • **epileptic** convulsions; with:
  • **irritability**; with:
  • **itching**; with:
  • **milk**; with the appearance of:
    : **copious:** puls$_{hnb}$

Pregnancy – imaginary: ...
  • **nest**; guarding:
  • **nest**; making a:
  • **restlessness**; with:
  • **thirst**; with increased:
    : **large** quantities; for:
  • **thirstlessness**; with: puls$_{hnb}$

PROESTRUS:
- **prolonged:** ust$_{brm}$

PROLAPSUS:
- **Uterus** (see pg 1086): Alet$_{dyc}$ Helon$_{dyc}$ Sec$_{dyc}$ Sep$_{dyc}$
  • **delivery**; after (see pg 1087): aur$_{hnb}$
  • **Vagina** (see pg 1087): alet$_{dyc,qqh}$ calc$_{qqh}$ helon$_{dyc}$
  murx$_{qqh}$ Nux-v$_{dyc}$ Sep$_{dyc}$

PUBERTY:
- **ailments** at (see pg 1087)

PULSATING (see pg 1087)

RELAXATION:
- **Pubis** and in pelvis; muscles around (see pg 1087)
- **Vagina**; sphincter of (see pg 1087)

RETENTION OF THE EGG: bell$_{ljyl}$ cham$_{ljyl}$ op$_{ljyl}$

SENSITIVENESS (see pg 1087)

SEXUAL DESIRE:
- **diminished:**
  • **old** people; in:
- **increased:**
  • **castration**; after:
  • **estrus**; during:
  • **ovariectomy**; after:
  • **ovariohysterectomy**; after:
- **violent:**
  • **estrus**; during: sep$_{brm}$
- **wanting** (see pg 1089)

SOFT, uterus (see pg 1089)

STERILITY (see pg 1089): Alet$_{dyc}$ apis$_{dyc}$ arist-cl$_{dyc}$
  Aur$_{dyc}$ bufo$_{dyc}$ calc-p$_{mld,mld5}$ cimic$_{dyc}$ cycl$_{itm,pkj1}$
  foll$_{bnfl.es,itm,mld1}$ ign$_{dyc,itm,pkj1}$ kali-c$_{dyc}$ Lach$_{dyc}$ murx$_{dyc}$
  pall$_{dyc}$ Phos$_{dyc}$ Plat$_{dyc}$ puls-vg$_{dyc}$ Sabin$_{dyc}$ Sep$_{dyc}$
  tub$_{dyc}$

SUBINVOLUTION (see pg 1090)

SWOLLEN (see pg 1090)

TUBERCLES (see pg 1090)

TUMORS:
- **Ovaries** (see pg 1091)
  • **cysts** (see pg 1091): aur-i$_{mld4}$ foll$_{bnfl.es,mld1}$
  ov$_{mld,mld4}$
    : **accompanied** by:
    : **sterility:**
      . **old** animals; in:
      . **young** animals; in:
    : **corpus** luteum; encysted:
    : **persistent:**

ULCERS:
- **Vulva** (see pg 1091): sep$_{brm}$

In this chapter only remedies from veterinary authors are printed

VAGINISMUS (see pg 1091)

VEINS, varicose (see pg 1091)

WORMS:
- pinworms (see pg 1092)

Larynx and trachea

ANESTHESIA of larynx (see pg 1093)

CANCER:
- **Larynx** (see pg 1093)

CATARRH (see pg 1093)

COLLAPSE OF TRACHEA: phos$_{brm}$

CONDYLOMATA:
- **Larynx** (see pg 1093)
- **Vocal** cords (see pg 1093)

CONSTRICTION (see pg 1093)

CROUP (see pg 1094)

DUST, as from (see pg 1095)

EDEMA:
- **Glottis** (see pg 1096)

FOOD drops into larynx (see pg 1096)

HEAT:
- **Larynx** (see pg 1096)
- **Trachea** (see pg 1096)

INFLAMMATION:
- **Larynx** (see pg 1096): arn$_{bnf1.es,itm,qqh}$ merc-cy$_{mld,mld4}$ sil$_{mld,qqh}$
- **Trachea** (see pg 1097)

INJURIES to air passages (see pg 1097)

INSENSIBILITY of larynx (see pg 1097)

IRRITATION (see pg 1097)

ITCHING:
- **Larynx** (see pg 1097)
- **Throat**-pit:

JERK, drinking (see pg 1098)

LARYNGISMUS stridulus (see pg 1098)

LIQUIDS pass into larynx (see pg 1098)

MEMBRANE (see pg 1098)

MUCUS:
- **Air** passages, in the (see pg 1098)
- **Larynx** (see pg 1098)
- **Trachea** (see pg 1099)

NECROSIS of cartilages of larynx (see pg 1099)

PAIN:
- **Larynx** (see pg 1099)
- **Throat**-pit (see pg 1102)
- **Trachea** (see pg 1102)

PARALYSIS:
- **Larynx** (see pg 1103): nux-v$_{brm}$

LARYNX AND TRACHEA – **Paralysis** – **Larynx**: ...
- **hemiplegia**:
- **Epiglottis** (see pg 1103)
- **Vocal** cord (see pg 1103)
  - **hemiplegia**: caust$_{dyc}$ lach$_{dyc}$ plb$_{dyc}$

PHTHISIS:
- **Larynx** (see pg 1103)
- **Trachea** (see pg 1103)

POLYPI:
- **Larynx** (see pg 1103)
- **Vocal** cords (see pg 1103)

RATTLING:
- **Larynx** (see pg 1103)
- **Trachea** (see pg 1103)

ROUGHNESS (see pg 1103)

SENSITIVE:
- **Larynx** (see pg 1104)
- **Trachea** (see pg 1104)

ULCERATION:
- **Larynx** (see pg 1106)

VOICE:
- **croaking**:
  - **morning**: lyc$_{brm}$
- **deep**:
  - **women**; like a men's voice in: aur$_{hnb}$
- **high**:
  - **deep** voice; becoming: aur$_{hnb}$
- **higher**:
  - **excited**; when: sulph$_{brm}$
- **hoarseness** (see pg 1107)
  - **coryza**:
    : **during** (see pg 1108)
- **lost** (see pg 1109): arn$_{bnf1.es,pkj1}$ aur$_{bnf1.es}$ calc$_{pkj1}$ Caust$_{dyc,mld5,pkj,qqh}$ coll$_{dyc,mld5}$ Gels$_{dyc,mld5}$ Merc$_{pkj,qqh}$ Phos$_{pkj,qqh}$ Rhus-t$_{pkj,qqh}$ sep$_{pkj1}$ sil$_{qqh}$
- **toneless** (see pg 1110): lyc$_{brm}$

WHISTLING (see pg 1110)

Respiration

ABDOMINAL (see pg 1113)

ACCELERATED (see pg 1113)

ANXIOUS (see pg 1113)

ARRESTED (see pg 1113)

ASPHYXIA (see pg 1114)
- **amniotic** fluid; because of aspiration of: am-i$_{hnb}$ ant-t$_{hnb,klp}$ laur$_{klp}$
  - **aspiration** pneumonia; to prevent: ant-t$_{hnb}$
- **anesthesia**; during: helo-h$_{klp}$
- **children**, newborns (see pg 1114): carb-v$_{elg}$

ASTHMATIC (see pg 1114): Lyc$_{brm}$ pert$_{klp}$ Phos$_{brm}$
- **allergic**:
  - **spring**; in: puls$_{brm}$

- **cats**; in: lyc$_{brm}$ pert$_{klp}$ phos$_{brm}$
- **spring**; in (see pg 1118): puls$_{brm}$

BLOWING (see pg 1119)

CATCHING (see pg 1119)

CHRONIC OBSTRUCTIVE PULMONARY DISORDER:
ant-t$_{dyc}$ ars$_{dyc}$ asperg-fu$_{dyc}$ bac$_{klp}$ bry$_{dyc}$ calc$_{dyc}$ dros$_{dyc}$ lob$_{dyc}$ lobl-m$_{dyc}$ lyc$_{dyc}$ phos$_{dyc}$ puls-vg$_{dyc}$ spong$_{dyc}$ tub$_{dyc}$

COLDNESS of breath (see pg 1119)

CROAKING (see pg 1119)

DEEP (see pg 1119)

DIFFICULT (see pg 1120): **Lyc** $_{fmx}$
- **night** (see pg 1121): *Lyc* $_{brm}$
- **children**; in:
  • **newborns**:
    ¦ **delivery**; after:
- **emphysema**, in (see pg 1123): arg-n$_{hnb}$
- **fever**; during (see pg 1124): ail$_{qqh}$
- **inspiration** (see pg 1124): lyc$_{fmx}$

FORCIBLE (see pg 1128)
- **expiration** (see pg 1128)

GASPING (see pg 1128)

HOT breath (see pg 1128)

IMPEDED, obstructed (see pg 1128)
- **chronic**:

IMPERCEPTIBLE (see pg 1129)

INTERMITTENT, unequal (see pg 1129)

INTERRUPTED (see pg 1130)

IRREGULAR (see pg 1130): *Nux-v* $_{brm}$

JERKING (see pg 1130)

LONG (see pg 1130)

LOUD (see pg 1130)

MOANING (see pg 1130)

PAINFUL (see pg 1131)

PANTING (see pg 1131)

PAROXYSMAL (see pg 1131)

PUFFING:
- **expiration** (see pg 1131)

RATTLING (see pg 1131)

ROUGH (see pg 1132)

SIGHING (see pg 1132)
- **sleep**:
  • **going** to sleep; on:
    ¦ **agg.**: nat-m$_{brm}$ sep$_{brm}$

SLOW (see pg 1132)

SNORING (see pg 1133): sil$_{brm}$
- **inspiration** (see pg 1133)
  • **sleep**; in (see pg 1133): sulph$_{brm}$
- **sleep**; during: calc-p$_{brm}$

RESPIRATION: ...

SOBBING (see pg 1133)

STERTOROUS (see pg 1133)

STRIDULOUS (see pg 1133): lyc$_{fmx}$

SUPERFICIAL (see pg 1133)

TREMULOUS (see pg 1133)

TUBE; as if through a metallic (see pg 1133)

WHEEZING (see pg 1134)

WHISTLING (see pg 1134)

Cough

COUGH in general: **Acon** $_{qqh}$ naphtin$_{qqh}$ **Nux-v** $_{qqh}$ *Sabad* $_{qqh}$ *Sil* $_{qqh}$ *Squil* $_{qqh}$

DAYTIME (see pg 1135)

MORNING (see pg 1135)

FORENOON (see pg 1135)

NOON (see pg 1136)

AFTERNOON (see pg 1136)

EVENING (see pg 1136)

NIGHT (see pg 1136)
- **midnight**:
  • **after**:
    ¦ **morning**, until (see pg 1137): phos$_{brm}$

ABDOMEN, seems to come from (see pg 1137)

ACIDS:
- **agg.** (see pg 1138)

AGITATION, from (see pg 1138)

AIR; IN OPEN:
- **amel.** (see pg 1138): lyc$_{fmx}$ **Puls** $_{fmx}$

ALTERNATING with:
- **eruptions** (see pg 1138)

ASCENDING STAIRS agg. (see pg 1139)

ASTHMATIC (see pg 1139)

BARKING (see pg 1139)

BLOOD:
- **rush** of blood to chest; cough from (see pg 1139)

BREATHING:
- **agg.** (see pg 1139)

BRIGHT objects (see pg 1140)

CELLARS, air of (see pg 1140)

CHILL:
- **after** (see pg 1140)
- **before** (see pg 1140)
- **during** (see pg 1140)

CHOKING (see pg 1140)

CHRONIC (see pg 1140)

CLOTHES AGG.; TIGHT (see pg 1140)

COITION; after (see pg 1140)

COLD:
- **air**:
  - **entering** cold air from a warm room agg. (see pg 1140)

COMPANY (see pg 1141)

CONSCIOUSNESS; with loss of (see pg 1141)

CONSOLATION agg. (see pg 1141)

CONSTANT (see pg 1141)

CONSTIPATION agg. (see pg 1141)

CONVULSIONS; with (see pg 1141)

COUGH agg.; during (see pg 1141)

CRAWLING, sensation of (see pg 1141)

CROUPY (see pg 1142)

CRYING agg. (see pg 1142)

DEEP (see pg 1142)

DEEP-SOUNDING (see pg 1142)

DELIVERY:
- **after** (see pg 1142): rhus-t$_{trj}$
- **during**: kali-c$_{trj}$

DENTITION; during (see pg 1142)

DESCENDING, on (see pg 1142)

DIFFICULT (see pg 1142)

DISTRACTING (see pg 1142)

DISTRESSING (see pg 1142)

DRY (see pg 1143)
- **fever**:
  - **during**:
    - agg. (see pg 1145): rhus-t$_{qqh}$

DUST, as from (see pg 1146)

EATING:
- **agg.** (see pg 1146)
- **amel.** (see pg 1146)

ELONGATED Uvula; from (see pg 1146)

EMOTIONS agg. (see pg 1146)

ERUCTATIONS:
- **amel.** (see pg 1146)
- **excite** cough; eructations (see pg 1146)

ERUPTIONS:
- **cough**; from suppressed (see pg 1146)
- **receding**; when eruptions are (see pg 1146)

EXCITEMENT (see pg 1146)

EXERTION:
- **agg.** (see pg 1146): *Lyc*$_{fmx}$ phos$_{brm}$ **Puls**$_{fmx}$

EXHAUSTING (see pg 1146)

EXPECTORATION:
- **amel.** (see pg 1146)

EXPIRATION agg. (see pg 1147)

EXPLOSIVE (see pg 1147)

FAT FOOD agg. (see pg 1147)

FIRE; when looking into (see pg 1147)

FISH, from eating (see pg 1147)

FLATUS; PASSING:
- **amel.** (see pg 1147)

FLUIDS; from loss of (see pg 1147)

FORCIBLE (see pg 1147)

FOREIGN body; sensation of a:
- **Larynx**; in (see pg 1147)
- **Trachea**; in (see pg 1147)

FRIGHT agg. (see pg 1147)

GASTRIC (see pg 1147)

GRIEF (see pg 1147)

HACKING (see pg 1147)

HAPPY surprise; from a (see pg 1148)

HEART affections, with (see pg 1149)

HEARTBURN, from (see pg 1149)

HEAT:
- **after** (see pg 1149)

HECTIC (see pg 1149)

HOARSE (see pg 1149)

HOLLOW (see pg 1149)

HUNGER:
- **from** (see pg 1149)
- **violent**, with (see pg 1149)

HYSTERICAL attack of:
- **followed** by crying, night (see pg 1149)
- **women** (see pg 1149)

ICE CREAM, at first amel., then agg. (see pg 1149)

INABILITY to (see pg 1149)

INFLUENZA:
- **after** (see pg 1149)
- **during** (see pg 1150)

INJURIES (see pg 1150)

INSPIRATION agg. (see pg 1150)

INTERRUPTED (see pg 1150)

IRREPRESSIBLE, sudden, violent:
- **evening**:
  - sitting agg. (see pg 1150)

IRRESISTIBLE:
- **short**, hawking (see pg 1150)

IRRITABLE (see pg 1150)

IRRITATING things (see pg 1150)

ITCH; after suppressed (see pg 1151)

JERKING of head forward and knees upward; with (see pg 1151): phos$_{qqh}$

KENNEL COUGH: bell$_{elg}$ cupr$_{hnb}$ dros$_{hnb}$ phos$_{klp}$

LACTATION; during (see pg 1151)

LIE DOWN:
- **not** lie down; sat bent forward could (see pg 1151)

LIGHT, looking at (see pg 1151)

LOOSE (see pg 1151)

MEAT agg. (see pg 1153)

MENTAL EXERTION:
- **agg.** (see pg 1153)

METALLIC (see pg 1153)

MILK agg. (see pg 1153)

MOTION:
- **beginning** of:
  - · **agg.** (see pg 1153)

MUCUS:
- **Chest;** in (see pg 1153)
- **Larynx** (see pg 1153)
- **Trachea** (see pg 1153)

MUSIC:
- **agg.** (see pg 1153)

NERVOUS (see pg 1153)

NOISE agg. (see pg 1154)

ODORS AGG.; STRONG (see pg 1154)

OLD people (see pg 1154)

OPPRESSION; from:
- **Chest;** in (see pg 1154)
- **Epigastrium** (see pg 1154)

OPPRESSIVE (see pg 1154)

PAIN:
- **Epigastrium**; cough from pain in (see pg 1154)
- **Larynx**; cough from pain in (see pg 1154)
- **Trachea**; cough from pain in (see pg 1154)

PAINFUL (see pg 1154)

PALPITATION; from tumultuous (see pg 1154)

PANTING (see pg 1154)

PAROXYSMAL (see pg 1154)

PERIODICAL (see pg 1155): syph$_{brm}$

PERSISTENT (see pg 1155)

PERSONS:
- **approaching** or passing, agg. (see pg 1156)
- **coming** into room; other persons (see pg 1156)
- **present**; when many persons are (see pg 1156)

PLEURITIS, in (see pg 1156)

PNEUMONIA, after (see pg 1156)

POTATOES agg. (see pg 1156)

PREGNANCY agg.; during (see pg 1156)

PRODROME, as a (see pg 1156)

PURRING (see pg 1156)

RACKING (see pg 1156)

RASPING (see pg 1156)

RATTLING (see pg 1156)

REFLEX (see pg 1157)

REMITTENT fever, during (see pg 1157)

REPOSE, amel. (see pg 1157)

RESONANT (see pg 1157)

RIDING agg. (see pg 1157)

ROOM agg. (see pg 1157)

ROUGH (see pg 1157)

RUNNING agg. (see pg 1157)

SALT food (see pg 1157)

SCARLATINA; following (see pg 1157)

SEASONS:
- **autumn** agg. (see pg 1158)
- **spring** agg. (see pg 1158)
- **summer** agg. (see pg 1158)
- **winter**; in (see pg 1158)

SERIES, in (see pg 1158)

SHARP (see pg 1158)

SHORT (see pg 1158)

SHRILL (see pg 1158)

SIBILANT (see pg 1158)

SITTING:
- **agg.** (see pg 1159)

SMOTHERED (see pg 1159)

SMOTHERING in throat; from (see pg 1159)

SNEEZING:
- **with** (see pg 1159): acon$_{qqh}$ naphtin$_{qqh}$ nux-v$_{qqh}$ sabad$_{qqh}$ sang$_{qqh}$ sil$_{qqh}$ squil$_{qqh}$

SNORING, with (see pg 1159)

SNOWFALL; cough in children from exposure to (see pg 1159)

SOLID food agg. (see pg 1159)

SONOROUS (see pg 1159)

SOUR FOOD agg. (see pg 1159)

SPASMODIC (see pg 1160)

SPLEEN:
- **complaints** of; from (see pg 1160)
- **enlarged** spleen or pain in spleen; with (see pg 1160)

SPLITTING (see pg 1160)

SPOKEN to, on being (see pg 1160)

STERTOROUS (see pg 1160)

STINGING or burning tickling in larynx; from (see pg 1161)

STOMACH:

- **come** from the stomach; seems to (see pg 1161)
- **fullness** in stomach rises to throat and triggers coughing (see pg 1161)

STOOL:
- **frequent**:
  · amel. (see pg 1161)

STRAINING (see pg 1161)

STRANGERS:
- **presence** of; in the (see pg 1161)

SUDDEN (see pg 1161)

SUFFOCATIVE (see pg 1161)

SUGAR:
- **agg.** (see pg 1161)
- **amel.** (see pg 1161)

SUN agg. (see pg 1162)

SWALLOWING:
- **agg.** (see pg 1162)
- **amel.** (see pg 1162)
- **empty**:
  · agg. (see pg 1162)

SWEETMEATS:
- **agg.** (see pg 1162)
- **amel.** (see pg 1162)

SWELLING:
- **larynx**; from swelling of (see pg 1162)

SYMPATHETIC (see pg 1162)

TALKING:
- **agg.** (see pg 1162)

TALL, slender, tuberculous subjects; in (see pg 1162)

TEA agg. (see pg 1162)

TEARING (see pg 1162)

TEDIOUS (see pg 1162)

TEMPERATURE, change of (see pg 1162)

THUNDERSTORM; before (see pg 1162)

TIGHT (see pg 1163)

TIRED; agg. when (see pg 1163)

TONELESS (see pg 1164)

TORMENTING (see pg 1164)

TOUCHED; from being (see pg 1164)

TUBE, sounds as if he coughed in a (see pg 1164)

TUBERCULOUS persons, in (see pg 1164)

ULCERATION deep in trachea; as if from an (see pg 1164)

VACCINATION; after (see pg 1164)

VEXATION; after (see pg 1164)

VINEGAR agg. (see pg 1164)

VIOLENT (see pg 1164)

VOMITING:

COUGH: ...

WAKING; on (see pg 1165)

WALKING:
- **agg.** (see pg 1165)

WARM:
- **room**:
  · **agg.** (see pg 1165): *Lyc* fmx
    : cold air, or vice versa; going from warm room to (see pg 1165)

WARM; BECOMING:
- **agg.** (see pg 1165)

WATER:
- **Trachea** from mouth; from water running into (see pg 1165)

WEATHER:
- **hot** (see pg 1165): sep brm

WET; GETTING:
- **agg.** (see pg 1165)
- **amel.**:
  · chest getting wet (see pg 1165)

WET room (see pg 1165)

WHINING, during (see pg 1165)

WHISPERING sound; has a (see pg 1165)

WHISTLING (see pg 1165): lyc fmx

WHOOPING (see pg 1166)

WIND; in (see pg 1166)
- **sea**, at the (see pg 1166)

WINE (see pg 1166)

WORMS (see pg 1167)

YAWNING agg. or excites the cough (see pg 1167)

Expectoration

MORNING (see pg 1169)

FORENOON (see pg 1169)

NOON (see pg 1169)

AFTERNOON (see pg 1169)

EVENING (see pg 1169)

NIGHT (see pg 1169)

ACRID (see pg 1169)

AIR agg. (see pg 1169)

AIR; IN OPEN:
- **agg.** (see pg 1169)

BALL and rushes into mouth; feels like a round (see pg 1169)

BALLS, in shape of (see pg 1169)

BILIOUS (see pg 1169)

BLACKISH (see pg 1169)

BLUISH (see pg 1171)

BRICK-DUST color (see pg 1171)

BROWNISH (see pg 1171)

BURNED; when dry on the floor looks as if (see pg 1171)

CHEESE, like (see pg 1171)

COLD:
- air:
  · **agg**. (see pg 1171)

CONSTANT, almost day and evening (see pg 1171)

COOL (see pg 1171)

COPIOUS (see pg 1171)

CORROSIVE (see pg 1171)

CREAM-LIKE, yellowish white (see pg 1171)

CRUMBLY (see pg 1171)

DARK (see pg 1171)

DIFFICULT (see pg 1171)

DIRTY-LOOKING (see pg 1171)

DRINKING amel. (see pg 1171)

DUST, as if mixed with (see pg 1171)

EASIER after each cough (see pg 1171)

EASY (see pg 1171)

EATING; after (see pg 1172)

EPITHELIUM; exfoliated (see pg 1172)

FLAKES (see pg 1172)

FLIES forcibly out of mouth (see pg 1172)

FREQUENT (see pg 1172)

FROTHY (see pg 1172)

GELATINOUS (see pg 1172)

GLAIRY (see pg 1172)

GLOBULAR (see pg 1172)

GRANULAR (see pg 1172)

GRAYISH (see pg 1172)

GREENISH (see pg 1172)

HARD (see pg 1172)

HAWKED up, mucus (see pg 1172)

HOUSE, in the (see pg 1172)

INFREQUENT (see pg 1172)

LIVER-COLORED (see pg 1173)

LUMPY (see pg 1173)

MASSES, in (see pg 1173)

MEMBRANOUS (see pg 1173)

MILKY (see pg 1173)

MUCOUS (see pg 1173)

MUDDY-LIKE pus, flies like batter (see pg 1173)

OLEAGINOUS (see pg 1174)

EXPECTORATION: ...

OPAQUE (see pg 1174)

PAINFUL (see pg 1174)

PALE (see pg 1174)

PASTY (see pg 1174)

PHOSPHORESCENT (see pg 1174)

PIECES, in (see pg 1174)

PRUNE juice (see pg 1174)

PURULENT (see pg 1174)

ROPY (see pg 1174)

RUSTY (see pg 1174)

SALIVA-LIKE (see pg 1174)

SCABS coughed up every few weeks (see pg 1174)

SCANTY (see pg 1174)

SEA BATHING, after (see pg 1174)

SKIN, like dead (see pg 1174)

SLATE-COLORED (see pg 1174)

SLIPS back again (see pg 1174)

SOAP-LIKE (see pg 1174)

SOAPSUDS, like (see pg 1174)

STARCH, like (see pg 1174)

STRINGY (see pg 1174)

SWALLOW what has been loosened; must (see pg 1174)

SYRUP-LIKE (see pg 1174)

THICK (see pg 1175)

THIN (see pg 1175)

TOUGH (see pg 1175)

TRANSPARENT (see pg 1176)

TUBERCLES (see pg 1176)

VISCID (see pg 1176)

WALKING:
- after:
  · **agg**. (see pg 1176)
- **agg**. (see pg 1176)

WATERY (see pg 1176)

WHITE (see pg 1176)

YELLOW (see pg 1176)

Chest

ABSCESS:
- **Lungs** (see pg 1177): carb-v$_{\text{mld1}}$

ADHESIONS:
- **pleuritis**; after (see pg 1177)
- **Pericardium**; of the (see pg 1177)

ANEURYSM of (see pg 1177)

ANGINA pectoris (see pg 1177)

ANXIETY in (see pg 1177)

AORTIC disease:

ATROPHY:
- **Mammae** (see pg 1179)
- **Nipples**; of (see pg 1179)

BLEEDING:
- **Mammae**:
  · **Nipples** (see pg 1179)

BRONCHIECTASIS (see pg 1179): ars$_{pkj1}$ ip$_{pkj1}$ samb$_{pkj1}$ stict$_{pkj1}$

CANCER:
- **Mammae** (see pg 1179): calc$_{fmx}$ calc-f$_{bnfl.es,pkj1}$ carc$_{mld3}$ coloc$_{brm}$ iod$_{mld,pkj1}$ thuj$_{ffd}$

CARIES:
- **Clavicles** (see pg 1180)
- **Sternum** (see pg 1180)

CATARRH (see pg 1180): bell$_{gsd,mjs,qqh,spk1}$ calc-p$_{qqh}$ gels$_{gsd,spk1}$ influ$_{qqh}$ oscilloc$_{qqh}$

CHRONIC OBSTRUCTIVE PULMONARY DISEASE (see pg 1181): led$_{brm}$ nux-v$_{brm}$ sulph$_{brm}$

CICATRICES; old:
- **suppurating** (see pg 1181)
- **Mammae**; in (see pg 1181)

CLOTHING agg. (see pg 1181)

CLUCKING sound (see pg 1181)

COLDNESS (see pg 1181)
- **Mammae**:
  · **Nipples** (see pg 1181): *Rhus-t*$_{brm}$

CONGESTION (see pg 1183): am-caust$_{mld,mld5}$ ant-t$_{mld,mld5}$ sang$_{mld5,qqh}$
- **Mammae** (see pg 1183): apis$_{itm,qqh}$ bell$_{itm,qqh}$ puls$_{itm,qqh}$

CONVULSIONS (see pg 1186)

CRACKING:
- **motion** agg. (see pg 1186)
- **Heart**, in region of (see pg 1186)
- **Sternum** (see pg 1186)

CRACKS:
- **Mammae**:
  · **Nipples** (see pg 1186): **Petr**$_{itm}$ puls$_{itm}$

CYANOSIS (see pg 1186)

DEFORMED (see pg 1186)

DILATATION of heart (see pg 1186)
- **Atrium**:
  · **right**: rhus-t$_{brm}$

Dilatation of heart – Atrium: ...
  · **left**:

DISCHARGE from nipple (see pg 1186)

DISCOLORATION:
- **spots** (see pg 1187)
- **Mammae**:
  · **bluish red** (see pg 1187)
  · **redness**:
    ⁞ **dark**:
    ⁞ **light**:

DISTENSION (see pg 1187)

DROPSY (see pg 1187)

DRUMMING heart sounds (see pg 1187)

DRYNESS (see pg 1187)

EDEMA; PULMONARY (see pg 1187): *Apis*$_{brm}$ kali-c$_{fmx}$
- **accompanied** by:
  · **anemia**; non-regenerative: kali-c$_{fmx}$
  · **Liver** complaints: kali-c$_{fmx}$

EMACIATION (see pg 1188)

EMPHYSEMA (see pg 1188): bry$_{itm,mld1}$

EMPYEMA (see pg 1188)

ERUPTIONS (see pg 1188)
- **vesicles** (see pg 1189)
- **Axillae**:
  · **bathing**; after: lyc$_{fmx}$
  · **swimming**; after: lyc$_{fmx}$

ERYSIPELAS of mammae (see pg 1190)

EXCORIATION:
- **Axillae** (see pg 1190)
- **Mammae**:
  · **rubbing**; from (see pg 1190)
  · **Nipples** (see pg 1190)

EXOSTOSIS:
- **Ribs**; on (see pg 1190)

EXUDATION:

FAT about the heart with nervous irritability (see pg 1190)

FATTY degeneration of heart (see pg 1190)

FISTULOUS openings:
- **Axillae**, in (see pg 1190)
- **Mammae**; in (see pg 1190)

FLABBY mammae (see pg 1190)

FLUTTERING (see pg 1190)

GANGRENE of lungs (see pg 1192)

GOUTY heart (see pg 1192)

HEART; complaints of the (see pg 1264): adon$_{itm,mld,mld,mld5}$ apis$_{itm,pkj1}$ apoc$_{itm,pkj1}$ *Arn*$_{mld5,pkj,qqh}$ carb-v$_{itm,mld,pkj1}$ conv$_{itm,mld,qqh}$ *Dig*$_{itm,mld,mld,mld5,pkj,qqh}$ *Iber*$_{itm,mld5,pkj1}$ kali-c$_{mld5,pkj,qqh}$ *Laur*$_{mld,pkj1}$ stroph-h$_{mld,mld,mld,mld5,qqh}$ verat-v$_{itm,mld,qqh}$

HEART failure (see pg 1192)

HEAT (see pg 1192)

HEAVES: puls$_{fmx}$
- **air** amel.; open: puls$_{fmx}$

HEMORRHAGE of lungs (see pg 1193): fic-r$_{mld1}$

HEPATIZATION of lungs (see pg 1194)

HYPERTROPHY (see pg 1194)
- **Heart**; of:
  - **Atrium**:
    - **left**: nat-m$_{brm}$

IMPULSE of heart; excessive (see pg 1195)

INDURATION:
- **Axillary** glands (see pg 1195)
- **Mammae** (see pg 1195)

INFLAMMATION:
- **Bronchial** tubes (see pg 1195): *Acon*$_{itm,mld,mld3}$ **Ant-t**$_{bnf1.es,itm,mld3}$ *Bell*$_{itm,qqh}$ **Bry**$_{itm,mld,mld3}$ calc-p$_{qqh}$ *Carb-v*$_{itm,mld3}$ *Coc-i*$_{itm,mld3}$ *Dros*$_{itm,mld1}$ *Dulc*$_{bnf1.es,mld1}$ **Ip**$_{bnf1.es,itm,mld3}$ merc-cy$_{mld,mld4}$ **Puls**$_{bnf1.es,itm}$ *Rumx*$_{itm,mld3}$ **Sil**$_{mld,qqh}$ **Spong**$_{bnf1.es,itm,mld3}$ *Squil*$_{itm,mld1}$ tub$_{itm}$
- **Heart** (see pg 1196): conv$_{mld,mld4}$
  - **Valves**: adon$_{mld4}$ conv$_{mld4}$ crat$_{mld4}$ laur$_{mld4}$ lyc$_{mld4}$ naja$_{mld4}$ spig$_{mld4}$ spong$_{mld4}$ stroph-h$_{mld4}$
- **Lungs** (see pg 1196): dros$_{mld,mld5}$ **Lyc**$_{fmx}$
  - **aspiration** pneumonia (see pg 1197): ant-t$_{elg,hnb}$
  - **children**; in:
    - **infants** (see pg 1197)
- **Mammae** (see pg 1198): *Acon*$_{dyc}$ *Apis*$_{dyc}$ arg-met$_{dyc}$ arn$_{ljy,mld,plr1}$ **Bell**$_{dyc}$ **Bry**$_{dyc}$ calc-f$_{bnf1.es,dyc,mld5}$ carc$_{dyc}$ *Cist*$_{dyc}$ *Con*$_{dyc}$ *Lach*$_{dyc}$ *Merc*$_{dyc}$ phel$_{dyc}$ **Phyt**$_{dyc}$ pyrog$_{bnf1.es,itm,mld,pkj1}$ sep$_{dyc}$ **Sil**$_{dyc}$ **Sulph**$_{dyc}$ tub$_{dyc}$ urt-u$_{dyc}$ viol-o$_{dyc}$
  - **alternating** sides:
  - **accompanied** by:
    - **milk** secretion:
      - **absent**:
      - **decreased**:
      - **quality** and quantity unchanged:
      - **quality** unchanged:
      - **quantity** unchanged:
    - **Veins**; swelling of:
  - **edematous**:
  - **induration**; with:
  - **liver** enzymes; with increased:
  - **nodular**:
  - **Nipples** (see pg 1198): arn$_{itm}$ bell$_{itm}$ con$_{itm}$ vip-a$_{itm}$
- **Pleura** (see pg 1198): lyc$_{fmx}$

INJURIES:
- **Mammae**; to (see pg 1199)
  - **Nipples**:
    - **step** of kick; from a: hyper$_{hnb}$

INSENSIBILITY of nipples (see pg 1199)

INVERSION:
- **Nipples**; of (see pg 1199)

ITCHING (see pg 1199)

- **Axillae** (see pg 1199): carc$_{brm}$ **Sulph**$_{fmx}$

JERKS (see pg 1199)

LUMPS:
- **Sternum**:

MAMMAE; complaints of:
- **menses**; before (see pg 1267)

MEALY coating nipples (see pg 1200)

MILK:
- **absent** (see pg 1200): **Calc**$_{klp}$ phyt$_{hnb}$ puls$_{hnb}$ Urt-u$_{elg,klp}$
  - **delivery**; after (see pg 1200): phyt$_{hnb}$ *Puls*$_{hnb}$
- **bitter** (see pg 1200): calc-p$_{qqh}$ phos$_{plr1}$ sulph$_{plr1}$
- **bloody** (see pg 1200): acon$_{bnf1.es,plr1}$ ip$_{bnf1.es,plr1}$ phos$_{mld5,plr1}$
  - **colostrum**: calc$_{hnb}$
  - **injuries** of mammae; after: arn$_{hnb}$
- **brown** colored:
- **cell** count too high:
- **constant** secretion:
  - **emaciation**; in spite of: phos$_{hnb}$
  - **illness**; in spite of a severe:
- **copious**:
- **decreased** (see pg 1200): acon$_{plr1}$ alf$_{mld5}$ apis$_{dyc}$ bell$_{plr1}$ bry$_{plr1}$ caul$_{dyc}$ cham$_{plr1}$ dulc$_{plr1}$ galeg$_{dyc}$ phyt$_{hnb}$ puls$_{hnb}$ puls-vg$_{dyc}$ ric$_{qqh}$ sabal$_{qqh}$ sec$_{dyc}$ sep$_{dyc}$ ser-ang$_{dyc}$ urt-u$_{dyc}$
- **disappearing** (see pg 1200): acon$_{plr1}$ alf$_{qqh}$ bell$_{plr1}$ bry$_{plr1}$ *Dulc*$_{plr1}$ *Lac-c*$_{elg}$ ric$_{plr1}$ sabal$_{plr1}$
  - **death** of loved ones: ign$_{hnb}$
  - **fear**; from:
  - **homesickness**; from: ign$_{hnb}$
  - **mastitis**:
    - **after**:
    - **before**:
  - **weakness**; from:
- **failing** to release the milk: urt-u$_{hnb}$
  - **fear**; from: acon$_{elg}$ ign$_{elg,hnb}$ puls$_{hnb}$
  - **milking** parlor; in: arg-n$_{hnb}$
  - **pain**; from:
- **fat**:
  - **high**; too:
  - **low**; too:
- **flowing** spontaneously (see pg 1200)
- **increased** (see pg 1201): alf$_{mld5}$ lac-c$_{mld5}$ *Ric*$_{qqh}$ sabal$_{bhf}$
- **nursing** the calf; always:
- **offensive**:
- **painful** secretion:
- **pale**:
- **pregnancy**; in women when not related to (see pg 1201): apis$_{mmj,pkj1}$ arist-cl$_{dyc}$ ars$_{mmj}$ atro$_{mmj}$ calc$_{fmx,mmj,pkj1}$ caul$_{mmj}$ cham$_{mld5,pkj1}$ con$_{mmj}$ croc$_{mmj,pkj1}$ helon$_{mmj}$ ign$_{bnf1.es,dyc,itm,klp,mmj,pkj,qqh}$ lac-c$_{bnf1.es,itm,mld5,mmj,pkj,qqh}$ lach$_{itm}$ nux-m$_{mmj,pkj,qqh}$ nux-v$_{itm,mmj,qqh}$ op$_{mmj}$ phyt$_{itm}$ **Puls**$_{hnb,klp}$ puls-vg$_{dyc}$ sabad$_{mmj}$ sep$_{qqh}$ sulph$_{brm,mmj,pkj1}$ thlas$_{mmj}$ thuj$_{itm,mmj,pkj1}$ Urt-u$_{dyc}$

- **pregnancy**; in women when not related to: ...
  · **bloody** milk:
  · **clotted**:
  · **copious**:
- **protein**:
  · **high**; too:
  · **low**; too:
- **purulent**:
- **putrid**:
- **red**:
- **scanty**:
- **sour** (see pg 1201): ant-t$_{plr1}$ phos$_{plr1}$ sulph$_{plr1}$
- **thin**:
  · **blue**; and (see pg 1201): nux-v$_{plr1}$
  · **watery**; and (see pg 1201): nux-v$_{bnfl.es}$
    Puls$_{bnfl.es,hnb}$
- **watery**:
- **white**:

MOISTURE from humor in axilla (see pg 1201)

MOVEMENT:
- **Heart** (see pg 1201)
- **Region** of heart (see pg 1201)

MURMURS:
- **cardiac** murmurs (see pg 1201): *Apis*$_{brm}$

NODULES, sensitive (see pg 1201)
- **Mammae** (see pg 1201): sep$_{ffd}$
  · **pregnancy** agg.:
    : **imaginary** pregnancy; during and after: lyc$_{ffd}$
    puls$_{ffd}$ sep$_{ffd}$

PAIN (see pg 1205)
- **cramping** (see pg 1209)
- **Mammae**:
  · **lying**:
    : **agg.**:
      : **painful** side amel.; lying on: bry$_{hnb}$
  · **palpation**; upon:
  · **pressure**:
    : **amel.** (see pg 1231): bry$_{hnb}$
  · **sore** (see pg 1231)
  · **touch** agg.:
    : **slightest** touch agg.: arn$_{hnb}$ bry$_{hnb}$ hep$_{hnb}$

PALPITATION of heart (see pg 1250): Acon$_{mld4}$
conv$_{mld4}$ crat$_{mld4}$ iber$_{mld,pkj1}$ *Lil-t*$_{mld4}$ *Lycps-v*$_{mld,pkj1}$
Naja$_{mld,pkj1}$ **Phos**$_{mld4}$ stroph-h$_{mld4}$ thyr$_{mld4}$
- **anxiety**:
  · **with** (see pg 1251): cham$_{brm}$
- **fever**:
  · **during**:
    : **agg.** (see pg 1253): lach$_{qqh}$
  - **irregular** (see pg 1253): cact$_{pkj1}$ *Crat*$_{pkj1}$ glon$_{pkj1}$
    Lyc$_{ffd}$ **Nat-m**$_{pkj1}$ stroph-h$_{pkj1}$

PARALYSIS:
- **Diaphragm** (see pg 1256)
- **Heart** (see pg 1256)
- **Lung** (see pg 1256)

PERSPIRATION (see pg 1256)
- **night**:
  · **sleep** (see pg 1256): phos$_{brm}$
- **Axillae**:
  · **sweetish** odor: sulph$_{qqh}$

PETECHIAE (see pg 1257)

PHTHISIS pulmonalis (see pg 1257)

POLLUTION; symptoms of heart and faintness are agg. after (see pg 1258)

PULSATION (see pg 1258)

PURPURA (see pg 1259)

RETRACTION of nipples (see pg 1259)

SENSITIVE (see pg 1259)

SHAKING of chest:
- **cough** agg.; during (see pg 1259)

SHOCKS (see pg 1259)

SMALL mammae:
- **one** mamma is smaller than the other (see pg 1260)

SPASMS of (see pg 1260)

STAGNATION:
- **blood** stagnated in chest; as if (see pg 1260)

STIFFNESS (see pg 1260)

STRAIN:
- **Heart**:
  · **violent** exertion; strain of the heart from (see pg 1260)

SWELLING (see pg 1260)
- **Mammae**:
  · **castration**; after: tub$_{brm}$
    : **men**; in:
    : **women**; in:
  · **edematous**:
    : **delivery**; during first: puls-vg$_{dyc}$ ser-ang$_{dyc}$
      urt-u$_{dyc}$
    : **liver** disease; from: card-m$_{hnb}$ lyc$_{hnb}$
    : **pain**; with: asaf$_{klp}$ ign$_{klp}$
    : **painless**: calc$_{klp}$ puls$_{klp}$
  · **secretion** of milk, with:
    : **non-pregnant** women; in: ign$_{klp}$ puls$_{klp}$
    : **large** quantities of milk: puls$_{klp}$

TREMBLING (see pg 1262)

TUMORS:
- **Axillae** (see pg 1262)
- **Mammae** (see pg 1262): calc$_{fmx}$
- **Mammary** gland; male:

ULCERS (see pg 1262)

WARTS (see pg 1263)
- **Mammae**; on:
  · **Nipples**:
    : **papillomatosis**: thuj$_{hnb}$

WEAKNESS (see pg 1263)

- **Heart**:
  - **Myocardium**:
    - **fever**; during (see pg 1264): lach$_{qqh}$

Back

AMPUTATION of the tail; ailments from:

CERVICAL STENOSIS: phos$_{fmx}$
- **accompanied** by:
  - **incoordination**: phos$_{fmx}$

COMPLAINTS of back:
- **Spinal** cord:
  - **accompanied** by:
    - **urination**; frequent: phos$_{fmx}$

COMPRESSION:
- **Lumbosacral** region (see pg 1272): nux-v$_{brm}$ phos$_{brm}$ sulph$_{brm}$

CURVATURE of spine (see pg 1273)
- **kyphosis**:
- **lordosis**:
- **scoliosis**:

DANDRUFF:
- **Tail**:

DYSPLASIA:
- **Intervertebral** disks: ang$_{bnfl.es}$ arn$_{bnfl.es}$ calc-f$_{bnfl.es}$ hyper$_{bnfl.es}$

EMACIATION (see pg 1274): mag-c$_{brm}$
- **Cervical** region (see pg 1274): mag-c$_{brm}$ sulph$_{brm}$

ERUPTIONS:
- **dry**:
  - **Tail**:
- **erythema**:
  - **Tail**:
- **itching**:
  - **Tail**:
- **scales**:
  - **Tail**:
- **Tail**:

HAIR:
- **falling**: sep$_{brm}$
  - **Lumbar** region: lyc$_{hnb}$
  - **Neck**:
  - **Scapulae**; between:
  - **Tail**:

HEAT:
- **Dorsal** region:
  - **Scapulae**:
    - **Between** (see pg 1277):

HERNIATED DISK: allox$_{pkj1}$ arn$_{pkj1}$ bry$_{pkj1}$ cimic$_{pkj1}$ oxal-a$_{pkj1}$ rad-met$_{pkj1}$ rhus-t$_{pkj1}$

INDURATIONS:
- **saddle**; under the: calc$_{brm,hnb}$

BACK: ...

INFLAMMATION:
- **Joints**:
  - **rheumatic** (see pg 1278): caust$_{itm}$ hyper$_{itm}$ kalm$_{itm}$ nux-v$_{itm}$ plb$_{itm}$ rauw$_{itm}$ thal$_{itm}$ tub$_{itm}$
- **Spinal** cord (see pg 1279): con$_{mld4}$
  - **Cervical** region (see pg 1279): lath$_{mld4}$
- **Tail**:
  - **Viol's** gland: sil$_{brm}$
- **Vertebrae** (see pg 1279): calc$_{mld3}$ calc-f$_{mld3}$ hecla$_{mld3}$ hyper$_{mld3}$ ruta$_{mld3}$

INJURIES (see pg 1279)
- **Sacroiliac** symphyses:
  - **delivery**; ailments from: symph$_{hnb}$
- **Tail**:
  - **accompanied** by:
    - **paralysis**: hyper$_{hnb}$

ITCHING:
- **Cervical** region (see pg 1279): Puls$_{brm}$
- **Lumbar** region (see pg 1280): sulph$_{brm}$

LONG BACK: calc-f$_{hnb}$ nux-v$_{hnb}$

NECROSIS:
- **Muscles**: arn$_{hnb}$
- **Tail**:
  - **offensive** smelling:
  - **paroxysmal**:
  - **Base**:
  - **Middle**:
  - **Tip**:

OPISTHOTONOS (see pg 1281): Cic$_{elg}$
- **accompanied** by:
  - **Brain**; inflammation of the:
  - **Meninges**; inflammation of the:
- **infants**; in:
  - **labor**; after prolonged: cupr$_{hnb}$
- **sexual** excitement; during: chin$_{brm}$

PAIN (see pg 1282)
- **lying**:
  - **hard**; on something:
    - **amel.** (see pg 1287)
- **motion**:
  - **agg.** (see pg 1288)
  - **beginning** of:
    - **agg.** (see pg 1288)
  - **must** move (see pg 1288)
- **Lumbar** region (see pg 1315): Berb$_{qqh}$ hecla$_{dyc1}$ Ruta$_{dyc1}$ solid$_{qqh}$
- **Spine**:
  - **sore** (see pg 1336): lyc$_{qqh}$
- **Tail**:
  - **motion**:
    - **agg.**:

PARALYSIS (see pg 1338): arn$_{klp}$ nux-v$_{klp}$ plb$_{klp}$ syph$_{klp}$
- **warts**; from suppressed: med$_{hnb}$

- **Sacroiliac** joints:
- **Sacrum:**
  - **painful:**
    - **crying** day and night: plb$_{hnb}$
- **Tail:**
  - **watertail:**

PERSPIRATION (see pg 1338)
- **Cervical** region:
  - **sweetish** odor: calc$_{qqh}$ sil$_{qqh}$

PROLAPSUS:
- **Intervertebral** disk (see pg 1339): arn$_{brm}$ kali-c$_{brm}$ lyc$_{brm}$ nux-v$_{brm}$ rhus-t$_{brm}$ sep$_{brm}$

SENSITIVE:
- **rider;** under the:

SPASMS:
- **Cervical** region (see pg 1341): nux-v$_{qqh}$

STIFFNESS:
- **Lumbar** region (see pg 1343): lyc$_{fmx,qqh}$ sulph$_{fmx}$

STRAINING; easily (see pg 1344): **Lyc**$_{brm}$

TWITCHING (see pg 1346): tub$_{brm}$

WAGGING one's tail:
- **absent:**
- **constant:**
- **fear;** with:
- **often:**
- **strongly:**
- **weakly:**

Extremities

ABSCESS:
- **shoeing;** after: hep$_{fmx}$ led$_{fmx}$

ANKYLOSIS (see pg 1351): calc$_{qqh}$ carbn-s$_{qqh}$ eup-per$_{qqh}$ rhus-t$_{qqh}$

ARTHROSIS (see pg 1352): arn$_{elg}$ bry$_{pkj1}$ calc$_{elg}$ calc-f$_{pkj1}$ calc-p$_{elg}$ caust$_{pkj1,qqh}$ dulc$_{pkj1}$ kali-c$_{pkj1}$ lyc$_{pkj1}$ med$_{pkj1}$ nat-s$_{pkj1}$ phos$_{elg}$ sulph$_{pkj1}$ thuj$_{pkj1}$ tub$_{pkj1}$
- **Ankle** joints: lyc$_{brm}$
- **Fingers:** act-sp$_{pkj1}$
- **Knees** (see pg 1352): kali-c$_{pkj1}$ led$_{pkj1}$ phos$_{brm}$
- **Shoulders:** lith-c$_{pkj1}$ rhod$_{pkj1}$ rhus-t$_{pkj1}$
  - **right:** staph$_{brm}$

AWKWARDNESS (see pg 1352): lyc$_{brm}$
- **Hands:**
  - **drops** things (see pg 1352)
- **Lower** limbs (see pg 1352)

BLOOD CIRCULATION; complaints of:
- **failure** of:
  - **Hooves;** in:
- **Corium:**

BURSAE:
- **Elbows:** lyc$_{brm}$

EXTREMITIES: ...

CALLUS of fractured bones:
- **absent:** calc$_{hnb}$
- **delayed:**
- **excessive:** calc-p$_{hnb}$

CARIES of bone (see pg 1354): arn$_{itm}$ hecla$_{bnfl.es}$ kreos$_{mld4}$ lach$_{itm}$ ust$_{mld3}$

CLAWS AND HOOVES; complaints of:
- **penetrated,** punctured:

CLUBFOOT (see pg 1356): sulph$_{brm}$

COLDNESS (see pg 1356)
- **fever;** during (see pg 1357): lach$_{qqh}$ sil$_{qqh}$
- **snake** bite; after a:
- **Feet:**
  - **night:**
    - **bed** agg.; in (see pg 1358): sulph$_{fmx}$
  - **one** cold:
    - **other** hot; the (see pg 1359)
- **Hands:**
  - **one** hand:
    - **hot;** and the other (see pg 1360): lyc$_{hnb}$

CRACKED skin:
- **Feet:**
  - **Soles** (see pg 1369): lyc$_{brm}$ sep$_{brm}$
    - **bleeding:** lyc$_{brm}$

CURVING and bowing (see pg 1377): *Calc*$_{bnfl.es,pkj,qqh}$ calc-f$_{bnfl.es}$ *Calc-p*$_{bnfl.es,pkj,qqh}$ cupr$_{bnfl.es}$ mang$_{bnfl.es}$ nat-m$_{bnfl.es,pkj,qqh}$ *Sil*$_{pkj1}$ zinc$_{bnfl.es}$

DISCOLORATION:
- **foul-in-the-foot:** gink-b$_{dyc}$ hep$_{dyc}$ kreos$_{dyc}$ pyrog$_{elg}$
  - **purple:** tarent-c$_{dyc}$
- **Toes:**
  - **Between** toes:
    - **right:**
    - **left:**
    - **redness:**

DISLOCATION:
- **Foot:**
  - **dew** claw:
- **Knees:**
  - **Patella** (see pg 1383): anac$_{klp}$ arn$_{pkj1}$ calc$_{elg}$ calc-f$_{hnb,klp,pkj1}$ gels$_{brm,elg}$ ign$_{brm}$ phos$_{brm}$ rhus-t$_{brm,klp}$ ruta$_{elg,pkj1}$ sep$_{brm}$
    - **right:** phos$_{brm}$
    - **recurrent:**

DISLOCATION; EASY (see pg 1383): arn$_{bnfl.es,itm,ljy,pkj1}$ calc-f$_{itm,qqh}$ calc-p$_{mld5}$ coloc$_{mld5}$ hecla$_{pkj1}$ hyper$_{pkj1}$ led$_{pkj1}$ nat-c$_{qqh}$ rhus-t$_{bnfl.es,itm,ljy,pkj,qqh}$ ruta$_{bnfl.es,itm,ljy,pkj,qqh}$ symph$_{bnfl.es}$

DRYNESS:
- **Feet:**
  - **Soles** (see pg 1384): lyc$_{brm}$

ERUPTIONS:
- **itching:**
  - **atopy:** thuj$_{brm}$

- **mud** fever: calc-sil$_{brm}$ calen$_{dyc}$ graph$_{dyc}$ hyper$_{dyc}$
maland$_{dyc,klp}$ sil$_{elg}$ sulph$_{brm,dyc}$
- **Feet**:
  - **Sole** of (see pg 1387): lyc$_{brm}$
- **Hands**:
  - **Between** the fingers (see pg 1391): nux-v$_{brm}$
    - **right**:
    - **left**: nat-m$_{brm}$
    - **blisters**: ruta$_{brm}$
    - **boils**: ars$_{brm}$ calc$_{brm}$
- **Joints**:
  - **Bends** of (see pg 1392)
- **Lower** limbs:
  - **left**:
    - **scratching**; from: sep$_{brm}$
- **Thighs**:
  - **Between** (see pg 1396): sil$_{fmx}$
- **Toes**:
  - **Between** (see pg 1396): ars$_{brm}$ calc$_{brm}$ graph$_{brm}$
  gunp$_{klp}$ hep$_{klp}$ lyc$_{brm}$ merc$_{klp}$ phos$_{brm}$ puls$_{brm}$ sep$_{brm}$
  sil$_{hnb,klp}$
    - **right**:
    - **left**:
    - **boils**: anac$_{brm}$ ars$_{brm}$ calc$_{brm}$ nat-m$_{brm}$ ruta$_{brm}$
      - **blue** discoloration; with:
      - **recurrent**: sil$_{hnb}$
      - **redness**: fl-ac$_{klp}$
- **Upper** limbs:
  - **mud** fever: sep$_{kgc}$

EXCORIATION:
- **Elbow**:
  - **lying** on lateral side; from: lyc$_{brm}$

EXOSTOSIS (see pg 1399): calc-p$_{qqh}$ hecla$_{qqh}$
- **injuries**; after:

FALL, liability to:
- **down** from high objects; falling: sulph$_{brm}$
- **hurry**; from: cham$_{brm}$
- **walking**:
  - **backward** agg.: phos$_{fmx}$

FELON:
- **Claws** and hooves:
- **Nail**; beginning in:
  - **runaround**:
    - **Lymphatics**, inflamed (see pg 1400)

FRACTURES (see pg 1403): arn$_{pkj1}$ **Calc-p** $_{bnfl.es,itm,pkj1}$
chin$_{pkj1}$ hecla$_{bnfl.es}$ **Ruta** $_{bnfl.es,pkj1}$ sul-ac$_{bnfl.es}$
Symph $_{bnfl.es}$

GANGRENE (see pg 1404): arn$_{itm}$ bapt$_{bnfl.es}$
pyrog$_{bnfl.es}$

HAIR:
- **falling**:
  - **Feet**:
  - **Forearms**:
  - **Hands**:
  - **Legs**:
  - **Lower** limbs:
  - **Shoulders**:
  - **Thighs**:
    - **Inner** side:
  - **Upper** arms:
  - **Upper** limbs:

HANG DOWN, letting:
- **Limbs**:
  - **amel.** (see pg 1404): puls$_{brm}$

HEAT:
- **Hands** (see pg 1406): nat-m$_{ffd}$

HEMATOMA:
- **Thigh**:
  - **left**: ham$_{dyc}$ lach$_{dyc}$

HIP JOINT disease (see pg 1413): all-s$_{pkj,qqh}$ arn$_{pkj1}$
Bry$_{pkj1}$ **Calc** $_{qqh}$ *Lyc* $_{brm}$ *Rhus-t* $_{pkj1}$ **Sil** $_{brm}$
- **right** (see pg 1413): lyc$_{brm}$
- **accompanied** by:
  - **Feet**; offensive perspiration of: med$_{dvr}$

HORNY:
- **breaking** off; walls:
- **brittle**:
  - **Hind** hand: ant-c$_{qqh}$ calc$_{frc}$ calc-f$_{mld5}$ fl-ac$_{qqh}$
  graph$_{qqh}$ hep$_{mld5}$ kreos$_{mld5}$ sep$_{frc}$ sil$_{frc}$ thuj$_{qqh}$
- **crumbling**:
- **deformed**:
- **foul**-in-the-foot:
- **poor** quality:
- **thin**:

INFLAMMATION (see pg 1413): arn$_{ljy1}$
- **Bones** (see pg 1413): hecla$_{qqh}$ ruta$_{qqh}$
  - **Navicular** bones: apis$_{bnfl.es}$ calc$_{brm}$ calc-p$_{brm}$
  crot-h$_{bnfl.es}$ phos$_{brm}$ rhus-t$_{bnfl.es}$ ruta$_{bnfl.es}$ vip$_{bnfl.es}$
  - **Periosteum** (see pg 1413): apis$_{mld4}$ arn$_{mld4}$ bry$_{mld4}$
  calc-f$_{mld4}$ ruta$_{mld4}$ sil$_{mld4}$
  - **Sesamoid** bones: arn$_{mld4}$ calc-f$_{mld4}$ hecla$_{mld5}$
  ruta$_{mld,mld5}$ sil$_{mld4}$
- **Claws** and hooves:
  - **foot** rot: kreos$_{dyc}$ sil$_{dyc}$
- **Feet**:
  - **ringbone**:
  - **Cartilage**; lateral: arn$_{mld4}$ hep$_{mld4}$ hyper$_{mld4}$ led$_{mld4}$
  sil$_{mld4}$
- **Fingers**:
  - **dermatitis** digitalis:
  - **mortellaro**: bell$_{elg}$ pyrog$_{elg}$
  - **Between**: apis$_{elg}$ bell$_{elg}$ myris$_{elg}$ tarent-c$_{elg}$ thuj$_{elg}$
- **Hands**:
  - **Bones**:
    - **Periosteum**: apis$_{mld4}$ arn$_{mld4}$ calc-f$_{mld4}$ rhus-t$_{mld4}$
    ruta$_{mld4}$

- **Hoof:**
- **Joints** (see pg 1414): arg-met$_{mld5}$ cimic$_{pkj1}$ med$_{itm,pkj1}$ nux-m$_{pkj1}$
  - **fever**; with: aethi-a$_{rms}$ apis$_{brm}$ *Nat-m*$_{brm}$
  - **synovitis** (see pg 1414): colch$_{bnfl.es}$ eup-per$_{mld5}$ kali-bi$_{mld4}$ ruta$_{mld5}$
- **Knees** (see pg 1414): ruta$_{mld4,mld4}$ symph$_{mld1}$
  - **Bursae** (see pg 1414): *Apis*$_{mld4}$ bry$_{mld4}$ calc-f$_{mld4}$ hep$_{mld4}$ ruta$_{mld4}$ sil$_{mld4}$
- **Laminae:** agar$_{dyc}$ alum$_{dyc}$ arn$_{dyc}$ bell$_{dyc}$ fl-ac$_{brm,dyc}$ gink-b$_{dyc}$ graph$_{dyc}$ hyper$_{dyc}$ lol$_{dyc}$ nux-v$_{dyc,srg}$ puls-vg$_{dyc}$ rhus-t$_{brm}$ sabad$_{dyc}$ sars$_{dyc}$ sec$_{dyc}$ sil$_{dyc}$ tritic$_{dyc}$
  - **accompanied** by:
    - **Feet**; swelling of: phyt$_{dyc}$
  - **acute**: bell$_{dyc}$ bry$_{elg}$ gink-b$_{dyc}$ hyper$_{dyc}$ sabad$_{dyc}$ sars$_{dyc}$ sec$_{dyc}$
  - **chronic**: alum$_{dyc}$ fl-ac$_{dyc}$ graph$_{dyc}$ puls-vg$_{dyc}$ sil$_{dyc}$
    - **accompanied** by:
      - **Hooves**; deformed: calc-f$_{dyc}$ fl-ac$_{dyc}$ graph$_{dyc}$ sil$_{dyc}$ thuj$_{dyc}$
  - **cold** applications agg.:
  - **eating**; from:
    - **overeating**:
  - **heat** agg.: sars$_{dyc}$
  - **injuries**; from:
  - **motion** agg.:
  - **retentio** secundinarum; from:
  - **rich** food; from:
  - **weather** agg.; frosty: agar$_{dyc}$ sabad$_{dyc}$
  - **Forelimb** nails: acon$_{mld,mld,mld5}$ bell$_{mld,mld,mld5}$ calc-f$_{mld,mld,mld5}$ hep$_{mld4}$ nux-v$_{mld,mld4}$ sil$_{mld4}$
- **Ligaments** (see pg 1415): arn$_{mld4}$ rhus-t$_{mld4}$ ruta$_{mld4}$ sil$_{mld4}$
- **Lymphatics** (see pg 1415): ars$_{itm}$ bell$_{itm}$ calc$_{itm}$ echi$_{itm}$ hep$_{itm}$ iod$_{itm}$ puls$_{itm}$ pyrog$_{itm}$ sulph$_{itm}$
- **Tendons** (see pg 1415): apis$_{mld4}$ arn$_{bnfl.es,mld4}$ ruta$_{bnfl.es,mld4}$ sil$_{mld4}$
- **Wrists** (see pg 1415): calc-f$_{mld4}$ hecla$_{mld4}$ ruta$_{mld4}$

INJURIES:
- **Fingers:**
  - **Nails**, of (see pg 1415): hyper$_{brm}$
    - **splinter** of glass (see pg 1415)
- **Foot:**
  - **dew** claws:
    - **inflammation**; without:
    - **suppurating**:
- **Joints** (see pg 1415): apis$_{pkj1}$ arn$_{pkj1}$ bry$_{pkj1}$ led$_{pkj1}$ nit-ac$_{bnfl.es}$
- **Knees**: calc$_{elg}$
- **Ligaments**: arn$_{mld4}$ gels$_{mld4}$ rhus-t$_{mld4}$ ruta$_{mld4}$
- **Tendons** (see pg 1415): arn$_{mld4}$ rhus-t$_{mld4}$ ruta$_{mld4}$
- **Thumbs:**
  - **bite** of a cat (see pg 1415)
- **Toes:**
  - **nail** in toe; from: acon$_{ijy1}$ arn$_{ijy1}$ ars$_{ijy1}$ led$_{ijy1}$ sulph$_{ijy1}$

Injuries – Toes: ...
- **Nails:**
  - **Root:**

ITCHING:
- **Feet:**
  - **left**: lyc$_{brm}$
- **Thighs** (see pg 1421): **Sulph**$_{brm}$
- **Toes** (see pg 1422): calc-p$_{brm}$
  - **Between** (see pg 1422): lyc$_{brm}$ puls$_{brm}$

JERKING (see pg 1423): arn$_{mld,mld4}$ calc$_{mld4}$ cupr-ar$_{pkj1}$ cur$_{mld3}$ mag-p$_{mld4}$ nux-v$_{pkj1}$ stry$_{mld4}$

JOINTS; complaints of:
- **acute**: hep$_{dyc}$
- **chronic**: gunp$_{dyc}$ sil$_{dyc}$

JUMPING:
- **high** up with difficulty; jumping: sulph$_{brm}$

LIFTING:
- **aversion:**
  - **Hooves:**
    - **blacksmith**; for the: calc-p$_{brm}$ nux-v$_{brm}$
- **Lower** limbs:
  - **left:**
    - **jumping**; when: sil$_{brm}$

LIMPING (see pg 1427): puls$_{ijy,qqh}$ rhus-t$_{ijy,qqh}$
- **Lyme** disease; from: aur-arn$_{nnb}$ calc-p$_{brm}$ lyc$_{brm}$

NAILS; complaints of:
- **brittle** nails (see pg 1635): **Calc**$_{elg}$ **Graph**$_{dyc}$ *Sil*$_{dyc,fmx}$ thuj$_{dyc}$
  - **Fingernails:**
    - **crumbling** (see pg 1635): fl-ac$_{klp}$ graph$_{klp}$ sil$_{klp}$
  - **Forelimb** nails: ant-c$_{qqh}$ calc$_{frc}$ calc-f$_{mld5}$ fl-ac$_{qqh}$ graph$_{qqh}$ hep$_{mld5}$ kreos$_{mld5}$ sep$_{frc}$ sil$_{frc}$ thuj$_{qqh}$
  - **Toenails** (see pg 1635): ars$_{brm}$
- **exfoliation** of nails (see pg 1635): **Calc**$_{brm}$
- **growth** of nails:
  - **interrupted** (see pg 1636): anan$_{rkb}$
  - **rapid** (see pg 1636): calc-sil$_{brm}$
- **irregular**: ant-c$_{qqh}$ calc$_{frc}$ calc-f$_{mld5}$ fl-ac$_{qqh}$ graph$_{qqh}$ hep$_{mld5}$ kreos$_{mld5}$ sep$_{frc}$ sil$_{frc}$ thuj$_{qqh}$

NAVICULAR BONE DISEASE: calc$_{brm}$ calc-p$_{brm}$ phos$_{brm}$ sulph$_{elg}$

NECROSIS:
- **Thighs:**
  - **Femur:**
    - **Head** of the femur; aseptic necrosis of the:

OSTEOCHONDROSIS DISSECANS:
- **Elbows:** lyc$_{brm}$
- **Knees:** calc-p$_{brm}$

OSTEOPOROSIS (see pg 1437): calc$_{mld,mld5}$ calc-f$_{mld3}$ calc-p$_{mld,mld5}$ hecla$_{mld3}$ nat-m$_{mld3}$ sil$_{mld,mld5}$

OVEREXERTION; after: arn$_{mld5,qqh}$ calc-p$_{mld5}$ calc-s$_{qqh}$ ph-ac$_{mld5}$ rhus-t$_{itm}$ ruta$_{bnfl.es}$ sarcol-ac$_{itm}$
- **Tendons:** calc-s$_{qqh}$

PAIN (see pg 1437)

- **cold**:
  - **bathing**:
    - **agg.**: phos$_{brm}$ staph$_{brm}$
- **eating**:
  - **overeating**; from:
- **exhausting** disease; from:
- **fever**:
  - **during**:
    - **agg.** (see pg 1441)
- **frost** agg.:
- **motion**:
  - **agg.** (see pg 1441)
  - **beginning** of:
    - **agg.** (see pg 1442): calc$_{ffd}$
- **neuralgic** (see pg 1442): bell$_{qqh}$ kalm$_{qqh}$ verat$_{qqh}$
- **rheumatic** (see pg 1442): calc-f$_{mld3}$ con$_{ljyl}$ *Iod*$_{mld3}$ lith-c$_{mld3}$ **Sulph**$_{mld,mld4}$ verat-v$_{mld5}$
- **rich** food; from too:
- **Articulations**:
  - **gouty**: acon$_{ljyl}$ bry$_{ljyl}$ rhus-t$_{ljyl}$
- **Bones** (see pg 1451): *Fl-ac*$_{bnfl.es}$ hecla$_{bnfl.es}$ **Merc**$_{bnfl.es}$ sil$_{bnfl.es}$ sul-ac$_{itm}$
- **Cartilages**: fl-ac$_{itm}$
- **Elbows**:
  - **motion**:
    - **motion** agg.; beginning of: lyc$_{brm}$
  - **processus** coronoideus:
    - **isolated**: lyc$_{brm}$
  - **Olecranon** (see pg 1455): rhus-t$_{fmx}$
- **Hips** (see pg 1488): asaf$_{klp}$ *Bell*$_{qqh}$ *Bry*$_{klp}$ **Rhus-t**$_{klp}$ *Stront-c*$_{klp}$ *Syph*$_{klp}$ vermic$_{klp}$
  - **right** (see pg 1488): caust$_{brm}$ rhod$_{brm}$
  - **exertion** agg.; after (see pg 1491): rhod$_{brm}$
  - **motion**:
    - **beginning** of:
      - **agg.** (see pg 1491): *Lyc*$_{ffd}$ rhod$_{brm}$
  - **periodical** (see pg 1491): phos$_{brm}$
  - **Joints** (see pg 1495): caust$_{qqh}$
- **Joints** (see pg 1495): am-m$_{qqh}$ fl-ac$_{bnfl.es}$ hecla$_{bnfl.es}$ *Merc*$_{bnfl.es}$ *Sil*$_{bnfl.es}$ staphycoc$_{mld3}$ streptoc$_{mld3}$ sul-ac$_{itm}$
  - **accompanied** by:
    - **septic** fever:
- **Legs**:
  - **growing** pains (see pg 1513)
- **Lower** limbs:
  - **ascending** stairs agg. (see pg 1523): calc-p$_{brm}$
- **Muscles** (see pg 1530): acon$_{ljyl}$ bell$_{ljyl}$ bry$_{ljyl}$ caust$_{mld5,qqh}$ cham$_{ljyl}$ cimic$_{mld5}$ con$_{mld5}$ dulc$_{ljy,mld5,qqh}$ lith-c$_{mld5}$ nux-v$_{ljyl}$ op$_{ljyl}$ rhod$_{qqh}$ sul-ac$_{qqh}$ thal$_{mld5}$
  - **rheumatic** (see pg 1530): arn$_{bnfl.es,itm}$ *Cimic*$_{bnfl.es,itm}$ phyt$_{bnfl.es,itm}$
- **Shoulders**:
  - **right** (see pg 1532): phos$_{fmx}$

PARALYSIS (see pg 1579): hyper$_{itm,pkj1}$ lath$_{bnfl.es,mld5,pkj1}$ phys$_{bnfl.es,mld5,pkj1}$ stry$_{ljyl}$
- **abdominal** symptoms, with (see pg 1579): plb$_{brm}$
- **pain**; from:
  - **abdomen**; in the: plb$_{brm}$
- **Lower** limbs (see pg 1581): *Con*$_{brm}$

Paralysis – Lower limbs: ...
- **delivery**; after (see pg 1581): arn$_{qqh}$ calc-p$_{mld3}$ *Caust*$_{qqh}$ mag-p$_{mld4}$
- **Nerves**:
  - **Femoral** nerve: arn$_{mld4}$ con$_{mld4}$ gels$_{mld4}$ plb$_{mld4}$
- **Upper** arms:
  - **Radial** side: cur$_{mld4}$ gels$_{mld4}$ plb$_{mld4}$ ruta$_{mld4}$

PERSPIRATION (see pg 1583)
- **Foot**:
  - **Ball**: calc$_{frc}$
- **Hand**:
  - **Ball**: calc$_{frc}$

PODOTROCHLEOSIS:

RUPTURE of ligaments:
- **Knees**:
  - **cruciate** ligaments: bry$_{brm}$ calc$_{brm}$ sep$_{brm}$ sulph$_{brm}$

SEPARATION of white line:
- **Hooves**; in:

SPAVIN: arn$_{mld4}$ calc$_{hnb}$ calc-f$_{mld4}$ con$_{ljyl}$ hecla$_{qqh}$ rhus-t$_{ljyl}$ sep$_{ljyl}$ sil$_{ljyl}$ sulph$_{ljyl}$

STIFFNESS:
- **morning** (see pg 1593): nat-m$_{brm}$
- **walking**:
  - **agg.**:
    - **fever**; during: pyrog$_{qqh}$
- **Lower** limbs (see pg 1596): *Calc*$_{ffd}$ *Caust*$_{ffd}$
  - **right** (see pg 1596): sulph$_{brm}$

SUPPURATION: aur$_{itm,qqh}$ bell$_{pkj,qqh}$ calc-f$_{mld5}$ calc-p$_{mld3}$ calc-s$_{qqh}$ hecla$_{itm}$ hep$_{itm,mld5,qqh}$ myris$_{pkj,qqh}$ pyrog$_{itm,qqh}$ sil$_{pkj,qqh}$ staph$_{qqh}$ symph$_{mld3}$

SWELLING:
- **Fingers**:
  - **Between**: thuj$_{dyc,elg}$
    - **accompanied** by:
      - **inflammation**: gink-b$_{dyc}$ hep$_{dyc}$
- **Hock**:
  - **subacute**: bry$_{elg}$ led$_{elg}$ ruta$_{elg}$ sil$_{elg}$
  - **suppurating**: arn$_{elg}$ hep$_{elg}$ lach$_{elg}$ pyrog$_{elg}$
- **Joints**:
  - **standing**; after: led$_{brm}$
- **Legs**:
  - **lymphatic** swelling:
    - **congenital**: berb$_{elg}$
    - **recurrent**: arn$_{elg}$ sulph$_{elg}$
- **Lower** limbs:
  - **injuries**; after:
    - **lymphatics**; of the: ser-ang$_{hnb}$
- **Muscles**; of: arn$_{itm}$ ruta$_{itm}$ symph$_{itm}$
- **Tendons**; of: arn$_{ljy,mld5}$ hyper$_{mld5}$ rhus-t$_{ljy,mld5}$ ruta$_{mld5}$
- **Toes**:
  - **Joints** (see pg 1603): led$_{brm}$

THIN:
- **Skin**:
  - **Feet**:
    - **Soles**: calc$_{brm}$

THROMBOSIS: arn_{qqh} both_{mld,mld5} calc-f_{mld4} crot-h_{mld5} lach_{mld,mld5} sec_{mld5} vip_{mld,mld5}

TOTTERING GAIT (see pg 1610)

TREMBLING:
- **Lower** limbs (see pg 1614): phos_{brm}

TWITCHING:
- **Feet** (see pg 1616): nat-m_{brm}

ULCERS:
- **Feet**:
  - **Claws**:
  - **Soles** (see pg 1620): sil_{dyc}
  - **Toes**:
    - **Between**: kali-bi_{hnb}

WALKING:
- **backwards**:
  - **impossible**; walking backward: phos_{fmx}
- **gressus** gallinaceous (see pg 1623): sep_{brm}
- **infirm** (see pg 1623): arg-n_{qqh} ign_{qqh}
- **tarsal** joint; on feet until: calc_{hnb} op_{brm}

WEAKNESS:
- **Lyme** disease; during: anac_{brm}
- **Legs**:
  - **accompanied** by:
    : **sexual** desire; diminished:
- **Lower** limbs:
  - **accompanied** by:
    : **sexual** desire:
      : **increased**: gels_{dyc} pic-ac_{dyc}
      : **wanting**: cann-i_{dyc} con_{dyc}
  - **rising**:
    : **sitting**; from:
      : **agg.** (see pg 1630): sulph_{brm}

Sleep

COLD PLACES:
- **desire** to sleep in cold places:
  - **pregnancy**; during imaginary: asaf_{brm}

FALLING ASLEEP:
- **standing** agg. (see pg 1647): nat-m_{brm}

NEED OF SLEEP:
- **great** (see pg 1648): calc_{frc,qqh}

POSITION:
- **back**; on (see pg 1648): *Lyc*_{ffd}
  - **impossible** (see pg 1648): sep_{brm}
- **face**; on the (see pg 1649): puls_{brm}
- **head**:
  - **covered** with sheet (see pg 1649): calc_{brm}
- **knees**:
  - **chest** position; knee (see pg 1649): **Med**_{frc}
- **leaning** on the walls: sulph_{brm}
- **limbs**, lower:
  - **stretched** out (see pg 1649): aur_{brm}
- **side**; on:
  - **left** side; on (see pg 1649): lyc_{brm}

SLEEP – Position – side; on: ...
- **right** side; on:
  : **impossible** (see pg 1649): *Borx*_{hnb}
- **sink**; sleeping in the: sulph_{brm}
- **sitting**:
  - **riding** in a car; when: arn_{brm}

SLEEPINESS (see pg 1652): **Lach**_{frc,qqh}
- **daytime** (see pg 1652): apis_{brm}
- **morning** (see pg 1652): lyc_{ffd}
- **fever**:
  - **during**:
    : **agg.** (see pg 1656): echi_{qqh} gels_{qqh}
- **vaccination**; after: thuj_{brm}
- **vomiting**:
  - **after** (see pg 1658)

SLEEPLESSNESS (see pg 1658): **Nux-v**_{qqh}
- **night**:
  - **midnight**:
    : **after**:
      : **3** h (see pg 1660)
  - **walking** around: thuj_{brm}
- **hunger**; from (see pg 1663): *Cina*_{fmx}
- **warmth**, from (see pg 1667)
  - **bed**; of:

UNREFRESHING:
- **morning** (see pg 1667): arn_{brm} sil_{brm}

WAKING:
- **morning**:
  - **6** h (see pg 1668): nat-m_{brm}
- **evening**:
  - **falling** asleep, soon after (see pg 1668): lach_{frc,qqh}
- **difficult**:
  - **morning** (see pg 1669): lyc_{brm} sil_{brm}

YAWNING:
- **sleepiness**:
  - **during** (see pg 1674): ign_{frc,qqh}

Dreams

ACTIVE:
- **movements** during sleep; strong:

EVENTS:
- **previous**:
  - **day**, of the previous (see pg 1683)

WHIMPERING, whining:
- **sleep**; during: sulph_{brm}

Chill

AIR; DRAFT OF:
- **slightest** (see pg 1703)

CHILLINESS:

- **menses**:
  - **before**:
    - **agg.** (see pg 1705)

COLD:
- **agg.**:
  - **day** in the summer; on a (see pg 1706)

EXPOSURE, after (see pg 1707)
- **wet**:
  - **becoming**; from (see pg 1707): **Rhus-t**$_{fmx}$ sil$_{fmx}$

Fever

NOON (see pg 1717): ign$_{qqh}$

AFTERNOON (see pg 1718): *Lyc*$_{fmx}$

NIGHT (see pg 1718): ferr-p$_{qqh}$
- **midnight**:
  - **after** (see pg 1719): rhus-t$_{qqh}$

AIR; IN OPEN:
- **amel.** (see pg 1719): apis$_{qqh}$ puls$_{qqh}$

CHILL; with (see pg 1722): arn$_{qqh}$ **Calc**$_{qqh}$ calc-p$_{qqh}$ calc-s$_{qqh}$ dulc$_{qqh}$ eup-per$_{qqh}$ **Ign**$_{qqh}$ **Merc**$_{qqh}$ nat-m$_{qqh}$ **Nux-v**$_{qqh}$ phos$_{qqh}$ *Puls*$_{qqh}$ sil$_{qqh}$ **Sulph**$_{qqh}$

COLD:
- **air** agg.: bell$_{qqh}$ caps$_{qqh}$ nux-v$_{qqh}$ rhus-t$_{qqh}$
- **bathing**:
  - **amel.**: apis$_{qqh}$

DARKNESS agg. : stram$_{qqh}$

DRINKING:
- **cold** water:
  - **agg.**: rhus-t$_{qqh}$

DRY heat:
- **alternating** with:
  - **perspiration** (see pg 1724): apis$_{qqh}$

EATING:
- **after**:
  - **agg.** (see pg 1724): caps$_{qqh}$

HEAT:
- **radiating** (see pg 1725): bell$_{qqh}$
  - **not** radiating: acon$_{qqh}$ caps$_{qqh}$ eup-per$_{qqh}$

INTERMITTENT (see pg 1726): *Puls*$_{qqh}$

MOTION:
- **agg.** (see pg 1727): caps$_{qqh}$ verat-v$_{qqh}$
- **amel.** (see pg 1727): ars$_{qqh}$
- **must** move: rhus-t$_{qqh}$

PAROXYSMAL fever (see pg 1727): acon$_{qqh}$ ail$_{qqh}$ ars$_{qqh}$ bell$_{qqh}$

PERSPIRATION:
- **amel.** (see pg 1728): bry$_{qqh}$
- **heat**; with (see pg 1728): ars$_{qqh}$ *Bell*$_{qqh}$ **Caps**$_{qqh}$ Merc$_{qqh}$ **Sulph**$_{qqh}$

FEVER: ...

PUERPERAL FEVER (see pg 1728): *Acon*$_{ljy,mld,plr1}$ bell$_{ljy,mld,plr1}$ bov$_{bnf1.es}$ carb-ac$_{bnf1.es}$ cham$_{ljy,plr1}$ **Crot-h**$_{mld5}$ **Echi**$_{ljy,mld,mld5}$ **Lach**$_{bnf1.es,frc,ljy,mld,mld5}$ nux-v$_{plr1}$ sabin$_{mld1}$
- **lochia**; from suppressed (see pg 1728): sabin$_{brm}$

SEPTIC FEVER (see pg 1729)

SLEEP, heat comes on:
- **during** (see pg 1729): bell$_{qqh}$

SUCCESSION of stages:
- **chill**:
  - **followed** by:
    - **heat** (see pg 1730): Acon$_{qqh}$ ars$_{qqh}$

TYPHOID FEVER:
- **accompanied** by:
  - **urination**:
    - **involuntary**: gels$_{pkj1}$

WARM:
- **room**:
  - **intolerable**; heat of the room is (see pg 1732): **Apis**$_{qqh}$

WEATHER:
- **wet**:
  - **agg.**: dulc$_{qqh}$

Perspiration

RIGHT side:

LEFT side:

MORNING:
- **waking**:
  - **after**:
    - **agg.**: thuj$_{qqh}$

NIGHT:
- **fever**; during: calc$_{qqh}$ calc-p$_{qqh}$

COLD:
- **night**:
  - **fever**; during: calc-p$_{qqh}$
- **fever**; during: verat$_{qqh}$

COVERED parts:
- **fever**; during: acon$_{qqh}$

ESTRUS:
- **before**: verat$_{qqh}$
- **during**: verat$_{qqh}$

HOT:
- **fever**; during: verat-v$_{qqh}$

ILLNESS; in case of:

INTERMITTENT: bell$_{qqh}$

LONG-LASTING: nux-v$_{brm}$
- **perspiration**; cold: led$_{brm}$
- **strain**; after:

ODOR:
- **offensive:** calc-s$_{qqh}$
  - **bathing** in summer; after: nux-v$_{brm}$ sulph$_{brm}$
- **sour:** Arn$_{qqh}$ calc$_{qqh}$ **Lyc**$_{brm}$ Sil$_{qqh}$ **Sulph**$_{qqh}$ **Verat**$_{qqh}$

PAINFUL parts: kali-c$_{qqh}$

PAINS:
- **from:**

SCANTY SWEAT: acon$_{qqh}$ caust$_{qqh}$ nat-m$_{qqh}$ staph$_{qqh}$

SINGLE parts: **Puls**$_{qqh}$

STICKY: nux-v$_{brm}$

WALKING:
- **agg.:** verat$_{qqh}$

Skin

ACTINOMYCOSIS (see pg 1747)
- **accompanied** by:
  - **Mammae;** inflammation of:

ALLERGY:
- **fleas;** to:

CICATRICES (see pg 1748)

COMPLAINTS of skin:
- **castration;** after:
  - **men;** in:
  - **women;** in:
- **ovariectomy;** after:

CRACKS:
- **winter** agg. (see pg 1750): calc-p$_{brm}$

DIRTY (see pg 1751)

DISCOLORATION:
- **blackish** (see pg 1751): nat-m$_{brm}$
  - **scratching;** from:
- **red:**
  - **bright** red:
  - **dark** red (see pg 1752): merc$_{klp}$ syph$_{klp}$
- **yellow** (see pg 1753)

DRY:
- **fever;** during (see pg 1754): acon$_{qqh}$ sulph$_{qqh}$

ECCHYMOSES:
- **fever;** during: lach$_{qqh}$

ERUPTIONS:
- **boils:**
  - **periodical** (see pg 1756): calc$_{brm}$ **Sulph**$_{brm}$
- **corticosteroids;** after use of: nat-m$_{elg}$
- **crusty** (see pg 1757): **Lyc**$_{fmx}$ **Rhus-t**$_{fmx}$
- **demodicidosis:** chin$_{brm}$ sulph$_{elg}$
  - **spots;** in single: puls$_{brm}$ sulph$_{brm}$
- **dermatomycosis:** bac$_{dyc}$ graph$_{dyc}$ maland$_{dyc}$ rhus-t$_{dyc}$ sulph$_{dyc}$
- **discharging** (see pg 1758): **Rhus-t**$_{fmx}$
- **dry** (see pg 1758): **Sil**$_{fmx}$
- **ecthyma:**
  - **contagious:** thuj$_{dyc}$

SKIN – Eruptions: ...
- **ectoparasitism:**
  - **fleas:**
- **eczema:**
  - **licking;** from: merc$_{klp}$
- **fleabites:** led$_{hnb,klp}$ staph$_{klp}$
- **granuloma;** eosinophilic: canth$_{elg}$ fl-ac$_{klp}$ nat-m$_{elg}$ nit-ac$_{klp}$ phos$_{brm,hnb}$ sil$_{klp}$
  - **linear** granuloma:
  - **plaque;** eosinophilic:
  - **ulcer;** eosinophilic: caps$_{hnb}$
  - **vaccination;** after: phos$_{hnb}$
- **herpetic:**
  - **circinate** (see pg 1760): lach$_{brm}$ **NAT-M**$_{ffd}$ sulph$_{fmx}$
- **homesickness;** from: ign$_{hnb}$
- **hot spot:** calc$_{ffd}$ lyc$_{ffd}$ phos$_{brm}$
- **lice;** from: thuj$_{elg}$
- **miliary** (see pg 1763): bac$_{klp}$ ign$_{klp}$ nat-m$_{klp}$
- **offensive** (see pg 1763): lyc$_{fmx}$ sulph$_{fmx}$
- **pemphigus** (see pg 1763): **Lyc**$_{brm}$ **Rhus-t**$_{fmx}$
- **petechiae:**
  - **fever;** during: lach$_{qqh}$
- **protein** food; from too much:
- **pustules:**
  - **contagious:**
- **rhus** poisoning (see pg 1766): rhus-t$_{fmx}$
- **ringworm:**
  - **left:**
    - **then** right: bac$_{elg}$ lach$_{elg}$
- **summer** (see pg 1768): anac$_{brm}$ calc-p$_{brm}$ cic$_{brm}$ lyc$_{brm}$ nat-m$_{brm}$ phos$_{brm}$ puls$_{elg,stan}$ sulph$_{brm}$
  - **sweat** itch: puls$_{elg}$ sep$_{elg}$
- **urticaria** (see pg 1769)
  - **fever:**
    - **during:**
      - **agg.** (see pg 1770): **Ign**$_{qqh}$
  - **food;** from: calc-p$_{brm}$ lyc$_{brm}$ med$_{brm}$
  - **milk** agg.: sep$_{brm}$
  - **soap;** from:
  - **warmth** and exercise (see pg 1771): anac$_{brm}$ calc-p$_{brm}$ cic$_{brm}$
- **winter:**
- **young** animals; in:
  - **females:**

ERYSIPELAS (see pg 1772): **Lach**$_{dyc}$ sec$_{dyc}$

EXCRESCENCES:
- **sarcoid** excrescences: ars$_{ags}$ aur$_{brm}$ calc$_{elg}$ caust$_{brm}$ lyc$_{dyc}$ nit-ac$_{dyc}$ nux-v$_{brm}$ sabin$_{dyc}$ sulph$_{brm}$ thuj$_{brm,dyc}$ tub$_{dyc}$
  - **sarcoid;** equine:

FEATHERS:
- **falling:**

FRECKLES (see pg 1774)

HAIR:
- **baldness:**
  - **castration;** after:
    - **hormonal** causes; from: lyc$_{brm}$ sulph$_{brm}$ tarent$_{brm}$

- **baldness – castration**; after: ...
  - **men**; in: lyc$_{brm}$ sulph$_{brm}$
  - **women**; in: tarent$_{brm}$
  - **generalized**:
  - **ovariectomy**; after:
  - **patches**:
    - **asymmetrical**:
      - **trichophytosis**: ars$_{dyc}$ bac$_{dyc}$ sep$_{dyc}$ tell$_{dyc}$ tub$_{dyc}$
    - **symmetrical**: syph$_{klp}$
- **brittle**:
- **broken**:
- **falling** out (see pg 1775): apis$_{brm}$ sep$_{brm}$ sulph$_{brm}$ thuj$_{klp}$
  - **excitement** agg. : sulph$_{brm}$
  - **hormonal** causes; from:
    - **Gonades**:
      - **Ovaries**:
      - **Testes**: lyc$_{brm}$
    - **Pararenal** glands:
    - **Thyroid** gland:
  - **indigestion**; after:
    - **accompanied** by:
      - **flatulence**; severe: lyc$_{hnb}$
  - **intoxication**; after:
  - **ovarian** dysfunction; from: lyc$_{brm}$ phos$_{brm}$
  - **scratching**:
    - **with** scratching:
    - **without** scratching:
- **molting** abnormalities: sulph$_{hnb,klp}$
  - **autumn**; in:
  - **constant**:
  - **incomplete**:
  - **long**; takes too:
  - **spring**; in:
- **shaggy**: calc-f$_{klp}$ calc-p$_{brm}$ fl-ac$_{klp}$ sulph$_{brm}$
- **tangles** easily: sep$_{brm}$

HEAT:
- **fever**; with (see pg 1775): sulph$_{qqh}$
- **fever**; without (see pg 1775): puls$_{frc,qqh}$

INDURATIONS, nodules, etc. (see pg 1776): **Calc**$_{brm}$ nux-v$_{brm}$
- **vaccination**; after: lyc$_{brm}$

INFLAMMATION:
- **Sebaceous** glands: lyc$_{brm}$

ITCHING (see pg 1776): **Tarent**$_{brm}$
- **night** (see pg 1777): lyc$_{brm}$ sep$_{brm}$
- **violent** (see pg 1779): mez$_{brm}$

OLD; becomes old:
- **prematurely**:

PURPURA:
- **fever**; during: lach$_{qqh}$

SENSITIVENESS:
- **light**; to:
  - **ultraviolet**: hyper$_{dyc}$

STINGS of insects (see pg 1783): anac$_{brm}$ *Apis*$_{fmx}$ *Lach*$_{fmx}$

SKIN: ...

TENSION (see pg 1784): med$_{brm}$

THICK:
- **scratching**; skin becomes thick after (see pg 1784): fl-ac$_{klp}$ graph$_{klp}$ maland$_{klp}$ sil$_{klp}$ thiosin$_{klp}$

UNHEALTHY (see pg 1789)

Generals

DAYTIME:
- **amel**. (see pg 1794)

MORNING:
- **6 h** (see pg 1794)
- **7 h** (see pg 1794)
- **8 h** (see pg 1794)
- **afternoon**; and:
- **evening**; and (see pg 1794)
- **night**; and:
- **amel**. (see pg 1794)
- **one** day and the afternoon of the next; morning of (see pg 1794)
- **sunrise**:
  - **after** (see pg 1794)
  - **before**:
- **waking**; on (see pg 1794)

FORENOON (see pg 1794)

NOON:
- **12-0 h** (see pg 1794)
- **increasing** till noon, then decreasing; symptoms (see pg 1794)

AFTERNOON (see pg 1794)

EVENING:
- **18 h** (see pg 1795)
- **19 h** (see pg 1795)
- **20 h** (see pg 1795)
- **21 h** (see pg 1795)
  - **21-5 h** (see pg 1795): merc$_{frc}$
  - **amel**. (see pg 1795)
- **air** agg.; in open (see pg 1795)
- **amel**. (see pg 1795)
- **every** other evening (see pg 1796)
- **sunset**:
  - **after** (see pg 1796)
  - **sunrise**; until (see pg 1796)
- **twilight**; in the:
  - **agg**. (see pg 1796)
  - **amel**. (see pg 1796)

NIGHT:
- **midnight**:
  - **before** (see pg 1796)
    - **23 h** (see pg 1796): acon$_{qqh}$

- midnight: ...
- · **after**:
  - : **0-1 h** (see pg 1796)
  - : **0-2 h** (see pg 1796)
  - : **0-4 h** (see pg 1796)
  - : **1 h** (see pg 1796)
  - : **2 h** (see pg 1796)
  - : **3 h** (see pg 1796)
  - : **4 h** (see pg 1797)
  - : **5 h** (see pg 1797)
  - : **amel.** (see pg 1797)
- **air** agg.; night (see pg 1797)
- **amel.** (see pg 1797)
- **periodical**:
  - · **alternate** nights; on (see pg 1797)

ABSCESSES (see pg 1797): tub$_{dyc}$
- **painful** (see pg 1797): hep$_{fmx}$ sulph$_{fmx}$
- **painless**: sil$_{brm}$

ACETONEMIA (see pg 1798): aceton$_{itm}$ calc$_{elg}$ lyc$_{bnfl.es,itm}$ phos$_{elg}$ *Senn* $_{bnfl.es,itm}$
- **delivery**; before: lyc$_{elg}$

ACRIDITY, excoriations, etc. (see pg 1798)

AGILITY (see pg 1799): lyc$_{frc}$

AGRANULOCYTOSIS (see pg 1799)

AILMENTS from:
- **castration**:
- **mother's** milk in nurslings; lack of: chin$_{brm}$ lac-c$_{hnb}$
- **weaned** too early; being: bar-c$_{klp}$ calc$_{klp}$ carc$_{klp}$ lac-c$_{hnb}$ puls$_{klp}$ sil$_{klp}$ syph$_{klp}$
- **Teeth**; the destruction of the:

AIR:
- **indoor** air:
  - · **agg.** (see pg 1799)
  - · **amel.** (see pg 1799)

AIR; DRAFT OF:
- **agg.** (see pg 1799)
- **amel.** (see pg 1799)
- **cold** draft of air:
  - · **agg.**:
    - : **perspiration**; during (see pg 1799)
- **warm** draft of air:
  - · **agg.** (see pg 1799)

AIR; IN OPEN:
- **agg.** (see pg 1799)
- **amel.** (see pg 1799): crat$_{qqh}$
- **exertion** in open air amel. (see pg 1800)

AIR; OPEN:
- **aversion** to open air (see pg 1800)
  - · **alternating** with desire for (see pg 1800)
- **desire** for open air:
  - · **but** draft agg. (see pg 1800)

ALLERGIC constitution (see pg 1800): bac$_{klp}$ calc$_{klp}$ carc$_{klp}$ lyc$_{klp}$ med$_{brm}$ merc$_{klp}$ nat-m$_{klp}$ phos$_{klp}$ psor$_{klp}$ thyr$_{klp}$ tub$_{klp}$
- **atopy**: thuj$_{brm}$

Allergic constitution: ...
- **fleas**; to:
- **flies**; to: bac$_{klp}$ calc$_{klp}$ lyc$_{klp}$ phos$_{klp}$ tub$_{klp}$
- **grass** pollen; to: nat-m$_{klp}$

ALUMINIUM poisoning (see pg 1801)

AMYOTROPHIC LATERAL SCLEROSIS (see pg 1801): bar-c$_{frc}$ plb$_{frc}$

ANALGESIA (see pg 1801): nat-m$_{brm}$
- **Affected** parts (see pg 1801)
- **Inner** parts (see pg 1801)

ANEMIA:
- **disease**; from exhausting (see pg 1801)
- **hemorrhage**; after (see pg 1802)
- **menorrhagia**, from (see pg 1802)
- **nursing** mothers (see pg 1802)
- **nutritional** imbalance; from (see pg 1802)
- **pernicious** (see pg 1802)

ANESTHESIA [=insensibility] :
- **right** side, of (see pg 1802)
- **Affected** parts, of (see pg 1802)

ANTHELMINTIC poison; complaints from: nux-v$_{elg}$ op$_{elg}$

ANXIETY, general physical (see pg 1802)

APOPLEXY:
- **threatened** (see pg 1803)

ARSENICAL poisoning (see pg 1803)

ARTERIOSCLEROSIS (see pg 1803)

ASCENDING:
- **agg.** (see pg 1803)
- **amel.** (see pg 1803)

ATROPHY:
- **Glands** (see pg 1803)
- **Muscles**; of (see pg 1803): abrot$_{mld4}$ acet-ac$_{mld4}$ arn$_{mld4}$ cur$_{mld4}$ lath$_{mld4}$ plb$_{mld4}$ thal$_{mld4}$

BATHING:
- **agg.** (see pg 1804)
- **amel.** (see pg 1804)
- **aversion** to bathing (see pg 1804)
  - · **legs** in the water; goes only with: phos$_{hnb}$
- **desire** for (see pg 1804)
- **lukewarm** bathing:
  - · **agg.** (see pg 1804)
- **sea**; bathing in the:
  - · **agg.** (see pg 1804)
  - · **amel.** (see pg 1804)
- **Affected** part; bathing the:
  - · **amel.** (see pg 1804)
- **Feet**; bathing:
  - · **cold** water; in:
    - : **amel.** (see pg 1804)
  - · **warm** water; in:

BENDING, turning:

BENT; holding the part:

BINDING UP, bandaging amel. (see pg 1805)

BITING:
- teeth together; biting:

BLACKNESS of external parts (see pg 1805)

BLOOD:
- **complaints** of the (see pg 1979)

BREATHING:

BRITTLE BONES (see pg 1806)

BROMIDES, abuse of (see pg 1806)

BRUSHING TEETH:

BURNS (see pg 1806)

BUTTERCUPS; intoxication by:

CACHEXIA (see pg 1806): phos$_{fmx}$

CANCEROUS affections:
- **cachectic** emaciation; with (see pg 1807)
- **cicatrices**, in old (see pg 1807)
- **contusions**, after (see pg 1807)
- **epithelioma** (see pg 1807)
- **lupus**; carcinomatous (see pg 1807)
- **melanoma** (see pg 1807)
- **sarcoma** (see pg 1807)
- **ulcers**:
  - **Glands** (see pg 1807)
- **Bones**, of (see pg 1807)
- **Glands** (see pg 1807)

CARIES:
- **Bone**, of (see pg 1808)
- **Periosteum**, of (see pg 1808)

CARTILAGES, affection of (see pg 1808)

CATALEPSY:
- **anger**; after (see pg 1808)
- **fright**; after (see pg 1808)
- **grief**; from (see pg 1808)
- **jealousy**; from (see pg 1808)
- **love**; from disappointed (see pg 1808)
- **sexual**:
  - **excitement** agg. (see pg 1808)
- **sexual** excesses; after:
- **worm** complaints; in (see pg 1808)

CAUTERY with argentum nitricum; antidote to (see pg 1808)

CHANGE:
- **position**:
  - **agg.** (see pg 1808)
  - **amel.** (see pg 1809)
  - **desire** for change of (see pg 1809)
- **symptoms**; change of:
  - **rapid** (see pg 1809)

CHEYNE-STOKES respiration (see pg 1809)

CHILDREN; complaints in:
- **delicate**, puny, sickly (see pg 1809)

CHILL, feels better before (see pg 1809)

CHLOROFORM; ailments from (see pg 1809)

CHLOROSIS (see pg 1809)

CHOREA (see pg 1810)

CHRONIC DISEASES, to begin treatment (see pg 1811)

CHRONICITY:

CIRCULATION; complaints of the blood:
- **fever**; during: verat-v$_{qqh}$

CLOTHING:
- **intolerance** of:
  - **woolen** (see pg 1811)

COAL GAS, from (see pg 1812)

COITION:
- **after** (see pg 1812)
  - **agg.** (see pg 1812)
  - **amel.** (see pg 1812): calc$_{klp}$ hep$_{klp}$ puls$_{klp}$
- **during**:
  - **agg.** (see pg 1812)
- **interrupted** coition agg. (see pg 1812)

COLD:
- **air**:
  - **desire** for:
    : **fever**; during: verat$_{qqh}$
- **bathing**:
  - **agg.** (see pg 1813)
  - **amel.** (see pg 1813)
  - **desire** for cold bathing (see pg 1813)

COLD; BECOMING:
- **agg.**:
  - **overheating**; after (see pg 1814): calc$_{frc}$ dulc$_{frc}$ rhus-t$_{frc}$
  - **perspiration**; during (see pg 1814): rhus-t$_{frc}$

COLD; TAKING A:
- **tendency** (see pg 1814): **Lyc**$_{brm}$ *Puls*$_{brm}$ **Sil**$_{brm}$

COLDNESS of affected parts (see pg 1815)

COLLAPSE:
- **diarrhea** agg.; after (see pg 1815)
- **needle**; from prick of a (see pg 1815)
- **paralysis**, at beginning of general (see pg 1815)
- **sudden** (see pg 1815)
- **vomiting**:
  - **after** (see pg 1815)
  - **during** (see pg 1815)

COMBING hair:
- **aversion** to comb hair: sep$_{brm}$ sulph$_{brm}$

COMPLEXION:
- **black**:
  - **completely**: stram$_{brm}$
  - **hair**:
    : **brown**; black hair turns: lyc$_{brm}$
- **red** hair (see pg 1817): lyc$_{a,brm}$

CONGESTION:

CONNECTIVE TISSUE; affections of (see pg 1817)

CONSTIPATION:

CONSTRICTION (see pg 1817)

CONTRACTIONS (see pg 1818)

CONTRADICTORY and alternating states (see pg 1818)

CONVALESCENCE; ailments during (see pg 1818)
- **castration**; after:
- **chemotherapy**; after (see pg 1819): op$_{brm}$
- **cortisone**; after use of: crat$_{hnb}$
- **piroplasmosis**: calc-p$_{brm}$
- **puberty**; after (see pg 1819)

CONVULSIONS (see pg 1819)
- **consciousness**:
  - **without** (see pg 1821)
- **epileptic** (see pg 1822): **Sulph**$_{brm}$
- **errors** in diet (see pg 1825): lyc$_{brm}$
- **heat**; during (see pg 1825): *Bell*$_{qqh}$ bry$_{qqh}$ calc$_{qqh}$ mur-ac$_{qqh}$ verat-v$_{qqh}$
- **injuries**; after:
  - **Head**, of the (see pg 1825): **Arn**$_{klp}$ nat-m$_{brm}$ *Nat-s*$_{klp}$ syph$_{klp}$
- **pregnancy** agg.; during (see pg 1826): *Acon*$_{mld3}$ *Bell*$_{bnfl.es,mld,mld5}$ calc$_{bnfl.es,qqh}$ calc-p$_{mld,mld5}$ *Cic*$_{bnfl.es}$ *Cupr*$_{bnfl.es}$ *Hyos*$_{mld3}$ lac-c$_{bnfl.es}$ *Oena*$_{bnfl.es}$ stram$_{mld3}$
- **sexual**:
  - **excitement** (see pg 1827): *Bufo*$_{bnfl.es}$
- **vaccination**; after (see pg 1828): **Sil**$_{brm}$

COPPER:
- **fumes** agg. (see pg 1828)
- **vessels** of copper agg. (see pg 1828)

CORYZA:

COVERS:
- **agg.** (see pg 1828)
- **amel.**:
  - **desire** for; and (see pg 1828): psor$_{dyc}$
- **aversion** to (see pg 1829)
- **kicks** off (see pg 1829)

CRACKLINGS, like tinsel (see pg 1829)

CROSSING A BRIDGE agg. :
- **narrow** bridge; a (see pg 1829)
- **running** water; over:

CROSSING OF LIMBS:

CYANOSIS (see pg 1829)

DARKNESS:

DEATH APPARENT (see pg 1829)

DEGENERATION OF TISSUES, tendency to (see pg 1829)

DERMATITIS PUSTULOSA CONTAGIOSA: nit-ac$_{dyc}$ thuj$_{dyc}$

DESCENDING:

DEVELOPMENT:

DIABETES MELLITUS (see pg 1830): acet-ac$_{mld,qqh}$ iris$_{mld5}$ *Lac-ac*$_{qqh}$ **Nat-s**$_{bnfl.es,mld5}$ ph-ac$_{mld,pkj1}$ **Syzyg**$_{bnfl.es,dyc,mld5,pkj,qqh}$ *Uran-n*$_{bnfl.es,dyc,mld,mld5,pkj,qqh}$

DIARRHEA:
- **amel.** (see pg 1831)

DISCHARGES:
- **bloody**:
  - **fever**; during: ail$_{qqh}$ anthraci$_{qqh}$
- **offensive**, fetid:
  - **fever**; during: ail$_{qqh}$ bapt$_{qqh}$ echi$_{qqh}$ pyrog$_{qqh}$

DOUBLING UP of the body (see pg 1833)

DRAWING UP the limb, flexing:

DRINKING:
- **after**:
  - **agg.** (see pg 1833)
  - **amel.** (see pg 1833)
- **agg.** (see pg 1833)
  - **rapidly** (see pg 1833)
- **amel.** (see pg 1833)
- **aversion** to drink in spite of thirst (see pg 1833)

DROPSY:
- **external** dropsy (see pg 1833)

DRYNESS of usually moist internal parts (see pg 1835)

DWARFISHNESS (see pg 1835)

DYSTROPHY:
- **Bones**; of: ars$_{mld3}$ calc$_{mld3}$ calc-f$_{mld,mld4}$ calc-p$_{mld,mld4}$ iod$_{mld3}$ phos$_{mld,mld4}$
- **Muscles**; of (see pg 1835): calc$_{mld3}$ cur$_{mld3}$ sel$_{mld3}$ sil$_{pkj1}$

EATING:
- **after**:
  - **agg.** (see pg 1835)
  - **long** time after; a (see pg 1835)
  - **amel.** (see pg 1835)
- **before**:
  - **agg.** (see pg 1836)
- **food** in the stomach:
  - **amel.** (see pg 1836)
- **overeating** agg.; after (see pg 1836)
- **satiety**; after eating to:
  - **amel.** (see pg 1836)
- **small** quantities:
  - **amel.** (see pg 1836)
- **untidily**: calc$_{brm}$ sulph$_{brm}$
- **while**:
  - **agg.** (see pg 1836)

EFFICIENCY:

ELECTRICITY of the atmosphere; ailments from (see pg 1836)

ELECTROSHOCK; ailments from (see pg 1836)

ELEPHANTIASIS (see pg 1836)

EMACIATION (see pg 1836): *Calc-p* $_{brm}$ **Iod** $_{dyc}$
Nat-m $_{dyc}$ **Phos** $_{dyc}$
- **appetite** with emaciation; ravenous (see pg 1837):
  Nat-m $_{klp}$ *Phos* $_{brm}$ *Sulph* $_{brm}$
- **grief**; after (see pg 1837): nux-v $_{brm}$

EMISSIONS SEMINAL:

ENERGY:
- **excess** of energy (see pg 1838): ars $_{dyc1}$ *Coff* $_{dyc1}$
  ign $_{dyc1}$ med $_{frc}$ nux-v $_{frc}$ phos $_{frc}$ tub $_{frc}$

EUTHANASIA; to induce (see pg 1838): ars $_{brm}$
carb-v $_{brm}$ phos $_{brm}$ pyrog $_{brm}$ sec $_{brm}$ tarent $_{brm}$

EXERTION; physical:

EXOSTOSIS (see pg 1839)

FAINTNESS:
- **excitement** agg. (see pg 1841): tab $_{brm}$
- **music**, on hearing (see pg 1842)
- **pregnancy** agg.; during (see pg 1842): *Nux-v* $_{qqh}$
- **tendency** to (see pg 1843): nux-v $_{frc}$
- **vomiting**:
  · **after** (see pg 1843): tab $_{brm}$

FANNED; being:
- **amel**. (see pg 1844)

FASTING:
- **agg**. (see pg 1844): nat-m $_{brm}$
- **amel**. (see pg 1844)

FATTY DEGENERATION (see pg 1844)

FEATHER BED agg. (see pg 1844)

FELINE IMMUNE DEFICIENCY VIRUS: calen $_{fmx}$
cham $_{fmx}$ hep $_{fmx}$ kali-c $_{fmx}$ lach $_{fmx}$ nux-v $_{fmx}$ sulph $_{fmx}$

FEVER:

FISTULAE (see pg 1845)
- **accompanied** by:
  · **ulcers**: sil $_{brm}$

FLATUS; PASSING:
- **agg**. (see pg 1845)
- **amel**. (see pg 1845)

FOOD and DRINKS:
- **almonds**:
  · **desire** (see pg 1846)
- **anchovies**:
  · **desire** (see pg 1846)
- **apples** (see pg 1846)
  · **desire** (see pg 1846): puls $_{brm}$
- **bacon**:
- **bananas**:
- **beef**:
- **biscuits**:
- **bitter** drinks:
- **bitter** food:
  · **desire** (see pg 1847): lac-c $_{brm}$

Food and drinks: ...
- **bones**:
  · **agg**.:
  · **amel**.:
  · **desire**:
- **bread**:
- **broth**:
- **buckwheat**:
  · **agg**. (see pg 1848)
- **buffalo**-skin bones:
  · **aversion**: sep $_{brm}$
- **butter**:
  · **desire** (see pg 1848): lyc $_{brm}$
- **canned** food:
  · **agg**.:
- **canned** fruit:
  · **agg**. (see pg 1848): lyc $_{brm}$:
- **carrots**:
  · **aversion**: coloc $_{brm}$
- **cereals**:
  · **aversion** (see pg 1848)
- **cheese**:
  · **aversion** (see pg 1848): calc-p $_{brm}$ puls $_{brm}$
  · **desire** (see pg 1848): verat $_{frc}$
- **chicken**:
- **chocolate**:
  · **desire**:
    ⋮ **white** chocolate: carc $_{brm}$
- **cloth** of cotton or wool:
  · **desire**:
- **cold** drink, cold water:
- **cold** food:
- **concentrates**:
  · **agg**.:
- **cooked** food:
- **corn**:
  · **desire**: bell $_{brm}$
- **delicacies**:
- **diet**:
  · **agg**.:
    ⋮ **errors** in diet (see pg 1851): lyc $_{brm}$
- **drinks**:
- **dry** commercial food:
  · **agg**.:
- **dry** food:
- **eggs**:
  · **desire** (see pg 1851): sulph $_{frc}$
- **everything**:
  · **desire** (see pg 1851): sulph $_{brm}$
- **farinaceous**:
  · **agg**. (see pg 1851): **Puls** $_{brm}$
  · **aversion** (see pg 1851): lyc $_{brm}$
- **fat**:
  · **desire** (see pg 1852): ant-c $_{frc}$
- **feces**:
  · **desire**:
- **fish**:
  · **aversion** (see pg 1852): *Colch* $_{fmx}$

- **food:**
  - **agg.:**
    - **smell** of (see pg 1852)
  - **aversion:**
    - **commercial** food:
      - **canned** meal:
      - **concentrates:**
      - **dry** meal:
      - **silage,** ensiled feed:
    - **eating:**
      - **sudden;** while eating (see pg 1853): sil_{frc}
    - **smell** of (see pg 1853)
  - **desire:**
    - **commercial** food:
      - **canned** meal:
      - **concentrates:**
      - **silage,** ensiled feed:
- **fried** food:
- **frozen:**
- **fruit:**
  - **aversion** (see pg 1853): $Puls_{brm}$
- **garbage:**
  - **desire:** $phos_{brm}$
- **garlic:**
  - **agg.** (see pg 1853): $calc_{brm}$
- **grapes:**
- **grass:**
  - **desire:** lyc_{brm} $mag-c_{brm}$ $phos_{brm}$ $puls_{brm}$ sep_{brm}
    - **broad** leafed: $tritic_{sxj}$
    - **vomit;** so it can: $tritic_{sxj}$
- **ham:**
- **hard** things:
  - **aversion:** tab_{brm}
- **hearty** food:
  - **desire** (see pg 1854)
- **heavy** food:
  - **agg.** (see pg 1854): $carb-v_{qqh}$ $nux-v_{frc}$
- **honey:**
- **ice:**
- **ice** cream:
- **indigestible** things:
  - **desire** (see pg 1854): $Calc_{brm,klp}$ $Calc-p_{klp}$ lyc_{klp} $puls_{klp}$
- **juicy** things:
- **kiwi:**
  - **desire:** $coloc_{brm}$
- **lard:**
  - **desire** (see pg 1854)
- **leek:**
  - **agg.:** $calc_{brm}$
- **lemonade:**
- **lemons:**
- **lime** [=derived from limestone]:
  - **desire** (see pg 1854): sil_{frc}
- **liquid** food:
- **liver:**
  - **desire** (see pg 1855): $nat-m_{brm}$

- **many** things:
  - **desire** (see pg 1855)
- **marinade:**
  - **desire** (see pg 1855)
- **meat:**
  - **agg.:**
    - **raw:** tab_{brm}
  - **aversion** (see pg 1855): $Kali-c_{frc}$ $Merc_{frc}$ $Nux-v_{frc}$
  - **desire** (see pg 1855): $Calc-p_{brm}$ sil_{frc}
    - **must** have (see pg 1855): $merc_{brm}$
- **melons:**
- **milk:**
  - **aversion** (see pg 1856): $bell_{brm}$
    - **mother's** milk (see pg 1856): $aeth_{qqh}$
      - **child** refuses (see pg 1856)
- **mustard:**
- **mutton:**
  - **aversion** (see pg 1856): $sulph_{brm}$
- **nuts:**
  - **desire** (see pg 1856): $sulph_{brm}$
- **onions:**
- **oranges:**
- **pasta:**
  - **aversion:** lyc_{brm}
  - **desire** (see pg 1857)
- **pastry:**
- **pears:**
- **pickles:**
- **pork:**
- **potatoes:**
- **poultry:**
  - **agg.** (see pg 1857)
- **pungent** things:
- **raw** food:
- **refreshing** things:
  - **desire** (see pg 1858): $sulph_{frc}$
- **rice:**
  - **aversion:** $calc-p_{brm}$
- **rich** food:
- **saffron:**
  - **desire:** $bell_{brm}$
- **salad:**
- **salt:**
  - **aversion** (see pg 1858): lyc_{brm}
    - **mineral** salt: lyc_{brm}
  - **desire** (see pg 1858): ign_{frc} sil_{fmx}
- **sand:**
  - **desire** (see pg 1858)
- **sauces** with food:
  - **desire** (see pg 1858)
- **sausages:**
  - **aversion:**
    - **raw:** lyc_{brm}
  - **desire** (see pg 1858): $calc-p_{brm}$

- **silage**:
  - **agg.**:
- **smoked** food:
- **snow**:
  - **desire** (see pg 1859)
- **soap**:
  - **desire** (see pg 1859): calc$_{ffd}$
- **soft** food:
  - **desire** (see pg 1859)
- **solid** food:
- **soup**:
  - **desire** (see pg 1859): lyc$_{frc}$
- **sour** food, acids:
- **spices**:
- **stones**:
  - **desire**: lyc$_{klp}$
- **strange** things:
  - **desire** (see pg 1860): alum$_{qqh}$ nux-v$_{frc}$
- **sugar**:
- **sweets**:
- **textile**:
  - **desire**:
- **valerian** tincture:
  - **desire**: lyc$_{brm}$
- **veal**:
- **vegetables**:
  - **desire** (see pg 1861): *Sulph*$_{fmx}$
- **vinegar**:
  - **desire** (see pg 1861): lach$_{frc}$
- **warm** drinks:
  - **aversion** (see pg 1861): sil$_{frc}$
- **warm** food:
- **water**:
  - **desire**:
    - **motion**; water in [e.g., health, spring]: calc$_{frc}$ phos$_{frc}$ puls$_{frc}$
- **weed**:
  - **aversion**: led$_{brm}$
- **wood**:
  - **desire** (see pg 1862): calc-p$_{klp}$ cann-i$_{hnb}$ lyc$_{klp}$
- **yoghurt**:

FOOD POISONING (see pg 1863)

FORCED through a narrow opening, as if (see pg 1863)

FROSTBITE, ailments from (see pg 1863)

GLANDERS (see pg 1864)

GRAYISH, dirty, etc. :

GREASY, oily, fatty (see pg 1864)

GREENISH:

GROWTH:
- **length** too fast; in (see pg 1864)

HAND on the part; laying one's:

HANG DOWN; letting limbs:

Hang down; letting limbs: ...
- **agg.** (see pg 1864)
- **amel.** (see pg 1864)

HARDNESS, induration (see pg 1865)

HEAT:
- **lack** of vital heat (see pg 1866)
  - **exertion** agg. (see pg 1867)
  - **menopause**; during (see pg 1867)
  - **nausea**; with (see pg 1867)
  - **warm** covering does not amel. (see pg 1867)
  - **warmth** agg.; and (see pg 1867)

HEATED, BECOMING (see pg 1868)

HEMATOMA:
- **painful**: arn$_{hnb}$

HEMORRHAGE (see pg 1868)
- **fever**; during paroxysmal (see pg 1869): lach$_{qqh}$

HEPATIC COMA: bell$_{hnb}$

HISTORY; personal:
- **death** of siblings when they are infants: syph$_{brm}$
- **diarrhea**; of recurrent (see pg 1870): ars$_{brm}$ sulph$_{brm}$
- **ear**:
  - **inflammation** (see pg 1871): lyc$_{brm}$
    - **External**; of recurrent: caust$_{brm}$ lyc$_{itm,qqh}$ med$_{itm,qqh}$ nat-m$_{itm,qqh}$ nux-v$_{brm}$ psor$_{itm,qqh}$ puls$_{brm,itm,pkj,qqh}$ sil$_{itm,qqh}$ sul-i$_{itm,qqh}$ sulph$_{itm,qqh}$ tub$_{pkj1}$
    - **Internal**; of recurrent (see pg 1871): sil$_{klp}$ thuj$_{klp}$ tub$_{klp}$
- **eyes**:
  - **recurrent** inflammation of the; of (see pg 1871): rhus-t$_{brm}$ syph$_{brm}$ thuj$_{brm}$
  - **infections**; of frequent: puls$_{brm}$
- **lids**; of recurrent tarsal tumors on the (see pg 1871)
- **tonsillitis**; of recurrent (see pg 1871): bell$_{brm}$ sulph$_{brm}$

HODGKIN'S disease (see pg 1871)

HUNGER:
- **agg.** (see pg 1872)

HYPERTENSION (see pg 1872)

HYPERTHYROIDISM (see pg 1872): ars$_{brl,qqh}$ calc-f$_{qqh}$ calc-i$_{qqh}$ *Iod*$_{bnfl.es,qqh}$ kali-i$_{bnfl.es,qqh}$ lach$_{brl}$ lyc$_{qqh}$ nat-m$_{qqh}$ phos$_{brm,qqh}$ puls$_{brm}$ sil$_{qqh}$ spong$_{bnfl.es,qqh}$ sul-i$_{qqh}$ tub$_{qqh}$
- **accompanied** by:
  - **diarrhea**: puls$_{brm}$

HYPOTENSION (see pg 1872)

HYPOTHERMIA (see pg 1872)
- **coldness**; with desire for:
  - **fever**; during: merc$_{frc}$

HYPOTHYROIDISM (see pg 1872): ars$_{qqh}$ bar-c$_{qqh}$ calc$_{qqh}$ flor-p$_{bnfl.es,qqh}$ puls$_{qqh}$ sulph$_{brm}$

INDOLENCE and luxury, ailments from (see pg 1872)

INDURATIONS (see pg 1873)

INFLAMMATION (see pg 1873)
- **Bursae**; of (see pg 1874): $apis_{mld4}$ arn_{mld4} $benz-ac_{mld4}$ bry_{mld4} $calc-f_{mld4}$ $hep_{mld,mld5}$ $hyper_{pkj1}$ iod_{mld5} $kali-m_{mld4}$ $Ruta_{mld,mld5}$ Sil_{mld4}
- **Joints**; of:
  - **osteoarthritis**: $rhus-t_{mld4}$
- **Muscles**; of (see pg 1875): $apis_{mld4}$ $Arn_{bnfl.es,itm,mld,pkj1}$ $caust_{pkj1}$ $cimic_{pkj1}$ $eup-per_{bnfl.es}$ hep_{mld4} $hyper_{pkj1}$ $phyt_{pkj1}$ $Rhus-t_{bnfl.es,itm}$ $ruta_{bnfl.es}$ $sarcol-ac_{bnfl.es,itm,pkj1}$
- **Nerves** (see pg 1875): $am-m_{frc}$

INFLUENZA (see pg 1876): $Acon_{mld,spk1}$ $ant-t_{mld4}$ $ars_{mld,spk1}$ $bapt_{mld,spk1}$ $Bell_{mld,spk1}$ $bry_{mld,spk1}$ $Eup-per_{mld5}$ $Gels_{mld,mld5,spk1}$ lyc_{mld4}

INJURIES (see pg 1876)
- **concussion** (see pg 1876): $gels_{frc}$ op_{frc}
- **sprains** (see pg 1877): $apis_{frc}$
- **Glands** (see pg 1877): $bar-c_{qqh}$ Iod_{qqh} Sil_{qqh}
- **Joints** (see pg 1877): $apis_{frc,qqh}$ $bell_{frc,qqh}$ $bry_{frc,qqh}$ $rhus-t_{frc,qqh}$
- **Nerves** (see pg 1877): $all-c_{frc}$ $am-m_{frc}$
- **Tendons**, of (see pg 1877): $Anac_{elg,hnb}$ sil_{frc} $staph_{hnb}$

IODINE, after abuse of (see pg 1878)

IRON, after abuse of (see pg 1878)

IRRITABILITY, physical:

ITCHING:

JAR, stepping:
- agg. (see pg 1878)
- amel. (see pg 1878)

JERKING (see pg 1879)

LABORATORY findings:
- **blood**:
  - **calcium**:
    - **decreased**:
      - **prevent** this condition; to: $calc_{elg}$
      - **rise**; can't: $calc_{elg}$
        - lying; after a few days: $rhus-t_{elg}$
  - **cholesterol**:
    - **decreased** (see pg 1880): sil_{hnb}
  - **kalium**:
    - **increased**: $kali-c_{hnb}$
    - **low**; too: $kali-c_{hnb}$
  - **magnesium**:
    - **decreased**: cic_{dyc} $mag-p_{dyc}$ $metald_{dyc}$ $nux-v_{dyc}$ $stry_{dyc}$
    - **increased**:
  - **natrium**:
    - **decreased**:
    - **increased**:
  - **phosphorus**:
    - **decreased**:
    - **increased**:

LAME feeling (see pg 1880)

LASSITUDE (see pg 1880)

LEAD poisoning; from (see pg 1881): $okou_{hnb}$

LEAN people (see pg 1881)

LEANING:
- **against** something:
  - amel. (see pg 1882)
- **desire** for leaning (see pg 1882): $sulph_{frc}$
- **hard**; against something:
  - amel. (see pg 1882)
- **sharp** edge; against a:
  - agg. (see pg 1882)
  - amel.:
- **side**; to:
  - agg.:

LEISHMANIASIS: $ars_{elg,hnb,sa}$ $calc_{lkk}$ $kali-c_{lkk}$ $lyc_{brm,lkk}$ med_{lkk} $phos_{brm,lkk}$ $sulph_{lkk}$ $syph_{lkk}$ tub_{lkk}

LEUKEMIA (see pg 1882): $apis_{brm}$ $Nat-m_{brm}$ $puls_{brm}$ $pyrog_{brm}$ $sulph_{brm}$
- **feline** leukemia: $apis_{brm}$ arn_{fmx} $kali-c_{fmx}$ $nat-m_{brm}$ $phos_{fmx}$ $puls_{brm}$ $pyrog_{brm}$ $sulph_{brm}$
- **seronegative**; getting: $bell_{brm}$ $sulph_{brm}$

LEUKORRHEA:
- amel. (see pg 1882)

LIE DOWN:
- **desire** to (see pg 1882)
  - **abdomen** in pregnancy, on (see pg 1882)
  - agg. thereby; but (see pg 1882)
  - **darkness** agg. (see pg 1882)
  - **eating**; after (see pg 1882)

LIFTING, straining of muscles and tendons (see pg 1882)

LIGHT; from:
- agg. (see pg 1882)

LISTERIOSIS: cic_{dyc}

LOSS:
- **blood**; of (see pg 1884)
- **fluids**, of (see pg 1884)

LOW-FEVER STATES (see pg 1884)

LYING:
- **abdomen**; on:
  - agg. (see pg 1884): lyc_{brm}
  - amel. (see pg 1884)
- **after**:
  - agg. (see pg 1884)
    - **immediately** after lying (see pg 1884)
  - amel. (see pg 1884)
- agg. (see pg 1884)
- amel. (see pg 1884)
- **back**; on:
  - agg. (see pg 1884)
  - amel. (see pg 1885)
  - **turn**; cannot (see pg 1885)
- **double**; bent:
  - agg.:
  - amel. (see pg 1885)
- **face**; on the:
  - amel. (see pg 1885)

- **hard** bed; on a:
  - **agg.** (see pg 1885)
  - **amel.** (see pg 1885)
- **head** high; with the:
  - **amel.** (see pg 1885)
- **head** low; with the:
  - **agg.** (see pg 1885)
  - **amel.** (see pg 1885)
- **head** towards wall; with: sulph$_{brm}$
- **knee** elbow position:
  - **amel.** (see pg 1885)
- **legs** drawn up; with:
  - **amel.** (see pg 1885): plb$_{brm}$
- **side**; on:
  - **agg.** (see pg 1885)
  - **amel.** (see pg 1885)
  - **left:**
    : **agg.** (see pg 1885)
    : **amel.** (see pg 1885): phos$_{brm}$
  - **pain** goes to side:
    : **Lain** on (see pg 1885)
    : **Not** lain on:
  - **painful** side:
    : **agg.** (see pg 1886): **Ruta**$_{brm}$
    : **amel.** (see pg 1886)
  - **painless** side:
    : **agg.** (see pg 1886)
    : **amel.** (see pg 1886)
  - **part** on which he is lying agg.:
  - **right:**
    : **agg.** (see pg 1886): arg-n$_{qqh}$ *Borx*$_{hnb}$
    : **amel.** (see pg 1886): naja$_{qqh}$
- **stretched** out; lying:
  - **agg.:**
  - **amel.:** puls$_{brm}$
- **wet** floor agg.; on a (see pg 1886)

LYME DISEASE (see pg 1886): anac$_{brm}$ aur-ar$_{hnb}$ calc-p$_{brm}$ lyc$_{brm}$ tarent$_{brm}$

MAGNETISM amel. (see pg 1886)

MANY SYMPTOMS (see pg 1886)

MASTURBATION; ailments from (see pg 1886)

MEDICINE:
- **allopathic:**
  - **oversensitive** to (see pg 1887): carc$_{klp}$ cortiso$_{klp}$ **Nux-v**$_{klp}$ phos$_{klp}$ **Sulph**$_{klp}$ thuj$_{klp}$
    : **antibiotics:** nux-v$_{klp}$ sulph$_{klp}$
    : **corticosteroids:** cortiso$_{klp}$ nat-m$_{elg}$ nux-v$_{klp}$ phos$_{klp}$ sulph$_{klp}$

MERCURY:
- **abuse** of (see pg 1888)

METASTASIS (see pg 1888)

MILK FEVER, veterinary condition: acet-ac$_{bnfl.es}$ agar$_{mld5}$ bell$_{mld5}$ calc$_{ljy,mld5}$ calc-p$_{mld5}$ nat-m$_{ljy1}$ puls$_{ljy1}$ ric$_{bnfl.es,pkj1}$ stram$_{mld5}$ sulph$_{ljy1}$

MOLTING period:
- **after** agg.:
- **during** agg.:

MOON:
- **full** moon:
  - **agg.** (see pg 1888): **Calc**$_{hnb}$ med$_{brm}$ *Merc*$_{klp}$
  - **new** moon agg.; and: med$_{brm}$
- **new** moon:
  - **agg.** (see pg 1888): med$_{brm}$

MOTION:
- **aversion** to:
  - **fever**; during: verat-v$_{qqh}$

MOUNTAIN:

MUCOUS MEMBRANES; complaints of:
- **dryness:**
  - **fever**; during: bell$_{qqh}$
- **serous** (see pg 1980)

MUCOUS SECRETIONS:
- **amel.** (see pg 1890): ign$_{frc}$
- **bloody** (see pg 1890): anthraci$_{qqh}$
- **corrosive** (see pg 1890): canth$_{qqh}$ med$_{frc}$ merc-c$_{frc}$ squil$_{qqh}$
- **frothy** (see pg 1890): calc$_{frc}$
- **greenish** (see pg 1891): merc-c$_{frc}$
- **purulent** (see pg 1891): arg-n$_{qqh}$ pareir$_{qqh}$
- **ropy**, tenacious (see pg 1891): sang$_{qqh}$
- **transparent** (see pg 1891): coc-c$_{qqh}$
- **watery** (see pg 1891): coc-c$_{qqh}$
- **yellow** (see pg 1891): merc-c$_{frc}$

MUSHROOM POISONING (see pg 1892)

MUSIC:

MYASTHENIA GRAVIS (see pg 1892)

MYATROPHY, progressive spinal (see pg 1892)

MYCOTOXIN:
- **poisoning** by: okou$_{hnb}$

MYOPATHIA (see pg 1892): cupr$_{mld4}$ pic-ac$_{mld4}$ sarcol-ac$_{mld4}$ thuj$_{mld4}$

MYXEDEMA (see pg 1892)

NARCOTICS:

NECROSIS (see pg 1892)

NOISES:

NURSING, suckling agg. (see pg 1894)

NURSLINGS (see pg 1894)

OBESITY (see pg 1894)
- **castration**; after: graph$_{brm}$
  - **men**; in:
  - **women**; in: graph$_{hnb}$ sep$_{hnb}$
- **ovariectomy**; after:

ODOR OF THE BODY:
- **offensive** (see pg 1895)

OLD AGE:
- **premature** (see pg 1895)

OSSIFICATION:
- **Cartilage**; lateral: arn_{mld4} $calc-f_{mld4}$ $ruta_{mld4}$ sil_{mld4}

OSTEOCHONDROSIS:
- **dissecans**: arn_{elg} $calc_{elg}$ $calc-f_{elg}$ $phos_{elg}$

OSTEO-FIBROSIS: $calc_{qqh}$

OSTEOMALACIA (see pg 1896): $calc_{qqh}$ $hecla_{mld3}$ $ph-ac_{mld3}$ sil_{mld3}

PAIN:
- **appear** gradually (see pg 1898)
- **appear** suddenly (see pg 1898)
- **cancerous** affections, in (see pg 1899)
- **growing** pains (see pg 1900): lyc_{brm}
- **Muscles**:
  - **fever**; during (see pg 1916): $bapt_{qqh}$ $eup-per_{qqh}$

PAINLESSNESS of complaints usually painful (see pg 1918)

PARALYSIS:
- **extending** to:
  - **Upward** (see pg 1920)

PERIODICITY (see pg 1920)
- **day**:
  - **fourth**; every (see pg 1921): $psor_{qqh}$
  - **third**; every (see pg 1921): $psor_{qqh}$
- **month**:
  - **six** months; every (see pg 1921): sep_{frc}
- **year**:
  - **every** (see pg 1921): sep_{frc}

PERSPIRATION:

PINCHING:
- **amel.** (see pg 1922)

PIROPLASMOSIS:

PLETHORA (see pg 1922)

POISONOUS plants; poisoning by: $hyos_{hnb}$ $nux-v_{klp}$ $okou_{klp}$ $phos_{klp}$

POLYPUS (see pg 1922)

PRESSURE:

PSORA (see pg 1923)

PUBERTY:
- **ailments** in (see pg 1924)

PULSE:
- **frequent**:
  - **fever**; with (see pg 1926): $acon_{qqh}$ bry_{qqh} $echi_{qqh}$ $ferr-p_{qqh}$ $pyrog_{qqh}$
- **hard**:
  - **slow**, and (see pg 1927): $bell_{qqh}$ bry_{qqh}
- **imperceptible** (see pg 1927): $mur-ac_{qqh}$
- **irregular** (see pg 1927): lyc_{brm}
  - **fever**; during: sil_{qqh}
- **slow** (see pg 1928): $Gels_{mld4}$ $Kalm_{mld,pkjl}$
  - **fever**; with (see pg 1928): $gels_{qqh}$

Pulse: ...
- **small**:
  - **frequent**; and: ars_{qqh} $phos_{qqh}$ sil_{qqh}
- **soft**:
  - **fever**; during: $ferr-p_{qqh}$
- **weak**:
  - **fever**; during: $mur-ac_{qqh}$

PUNISHMENT agg.: $calc_{frc}$ ign_{frc} lyc_{frc} $nux-v_{frc}$ $phos_{frc}$ $plat_{frc}$ $puls_{frc}$ sep_{frc} $sulph_{frc}$ $verat_{frc}$

PURGATIVES, abuse of (see pg 1930)

QUININE, abuse of (see pg 1930)

QUIVERING (see pg 1930)

RAGWORT; intoxication by:

REACTION (see pg 1930)

REDNESS (see pg 1931)

REFLEXES:

RELAXATION:

REMEDIES:

REST:
- **amel.** (see pg 1932): $grat_{qqh}$

RESTLESSNESS (see pg 1932)
- **travelling** by car; while:

RICKETS (see pg 1932)

RIDING:
- **car**, in a:
  - **after**:
  - **agg.**:

RISING:
- **aversion** to rise when lying: $calc_{brm}$

ROOM:
- **close** room:
  - **agg.** (see pg 1934)
- **full**:
  - **people** agg.; of (see pg 1934)

RUBBING:
- **agg.** (see pg 1934)
- **amel.** (see pg 1934)
- **gently**:
  - **agg.** (see pg 1934)

RUNNING:

SCURVY, scorbutus (see pg 1935)

SEASIDE; at the:
- **agg.** (see pg 1935)
- **amel.** (see pg 1935)

SEASONS:

SEDENTARY habits (see pg 1935)

SENSITIVENESS:

SEPTICEMIA, blood poisoning (see pg 1936)

SEWER-GAS poisoning (see pg 1936)

SHAVING:
- **agg.** (see pg 1937): bell$_{klp}$

SHINING objects; ailments from (see pg 1937)

SHOCK (see pg 1937)

SHORTENED muscles and tendons (see pg 1937)

SILICA; from overuse of (see pg 1939)

SITTING:

SLEEP:
- **during** sleep:
  • **amel.** (see pg 1940): phos$_{qqh}$

SMOG agg. (see pg 1941)

SMOKE:
- **inspiration** of:
  • **agg.** (see pg 1941)

SNEEZING:

SNOW, ailments from bright (see pg 1941)

SNOWY WEATHER:

SOFTENING bones (see pg 1941)

SOURNESS (see pg 1941)

STANDING:

STARVING (see pg 1942)

STASIS of the venous system (see pg 1942): puls$_{frc}$ sep$_{frc}$ sulph$_{frc}$

STIFFENING OUT of body (see pg 1942)

STIFFNESS (see pg 1942)

STOOL:

STOOP shouldered (see pg 1943)

STRANGLES: acon$_{qqh}$ ail$_{hnb}$ ars$_{qqh}$ bar-c$_{qqh}$ *Bell*$_{qqh}$ dulc$_{qqh}$ hep$_{qqh}$ lach$_{hnb}$ pilo-m$_{qqh}$ puls$_{qqh}$ rhus-t$_{qqh}$

STRETCHING:
- **amel.** (see pg 1943): phos$_{fmx}$ rhus-t$_{fmx}$ sep$_{frc}$

SUDDEN manifestation (see pg 1945)

SULPHUR, abuse of (see pg 1945)

SUN:
- **sunburn** (see pg 1945): apis$_{frc}$ ars$_{frc}$ canth$_{frc}$

SWELLING:

SYCOSIS (see pg 1948)

SYNALGIA (see pg 1948)

SYPHILIS (see pg 1948)

TEMPERATURE:
- **change** of (see pg 1949)
  • **cold** to warm (see pg 1949)

TENSION:
- **Joints**; of (see pg 1950)
- **Muscles**; of (see pg 1950)

TETANUS (see pg 1950): led$_{brl}$

THROMBOSIS (see pg 1950)

TOUCH:
- **agg.** (see pg 1951)
- **amel.** (see pg 1951)
- **slight** touch agg. (see pg 1951)
- **throat** agg.; touching (see pg 1951): arum-t$_{qqh}$ rumx$_{qqh}$ spong$_{qqh}$

TRAVELLING:
- **ailments** from (see pg 1952): **Cocc**$_{hnb,klp}$ nux-v$_{klp}$ tab$_{hnb,klp}$

TREMBLING:
- **Externally**:
  • **anxiety**:
    : **from** (see pg 1952): sulph$_{brm}$
  • **examination** table; on: nat-m$_{brm}$
  • **excitement**:
    : **emotional** excitement; after (see pg 1953): stram$_{brm}$
  • **fever**; during (see pg 1953): acon$_{qqh}$ gels$_{qqh}$
  • **injury** of the spine; after: cic$_{brm}$
  • **sleep**:
    : **during**:
      : **agg.** (see pg 1954): nat-m$_{brm}$

TUBERCULOSIS (see pg 1954)

TUMORS (see pg 1955)
- **fibrosarcoma** (see pg 1955): calc-p$_{brm}$ tub$_{brm}$

TURNING:
- **around** agg.; turning:
  • **impossible**: rhus-t$_{brm}$
- **bed**; in:
  • **agg.** (see pg 1956): arn$_{brm}$

TWITCHING:
- **night** (see pg 1956): puls$_{lkk}$

ULCERS:

UNCLEANLINESS agg. (see pg 1957)

UNCOVERING:
- **kicks** the covers of:
  • **coldest** weather; in (see pg 1957)

UNDRESSING agg.; after (see pg 1958)

UREMIA (see pg 1958): am-c$_{itm,pkj,qqh}$ apoc$_{itm,pkj,qqh}$ ars$_{pkj1}$ calc$_{bnfl.es}$ camph$_{pkj1}$ carb-v$_{pkj1}$ cupr$_{pkj1}$ *Hell*$_{pkj1}$ *Op*$_{bnfl.es,pkj1}$ phos$_{pkj1}$ ser-ang$_{bnfl.es,itm,pkj,qqh}$

URINATION:
- **after**:
  • **agg.** (see pg 1958): **Canth**$_{qqh}$ *Staph*$_{qqh}$
  • **amel.** (see pg 1958): berb$_{frc}$ led$_{qqh}$

VACCINATION; ailments after (see pg 1958)

VARICOSE veins:
- **blue** (see pg 1959)
- **congested** (see pg 1959)

VAULTS, cellars agg. (see pg 1959)

VENESECTION, ailments from (see pg 1959)

VIGOR (see pg 1959)

VIOLENT COMPLAINTS (see pg 1959)

VOMITING:

WAKING:
- **on** (see pg 1960)

WALKING:
- **after**:
  - **agg.** (see pg 1960)
- **agg.** (see pg 1960)
- **ailments** from walking (see pg 1960)
- **air**; in open:
  - **agg.** (see pg 1960)
  - **amel.** (see pg 1960)
- **amel.** (see pg 1961)
- **aversion** to (see pg 1961)
- **beginning** to walk (see pg 1961)
- **bent**:
  - **agg.**:
  - **amel.** (see pg 1961)
- **circle**, in a (see pg 1961)
- **desire** for (see pg 1961)
  - **night** (see pg 1961)
  - **air**, in open (see pg 1961)
- **easily** (see pg 1961)
- **learning** to walk:
  - **late** (see pg 1961): **Calc**_{ffd} lyc_{ffd}
    : **development** of bones; tardy (see pg 1961)
- **level** ground; on:
  - **agg.** (see pg 1961)
- **rapidly**:
  - **agg.** (see pg 1961)
  - **amel.** (see pg 1961)
- **slowly**:
  - **amel.** (see pg 1961): calc-f_{klp} nat-m_{brm} rhus-t_{klp} tub_{klp}
- **stone** pavement agg.; on a (see pg 1961)
- **uneven** ground agg.; on (see pg 1961)
- **wind**; in the:
  - **agg.** (see pg 1961)

WARM:
- **agg.** (see pg 1961)
- **air**:
  - **agg.** (see pg 1961)
  - **amel.** (see pg 1961)
- **amel.** (see pg 1962)
- **bathing**:
  - **agg.** (see pg 1962)
  - **amel.** (see pg 1962)
- **clothing**:
  - **desire** (see pg 1962)
- **desire** for warmth (see pg 1962): tritic_{sxj}
  - **alternating** with:
    : **coldness**; desire for:
      : **fever**; during: merc_{frc}
  - **fever**; during: bell_{qqh} merc_{frc}

Warm: ...
- **room**:
  - **agg.** (see pg 1962)
  - **amel.** (see pg 1962)
- **stove**:
  - **agg.** (see pg 1962)
  - **amel.** (see pg 1962): lyc_{brm}
  - **desire** (see pg 1963): *Sil*_{brm}
- **wraps**:
  - **agg.** (see pg 1963)
  - **amel.** (see pg 1963)

WARM; BECOMING:
- **agg.** (see pg 1963)
- **amel.** (see pg 1963)

WATER:
- **seeing** or hearing of running water agg. (see pg 1963)
- **working** in water:
  - **agg.** (see pg 1963)

WEAKNESS (see pg 1963)
- **children**; in:
  - **premature** infants: arn_{elg}
  - **twin**; in a too small: arn_{elg}
- **delivery**:
  - **after** (see pg 1967): arn_{hnb}
    : **prevent** this condition: arn_{elg}
- **fever**:
  - **during**:
    : **agg.** (see pg 1968): *Anthraci*_{qqh} *Arn*_{qqh} **Ars**_{qqh} *Bapt*_{qqh} *Bry*_{qqh} echi_{qqh} *Eup-per*_{qqh} lach_{qqh} pyrog_{qqh} *Rhus-t*_{qqh}
- **radiation** therapy; from: carc_{brm}
- **walking**:
  - **agg.** (see pg 1972): *Nat-m*_{qqh}

WEARINESS (see pg 1973): **Phos**_{elg}
- **morning** (see pg 1974)
  - **rising** agg. (see pg 1974)
  - **waking**; on (see pg 1974)
- **forenoon** (see pg 1974)
- **noon** (see pg 1974)
- **afternoon** (see pg 1974)
  - **16.30-19.30 h**:
  - **amel.** (see pg 1974)
- **evening** (see pg 1974)
  - **18 h**:
- **night** (see pg 1974)
- **agg.** (see pg 1974)
- **air**; in open:
  - **amel.** (see pg 1974)
- **ascending** stairs, from (see pg 1974)
- **coition**; after (see pg 1974)
- **diarrhea** agg.; after (see pg 1974)

- **eating**:
  - **after**:
    : agg. (see pg 1974)
  - **while**:
    : agg. (see pg 1974)
- **emissions**, after:
- **exertion**:
  - **amel.** (see pg 1974)
- **leukorrhea**:
  - **after** (see pg 1974)
  - **with** (see pg 1974)
- **menopause**; during (see pg 1974)
- **menses**:
  - **after**:
    : agg. (see pg 1974)
  - **before**:
    : agg. (see pg 1974)
  - **during**:
    : agg. (see pg 1974)
- **mental** exertion agg. (see pg 1974)
- **sexual** excitement, from (see pg 1974)
- **standing**:
  - **agg.** (see pg 1974): $puls_{frc}$ sep_{frc} $sulph_{frc}$
  - **amel.**:
- **waking**; on (see pg 1974)
- **walking**:
  - **after**:
    : agg. (see pg 1974)
  - **air**; in open:
    : agg. (see pg 1974)

WEATHER:
- **rainy**:
  - **agg.** (see pg 1975): sep_{brm}
  - **aversion** to walk in the rain: $calc_{klp}$ sep_{brm}
- **thunderstorm**:
  - **approach** of a (see pg 1976)
  - **lightning**; ailments from (see pg 1976)

WET:
- **applications**:
  - **warm** wet applications:
    : amel. (see pg 1977): arn_{qqh}
- **getting** (see pg 1977): $seneg_{qqh}$

WHITENESS:
- **Parts** usually red; of (see pg 1977)

WOUNDS (see pg 1977): *Calen*$_{fmx}$ *Hyper*$_{fmx}$
- **bites** (see pg 1978): $acet\text{-}ac_{klp}$ $anthraci_{klp}$ *Arn*$_{klp}$ $calen_{frc}$ $gunp_{klp}$ *Lach*$_{klp}$ $pyrog_{frc,klp}$
  - **cats**; of (see pg 1978): *Hep*$_{brm}$ *Lach*$_{brm}$ *Led*$_{brm}$ $merc_{brm}$ $phos_{brm}$ *Sil*$_{brm}$ $sulph_{brm}$
  - **dogs**, of (see pg 1978): hep_{brm} *Lach*$_{elg}$ $rhus\text{-}t_{brm}$
  - **horses**; of: $lach_{elg}$
  - **poisonous** animals, of (see pg 1978): $anac_{brm}$ *Lach*$_{fmx}$
  - **ticks**; of:
    : **abundant** bites: $calc\text{-}p_{brm}$ $sulph_{brm}$
- **constitutional** effects of (see pg 1978): *Lach*$_{brm}$ lyc_{brm}

Wounds: ...
- **gangrene** of (see pg 1978): $carb\text{-}ac_{frc}$ $mur\text{-}ac_{frc}$ $pyrog_{frc}$
- **large**:
  - **scratching**; from:
- **penetrating**, punctured (see pg 1979): $calen_{fmx}$ *Hyper*$_{fmx}$ **Led**$_{fmx}$
  - **Palms** and soles, of (see pg 1979): arn_{elg} $bell_{dyc}$ $gunp_{dyc}$ hep_{dyc} **Hyper**$_{dyc,elg}$ **LED**$_{dyc}$ $ruta_{elg}$ sil_{dyc}
    : **acute** infection: $bell_{dyc}$ hep_{dyc}
    : **chronic** infection: sil_{dyc}
- **septic** (see pg 1979): $calen_{frc}$ hep_{frc} $lach_{frc}$ $pyrog_{frc}$
- **small**:
  - **scratching**; from: bac_{klp}

YAWNING:
- **after**:
  - **agg.**:
- **agg.** (see pg 1979)
- **amel.** (see pg 1979)

YEW; intoxication by:

In this chapter only remedies from veterinary authors are printed

ANY ANIMAL; symptoms and behavior of:
- **abortion**
  - → FEMA - Abortion - accompanied by - chills
  - → FEMA - Abortion - accompanied by - joint pain
  - → FEMA - Abortion - accompanied by - perspiration
  - → FEMA - Abortion - accompanied by - septicemia
  - → FEMA - Abortion - accompanied by - spasms
  - → FEMA - Abortion - accompanied by - weakness
  - → FEMA - Abortion - accompanied by - Uterus; swelling of
  - → FEMA - Inflammation - Uterus - abortion; after
  - → FEMA - Leukorrhea - abortion with history of
  - → FEMA - Leukorrhea - pregnancy agg.; during - abortion; with tendency to
  - → FEMA - Lochia - abortion after
  - → FEMA - Metrorrhagia - abortion - after
  - → FEMA - Metrorrhagia - abortion - during
  - → FEMA - Placenta - retained - abortion after
  - → FEMA - Veins varicose - accompanied by - abortion
  - → FEVE - Abortion; after
  - → GENE - Anemia - accompanied by - abortion
  - → GENE - Convalescence; ailments during - abortion; after
  - → GENE - History; personal - abortion; of
- **angry** in situations where anger is normal; not
  - → MIND - Ailments FROM - anger - suppressed
- **backward**; complaints extending
  - → GENE - Complaints - extending to - Downward
- **bad** treatment; after
  - → MIND - Ailments FROM - abused; after being
  - → MIND - Ailments FROM - abused; after being - physically
  - → MIND - Ailments FROM - abused; after being - sexually
- **biting**:
  - · **smaller** animals:
    - ∶ **larger** animals; with fear of
      - → MIND - Hard for inferiors and kind for superiors
- **castration**; after
  - → MIND - Ailments FROM - castration
  - → MIND - Anger - castration; after
  - → MIND - Behavior PROBLEMS - castration; after
  - → MIND - Dullness - castration; after
  - → MIND - Grief - castration; after
  - → MIND - Irritability - castration; after
  - → MIND - Offended easily - castration; after
  - → HEAD - Hair - baldness - castration; after
  - → BLAD - Urination - involuntary - castration; after - women; in
  - → MALE - Fistula - Spermatic cord - castration; after
  - → MALE - Sexual desire - increased - castrated animals; in
  - → FEMA - Leukorrhea - castration; after
  - → CHES - Swelling - Mammae - castration; after
  - → SKIN - Complaints of skin - castration; after

- **castration**; after...
  - → SKIN - Hair - baldness - castration; after - hormonal causes; from
  - → SKIN - Hair - falling out - hormonal causes; from
  - → SKIN - Hair - falling out - hormonal causes; from - Gonades
  - → SKIN - Hair - falling out - hormonal causes; from - Gonades - Ovaries
  - → SKIN - Hair - falling out - hormonal causes; from - Gonades - Testes
  - → SKIN - Hair - falling out - hormonal causes; from - Pararenal glands
  - → SKIN - Hair - falling out - hormonal causes; from - Thyroid gland
  - → GENE - Ailments from - castration
  - → GENE - Convalescence; ailments during - castration; after
  - → GENE - Obesity - castration; after
- **compulsive** behavior
  - → MIND - Biting - nails
  - → MIND - Gestures makes - repeating the same actions
  - → NOSE - Boring in nose with fingers
- **copulate** after sexual excesses; aversion to
  - → MIND - Ailments FROM - sexual excesses
  - → MALE - Sexual desire - diminished - sexual excesses; after
- **copulate**; aversion to
  - → MALE - Sexual desire - wanting
  - → FEMA - Sexual desire - wanting
- **copulate**; desire to
  - → MALE - Sexual desire - excessive
  - → MALE - Sexual desire - increased
  - → MALE - Sexual desire - violent
  - → FEMA - Sexual desire - increased
  - → FEMA - Sexual desire - insatiable
  - → FEMA - Sexual desire - violent
- **copulate** rarely; old animals
  - → MALE - Sexual desire - diminished - old people; in
  - → FEMA - Sexual desire - diminished - old people; in
- **copulate** with weakness in posterior limbs; aversion to:
- **demanding** too much while training or breaking in an animal
  - → MIND - Ailments from - abused; after being - demanding too much while training or breaking in a horse
  - → MIND - Ailments from - mental exertion
  - → MIND - Anger - abused; after being - demanding too much while training or breaking in a horse
- **diarrhea** from excitement
  - → RECT - Diarrhea - excitement agg.
- **dirty** mouth after eating
  - → MIND - Dirty
  - → MIND - Dirty - eating; when
  - → MOUT - Discoloration - Tongue - dirty

- **discharge** from the nose
  → NOSE - Discharge
  → NOSE - Discharge - clear
  → NOSE - Discharge - copious
  → NOSE - Discharge - dripping
  → NOSE - Discharge - gray
  → NOSE - Discharge - greenish
  → NOSE - Discharge - offensive
  → NOSE - Discharge - purulent
  → NOSE - Discharge - thick
  → NOSE - Discharge - thin
  → NOSE - Discharge - viscid tough
  → NOSE - Discharge - watery
  → NOSE - Discharge - white
  → NOSE - Discharge - yellow
  → NOSE - Discharge - yellowish green
- **dreaming** a lot
  → DREA - Events - previous
  → DREA - Events - previous - day of the previous
- **eating** during fever; still
  → STOM - Appetite - increased - fever - during
- **ectoparasitism**
  → SKIN - Eruptions - demodicidosis
  → SKIN - Eruptions - demodicidosis - spots; in single
  → SKIN - Eruptions - fleabites
- **emaciation**
  → BACK - Emaciation
  → BACK - Emaciation - Cervical region
- **endoparasitism**
  → RECT - Worms - complaints of worms - roundworm
  → RECT - Worms - complaints of worms - tapeworm
- **estrus**
  → GENE - Menses - after
  → GENE - Menses - before
  → GENE - Menses - during
- **expression** of face
  → FACE - Expression
- **extremities**; symptoms of
  → EXTR
  → EXTR - Inflammation - Laminae - Forelimb nails
  → EXTR - Inflammation - Laminae - Hind limb nails
  → EXTR - Nails; complaints of - brittle nails - Forelimb nails
  → EXTR - Nails; complaints of - brittle nails - Hind limb nails
  → EXTR - Pain - kneeling agg.
  → EXTR - Pain - Ankles
  → EXTR - Pain - Elbows
  → EXTR - Pain - Feet
  → EXTR - Pain - Fingers
  → EXTR - Pain - Forearms
  → EXTR - Pain - Hands
  → EXTR - Pain - Hips
  → EXTR - Pain - Legs
  → EXTR - Pain - Lower limbs

- **extremities**; symptoms of...
  → EXTR - Pain - Nates
  → EXTR - Pain - Shoulders
  → EXTR - Pain - Thighs
  → EXTR - Pain - Toes
  → EXTR - Pain - Upper arms
  → EXTR - Pain - Upper limbs
  → EXTR - Pain - Wrists
- **fear** in between animals of their own species
  → MIND - Fear - animals of - own species; fear of
  → MIND - Fear - crowd in a
- **fear** of new things lying around
  → MIND - Conscientious about trifles
  → MIND - Fastidious
  → MIND - Fear - trifles of
  → MIND - Starting - trifles at
- **fear** of people
  → MIND - Fear - animals of
  → MIND - Fear - people; of
- **feet** only for a very short time on the ground
  → EXTR - Restlessness - Feet
  → EXTR - Sensitive - Feet - Soles
- **flea**-collar allergy
  → EXTE - Clothing agg.
  → EXTE - Eruptions - flea-collars; from
- **food** desires and aversions
  → GENE - Food and drinks
- **forefoot**
  → EXTR - Hands; complaints of
  → EXTR - Pain - Hands
- **forelimb**
  → EXTR - Pain - Upper limbs
  → EXTR - Upper limbs; complaints of
- **fore** toes
  → EXTR - Fingers; complaints of
  → EXTR - Pain - Fingers
- **foreward**; complaints extending
  → GENE - Complaints - extending to - Upward
- **freckles**
  → SKIN - Freckles
- **furniture** has been moved ; uncomfortable when
  → MIND - Conscientious about trifles
- **hind** foot
  → EXTR - Feet; complaints of
  → EXTR - Pain - Feet
- **hind** limb
  → EXTR - Lower limbs; complaints of
  → EXTR - Pain - Lower limbs
- **hind** toes
  → EXTR - Pain - Toes
  → EXTR - Toes; complaints of
- **jealousy**
  → MIND - Ailments from - jealousy
  → MIND - Envy
  → MIND - Jealousy

- **kidneys**; size or texture of
  → KIDN - Irregular surface
  → KIDN - Large kidneys
  → KIDN - Polycystic kidneys
  → KIDN - Small kidneys
- **looking** at owners after these have been absent for some days; not
  → MIND - Dwells - past disagreeable occurrences on
  → MIND - Looking - not looking - owner; at the - absent; when he has been - days; for some
  → MIND - Looking - not looking - owner; at the - absent; when he has been - hours; for some
- **loosing** food when eating
  → EXTR - Awkwardness
- **mastitis**
  → CHES - Discoloration - Mammae - blue
  → CHES - Discoloration - Mammae - redness - dark
  → CHES - Discoloration - Mammae - redness - light
  → CHES - Inflammation - Mammae
- **milk** for her young animal; the female has not enough
  → CHES - Milk - decreased
  → CHES - Milk - disappearing
- **nose** saddle; all discolorations and alterations of the
  → NOSE - Discoloration - yellow - saddle
- **offspring**
  → MIND - Anger - children; towards - own children; towards one's
  → MIND - Aversion - children to - own; her
  → MIND - Biting - children; her own
  → MIND - Children - flies from her or his own children
  → MIND - Estranged - children; flies from her own
  → MIND - Forsaking - children; his own
  → MIND - Irritability - children towards - own; his
  → MIND - Kill; desire to - child the own
  → MIND - Striking - children; striking one's own
  → MIND - Touched - aversion to be - children; by her own
  → GENE - Children; complaints in
- **ovariectomy**; after
  → MIND - Anger - ovariectomy; after
  → MIND - Behavior problems - ovariectomy; after
  → MIND - Dullness - ovariectomy; after
  → MIND - Grief - ovariectomy; after
  → MIND - Irritability - ovariectomy; after
  → MIND - Offended easily - ovariectomy; after
  → HEAD - Hair - baldness - ovariectomy; after
  → BLAD - Urination - involuntary - ovariectomy; after
  → FEMA - Sexual desire - increased - ovariectomy; after
  → SKIN - Complaints of skin - ovariectomy; after
  → SKIN - Hair - baldness - ovariectomy; after
  → GENE - Obesity - ovariectomy; after

- **ovaries**; complaints of
  → MIND - Mannish - women - ovaries; with tumors in
  → FEMA - Atrophy - Ovaries
  → FEMA - Pain - Ovaries - accompanied by - Heart; complaints of - difficult respiration; and
  → FEMA - Tumors - Ovaries - cysts - corpus luteum; encysted
- **perspiration** during illness
  → FEVE - Pers - heat; with
  → PERS - Diarrhea - during
  → PERS - Feve - after
- **poisoning**; after
  → GENE - Aluminium poisoning
  → GENE - Anthelmintic poison; complaints from
  → GENE - Buttercups; intoxication by
  → GENE - Lead poisoning; from
  → GENE - Mushroom poisoning
  → GENE - Poisonous plants; poisoning by
  → GENE - Ragwort; intoxication by
  → GENE - Sewer-gas poisoning
  → GENE - Yew; intoxication by
- **position** when awake; always remains in same
  → SLEE - Position
- **presence** of other people agg. symptoms
  → MIND - Company - aversion to
  → MIND - Sensitive - people; to presence of other
- **rachitis**
  → EXTR - Curving and bowing
- **scales** without an eruption
  → HEAD - Dandruff
- **scratching**
  → SKIN - Discoloration - blackish - scratching; from
  → SKIN - Discoloration - red - scratching; after
  → SKIN - Discoloration - spots - scratching; after
  → SKIN - Eruptions - bleeding - scratching; after
  → SKIN - Eruptions - scratching agg.; after
  → SKIN - Excoriation - scratching; after
  → SKIN - Thick - scratching; skin becomes thick after
  → GENE - Wounds - large - scratching; from
  → GENE - Wounds - small - scratching; from
- **shearing** animals; ailments after
  → NOSE - Coryza - cutting the hair from
  → GENE - Hair - cutting - agg.
- **shoes** are left at an unusual place ; uncomfortable when
  → MIND - Conscientious about trifles
- **sleep**; always the same position when going to
  → SLEE - Position
- **stand** still ; cannot
  → MIND - Restlessness - driving about
  → EXTR - Restlessness - Feet
- **suckling** her young
  → RECT - Diarrhea - nursing the child agg.; after
  → FEMA - Lochia - nursing the child agg.; when

→ FEMA - Metrorrhagia - nursing the child agg.; when

→ CHES - Pain - Mammae - Nipples - nursing the child - when - agg.

- **travelling**; doesn't tolerate
  → MIND - Anxiety - riding while - fast in a car
  → MIND - Fear - train; while travelling by
  → MIND - Fear - travelling of
  → MIND - Riding - carriage; in a - aversion to
  → STOM - Nausea - riding - carriage; in a - agg.
  → STOM - Vomiting - riding in a carriage agg. - while
  → GENE - Riding - car in a - agg.
  → GENE - Travelling - ailments from

- **urticaria**
  → SKIN - Eruptions - urticaria
  vertigo in old animals
  → EAR - Vestibular syndrome - old people; in

- **veterinarian**; angry towards the
  → MIND - Anger - veterinarian; towards the
  → MIND - Biting - people - veterinarian; the
  → MIND - Hysteria - veterinarian; when being at the
  → MIND - Kicking - veterinarian or the owner; the
  → MIND - Kicking - veterinarian or the owner; the - anger; from

- **weaning**
  → MIND - Ailments from - weaning too early
  → MIND - Forsaken feeling - weaning; when
  → MIND - Restlessness - weaning; after
  → RECT - Diarrhea - weaning after
  → SLEE - Sleelessness - children; in - weaning; after
  → SKIN - Eruptions - weaning; after
  → GENE - Ailments from - weaned too early; being

- **young** animals
  → MIND - Anxiety - children
  → MIND - Destructiveness - children; in
  → MIND - Dirty - urinating and defecating - everywhere - children
  → MIND - Disobedience - children in
  → MIND - Dullness - children in
  → MIND - Escape attempts to - waking; on - children
  → MIND - Excitement - alternating with - sleepiness - children; in
  → MIND - Fear - children in
  → MIND - Hiding - himself - children
  → MIND - Irritability - children in
  → MIND - Jumping - children; in
  → MIND - Laziness - children in
  → MIND - Playing - aversion to play - children; in
  → MIND - Restlessness - children in
  → MIND - Sadness - children in
  → MIND - Striking - children; in
  → MIND - Washing - aversion to wash - children in
  → EYE - Discharges - bloody - watery - children; in
  → EYE - Inflammation - children; in
  → EAR - Inflammation - Media - children; in

Any animals – **young** animals...
→ THRO - Inflammation - children; in
→ STOM - Vomiting - children; in
→ ABDO - Bleeding - Umbilicus - children; in - infants
→ RECT - Constipation - children; in
→ RECT - Diarrhea - children; in
→ RECT - Eruptions - Anus; about - children; in
→ RECT - Hemorrhage from anus - children; in
→ BLAD - Urination - involuntary - children; in
→ MALE - Erections - children; in
→ RESP - Difficult - children; in
→ CHES - Inflammation - Lungs - children; in
→ SKIN - Erysipelas - children; in
→ GENE - Children; complaints in
→ GENE - Convulsions - children; in
→ GENE - Emaciation - children; in
→ GENE - Obesity - children; in

ANY CARNIVORES; symptoms and behavior of:
- **fish**; aversion to canned or dried
  → GENE - Food and drinks - fish - aversion
- **fish**; desire for canned or dried
  → GENE - Food and drinks - fish - desire

ANY MAMMALS ; symptoms and behavior of:
- **biting** his paws
  → MIND - Biting - fingers
  → MIND - Biting - hands
- **black** dots in face or mucous membranes of facial region
  → NOSE - Freckles
  → FACE - Freckles
  → SKIN - Freckles
- **sucklings**
  → EYE - Inflammation - children; in - newborns
  → EYE - Ulceration - Cornea - children; in - newborns
  → FACE - Wrinkled - children; in - newborns
  → STOM - Vomiting; type of - blood - children; in - newborns; in
  → ABDO - Discharge from umbilicus - children; in - newborns
  → ABDO - Ulcers - Umbilicus about - children; in - newborns
  → RECT - Constipation - children; in - newborns
  → RECT - Diarrhea - children; in - newborns
  → STOO - Bloody - children; in - newborns
  → RESP - Difficult - children; in - newborns
  → SKIN - Eruptions - children; in - newborns; in
  → GENE - Children; complaints in - newborns
  → GENE - Convulsions - children; in
  → GENE - Emaciation - children; in - newborns; in
  → GENE - Weakness - children; in - newborns; in

BIRDS; symptoms and behavior of:
- **picking** feathers
  → MIND - Ailments from - grief
  → MIND - Company - desire for - alone agg.; when

- **picking** feathers...
  - → MIND - Monomania
  - → MIND - Picking with the beak - feathers - others; of
  - → MIND - Picking with the beak - feathers - own; his
  - → MIND - Pulling - hair
  - → MIND - Pulling - hair - desire to pull - her own hair
  - → HEAD - Hair - falling - grief; from

CATTLE; symptoms and behavior of:
- **bull**-like behavior in cows
  - → MIND - Mannish - behavior - women; in
  - → MIND - Mannish - women
- **fore** hoof
  - → EXTR - Fingers; complaints of
  - → EXTR - Hands; complaints of
  - → EXTR - Pain - Fingers
  - → EXTR - Pain - Hands
- **hind** hoof
  - → EXTR - Feet; complaints of
  - → EXTR - Pain - Feet
  - → EXTR - Pain - Toes
  - → EXTR - Toes; complaints of
- **hooves** and claws breaking off
  - → EXTR - Nails; complaints of - brittle nails
- **hyperplasia;** interdigital
  - → EXTR - Swelling - Fingers - Between
- **milk** producing cows
  - → CHES - Milk - flowing spontaneously
- **pointy** things and nails ; after standing in
  - → EXTR - Injuries - Fingers - Nails of
  - → EXTR - Injuries - Toes - Nails - Root
- **Rusterholz'**ulcera in soles
  - → GENE - Wounds - penetrating punctured - Palms and soles of
- **side** is dirtier; one
  - → SLEE - Position
- **snow;** licking
  - → GENE - Food and drinks - cold drink cold water - desire

CATS; symptoms and behavior of:
- **biting:**
  - • **family;** her
    - → MIND - Biting
    - → MIND - Biting - people - family; her
- **constipation** in cats who only live inside the house
  - → RECT - Constipation - sedentary habits agg.
- **constipation** in older cats that cannot go outdoors
  - → RECT - Constipation - sedentary habits agg.
- **eyes,** brown spots on iris
  - → SKIN - Discoloration - spots - dark spots - old people; in
- **fear** of climbing trees
  - → MIND - Fear - high places of
  - → VERT - High - places

Cats; symptoms and behavior of...
- **feline** urological syndrome (FUS)
  - → URIN - Sediment - oxalate of calcium lime
  - → URIN - Sediment - phosphates
  - → URIN - Sediment - sand - gravel
- **fish;** aversion to canned or dried
  - → GENE - Food and drinks - fish - aversion
- **fish;** desire for canned or dried
  - → GENE - Food and drinks - fish - desire
- **fore** claw
  - → EXTR - Fingers; complaints of
  - → EXTR - Hands; complaints of
  - → EXTR - Pain - Fingers
  - → EXTR - Pain - Hands
- **hind** claw
  - → EXTR - Feet; complaints of
  - → EXTR - Pain - Feet
  - → EXTR - Pain - Toes
  - → EXTR - Toes; complaints of
- **holiday** flats or houses; loves
  - → MIND - Travelling - desire for
- **indented** tongue
  - → MOUT - Indented - Tongue
- **lap,** but seeks to be near the owners; never sits on the
  - → MIND - Company - aversion to - fear of being alone; yet
- **lap;** doesn't want to be on the
  - → MIND - Company - aversion to
- **leukemia;** feline
  - → EYE - Pupils - insensible to light
  - → EYE - Pupils - unequal
  - → GENE - Leukemia
  - → GENE - Leukemia - feline leukemia
  - → GENE - Leukemia - seronegative; getting
- **lying** next to other animals; aversion of
  - → MIND - Aversion - persons - certain to - bed; lying next to him in
- **marking,** urinating indoors
  - → MIND - Dirty - urinating and defecating - indoors
  - → MIND - Dirty - urinating deliberately - indoors
  - → MIND - Dirty - urinating deliberately - urine spraying in the house or flat
- **pupils;** unequal
  - → EYE - Pupils - unequal
- **snow;** licking
  - → GENE - Food and drinks - cold drink cold water - desire
- **tickled** on the tummy; aversion to be
  - → ABDO - Clothing; sensitive to
- **trembling** of tongue
  - → MOUT - Trembling of tongue
- **vomiting** during stool
  - → STOM - Vomiting - stool - during
- **wrinkled** forehead
  - → FACE - Wrinkled - Forehead

DOGS; symptoms and behavior of:
- **abscesses** between the toes
  - → EXTR - Eruptions - Hands - Between the fingers - boils
  - → EXTR - Eruptions - Toes - Between - boils
  - → SKIN - Eruptions - boils - periodical
- **biting** people
  - → MIND - Biting
  - → MIND - Biting - people - approached; when being
  - → MIND - Biting - people - approached; when being - bed; while lying in the owner's bed
  - → MIND - Biting - people - approaching; when someone is - owner's bed; the
  - → MIND - Biting - people - approaching; when someone is - sleeping place; the
  - → MIND - Biting - people - disturbs him; bites everyone who
  - → MIND - Biting - people - owners - trifles; because of
  - → MIND - Rage - biting with
- **bleeding** gums when playing with sticks
  - → MOUT - Bleeding - Gums - cleaning them when
- **cleaning** branches
  - → MIND - Branches - chew branches vigorously; must
  - → MIND - Cleanness - mania for - branches wooden sticks; cleaning
  - → MIND - Tidy - branches in the fur coat are extremely disturbing when walking
- **cough** after drinking
  - → COUG - Drinking - after
- **covers**; desire for
  - → GENE - Covers - amel. - desire for; and
- **dropping** food in puppies
  - → MIND - Awkward - young animals; in
  - → GENE - Walking - learning to walk - late
- **ear**; hematoma of
  - → EAR - Swelling - Lobes
  - → EAR - Swelling - Lobes - hematoma
  - → EAR - Swelling - Lobes - hematoma - bluish
- **eversion** of eyelids
  - → EYE - Eversion of lids
- **everything**; eating
  - → GENE - Food and drinks - everything - desire
- **eyes** open when sleeping
  - → EYE - Open lids - sleep; during
- **fear** in between animals of their own species
  - → MIND - Fear - crowd in a
- **fear** of new things lying around
  - → MIND - Conscientious about trifles
  - → MIND - Fastidious
  - → MIND - Fear - trifles of
  - → MIND - Starting - trifles at
- **fore** paw
  - → EXTR - Fingers; complaints of
  - → EXTR - Hands; complaints of
- **fore** paw...
  - → EXTR - Pain - Fingers
  - → EXTR - Pain - Hands
- **forehead**; high
  - → HEAD - Domed forehead
- **forehead**; wrinkled
  - → FACE - Wrinkled - Forehead
- **growling** in sleep when disturbed
  - → MIND - Growling - sleep; when disturbed in
- **hiding** bones
  - → MIND - Avarice
  - → MIND - Delusions - poor; he is
  - → MIND - Fear - poverty of
  - → MIND - Fear - starving of
- **holes**; in
  - → MIND - Avarice
  - → MIND - Delusions - poor; he is
  - → MIND - Fear - poverty of
  - → MIND - Fear - starving of
- **not** eating one single bone
  - → MIND - Avarice
  - → MIND - Delusions - poor; he is
  - → MIND - Fear - poverty of
  - → MIND - Fear - starving of
- **hind** paw
  - → EXTR - Feet; complaints of
  - → EXTR - Pain - Feet
  - → EXTR - Pain - Toes
  - → EXTR - Toes; complaints of
- **inversion** of lids
  - → EYE - Inversion of lids
- **leukorrhea**
  - → FEMA - Leukorrhea
- **lip** eczema of spaniels
  - → FACE - Eruptions - Lips - Lower
  - → GENE - Family history of - eczema
- **lying** with head covered
  - → SLEE - Position - head - covered with sheet
- **masturbation** in isolated dogs
  - → MALE - Masturbation; disposition to
- **mouth**; excoriated corners of
  - → FACE - Excoriation - Mouth; corners of
- **mouth** open during sleep
  - → MOUT - Open - sleep agg.; during
- **nose**; warts on
  - → NOSE - Warts
- **puppies**:
  - **anger** towards her puppies
    - → MIND - Anger - children; towards - own children; towards one's
- **retinal** atrophy; progressive
  - → EYE - Atrophy - Retina - progressive
  - → VISI - Dim - night
- **rolling** in feces
  - → MIND - Rolling - feces or cow-dung; in

- **running** away for a long walk
  → MIND - Travelling - desire for
- **snow**; licking
  → GENE - Food and drinks - cold drink cold water - desire
- **stool** softer after walking
  → STOO - Hard - followed by - soft stool
- **tickled** on the tummy; aversion to be
  → ABDO - Clothing; sensitive to
- **touched** ; aversion to being
  → MIND - Touched - aversion to be - sleep; during
- **vestibular** syndrome
  → VERT - Fall tendency to - right to
  → VERT - Old animals; in - vestibular syndrome
  → VERT - Swaying - right to
  → VERT - Walking - circle; in a
  → EYE - Movement - involuntary
  → EAR - Vestibular syndrome - old people; in
  → MOUT - Salivation
  → GENE - Walking - circle in a
- **vomiting** food
  → STOM - Vomiting - cough - during - agg.
  → STOM - Vomiting; type of - food - cough agg.

GUINEA PIGS; symptoms and behavior:
- **paralysis**
  → EXTR - Paralysis - ascending
  → EXTR - Paralysis - Lower limbs

HORSES; symptoms and behavior of:
- **barn** doors; fear when walking through
  → MIND - Fear - narrow place in
- **demanding** too much while training or breaking in a horse
  → MIND - Ailments from - abused; after being - demanding too much while training or breaking in a horse
  → MIND - Ailments from - mental exertion
  → MIND - Anger - abused; after being - demanding too much while training or breaking in a horse
- **fear** in between animals of their own species
  → MIND - Fear - horses; of - herd of horses; in a
- **fear** of new things lying around
  → MIND - Conscientious about trifles
  → MIND - Fastidious
  → MIND - Fear - trifles of
  → MIND - Starting - trifles at
- **fore** hoof
  → EXTR - Fingers; complaints of
  → EXTR - Hands; complaints of
  → EXTR - Pain - Fingers
  → EXTR - Pain - Hands
- **girth** is fastened; don't like that the
  → ABDO - Clothing; sensitive to
  → ABDO - Pain - pressure - agg.
  → CHES - Clothing agg.
- **headshakers**
  → HEAD - Headshaker

- **Horses**; symptoms and behavior of – **headshakers**...
  → HEAD - Jerking of the head - headshaker
  → FACE - Pain - Nerves - Trigeminal neuralgia
- **heaves**
  → CHES - Heaves
  → CHES - Heaves - air amel.; open
- **hind** hoof
  → EXTR - Feet; complaints of
  → EXTR - Pain - Feet
  → EXTR - Pain - Toes
  → EXTR - Toes; complaints of
- **hyperplasia**; interdigital
  → EXTR - Swelling - Fingers - Between
- **laminitis**
  → EXTR - Inflammation - Laminae
- **moonblindness**
  → EYE - Inflammation - Iridochoroiditis - recurrent
- **pointy** things and nails ; after standing in
  → EXTR - Injuries - Fingers - Nails of
  → EXTR - Injuries - Toes - Nails - Root
- **roaring**
  → LARY - Paralysis - Vocal cord - hemiplegia
- **Rusterholz´**ulcera in soles
  → GENE - Wounds - penetrating punctured - Palms and soles of
- **saddleback**
  → BACK - Curvature of spine - lordosis
  → BACK - Tuberculosis - Vertebrae; of - accompanied by - curvature of spine
- **saddled**; refuses to be
  → ABDO - Clothing; sensitive to
  → ABDO - Pain - pressure - agg.
  → CHES - Clothing agg.
  → BACK - Sensitive - rider; under the
  → BACK - Straining; easily
- **shoeing**; abscess after
  → EXTR - Abscess - shoeing; after
- **shoeing**; punctured wounds from
  → GENE - Wounds - penetrating punctured
- **side** is dirtier; one
  → SLEE - Position
- **smegma** ; increased
  → MALE - Smegma - increased
- **snow**; licking
  → GENE - Food and DRINKS - cold drink cold water - desire
- **transporter**; loves travelling with the
  → MIND - Travelling - desire for

PIGS; symptoms and behavior of:
- **atrophic** rhinitis
  → NOSE - Caries
  → NOSE - Inflammation - atrophic
  → NOSE - Ozena
- **banana** disease
  → BACK - Necrosis - Muscles

- **piglets**:
  - **anger** towards her piglets
    → MIND - Anger - children; towards - own children; towards one's

RABBITS; symptoms and behavior of

List of remedy abbreviations

10 (Paterson) = bacls-10.
7 (Paterson) = bacls-7.

a-dnitroph.	alpha-dinitrophenolum
abel.	abelmoschus
abies balsamea = abies-c.	
abies-c.	abies canadensis
abies-n.	abies nigra
abr.	abrus precatorius
abrom-a.	abroma augusta
abrom-a-r.	abroma augusta radix
abrot.	abrotanum
absin.	absinthium
acal.	acalypha indica
acanthia lectularia = cimx.	
acanthus mollis = bran.	
acer negundo = neg.	
acet-ac.	aceticum acidum
acetan.	acetanilidum
acetylch.	acetylcholine
acetylch-m.	acetylcholinum muriaticum
acetyls-ac.	acetylsalicylicum acidum
achil-m.	achillea moschata
achillea millefolium = mill.	
achy.	achyranthes calea
achy-a.	achyranthes aspera
acidum aceticum glaciale = acet-ac.	
acidum benzoicum = benz-ac.	
acidum boricum = bor-ac.	
acidum butyricum = but-ac.	
acidum cis aconiticum = acon-ac.	
acidum hydriodicum = iod-h.	
acidum hydrochloricum = mur-ac.	
acidum hydroiodicum = iod-h.	
acidum lacticum = lac-ac.	
acidum maleicum = mal-ac.	
acidum phosphoricum = ph-ac.	
acidum picronitricum = pic-ac.	
acidum salicylicum = sal-ac.	
acidum silicicum = sil.	
acidum tartaricum = tart-ac.	
acokanthera schimperi = car.	
acon.	aconitum napellus
acon-a.	aconitum anthora
acon-ac.	aconiticum acidum
acon-c.	aconitum cammarum

acon-f.	aconitum ferox
acon-l.	aconitum lycoctonum
acon-s.	aconitum septentrionale
aconin.	aconitinum
acorus calamus = calam.	
act-sp.	actaea spicata
actaea racemosa = cimic.	
actea racemosa = cimic.	
actea spicata = act-sp.	
ACTH = cortico.	
adam.	adamas
adax.	adaxukah
adel.	Adelheid aqua
Adelheid quelle = adel.	
adelpha bredowii = limen-b-c.	
adeps suillus depuratus = adeps-s.	
adeps suillus = adeps-s.	
adeps-s.	adeps suis
adhatoda vasika = just.	
adhatoda = just.	
adlu.	adlumia fungosa
adn = des-ac.	
adon.	adonis vernalis
adon-ae.	adonis aestivalis
adonin.	adonidinum
adox.	adoxa moschatellina
adren.	adrenalinum
adrenocorticotropinum = cortico.	
aegle-f.	aegle folia
aegle-m.	aegle marmelos
aesc.	aesculus hippocastanum
aesc-c.	aesculus carnea
aesc-g.	aesculus glabra
aeth.	aethusa cynapium
aethanolum = alco.	
aether aethylicus = aether	
aether sulphuricus = aether	
aether	aether
aethi-a.	aethiops antimonialis
aethi-m.	aethiops mineralis
aethyl alcohol = alco.	
aethyl.	aethylium
aethyl-act.	aethylium aceticum
aethyl-n.	aethylium nitricum
aethyl-s-d.	aethylium sulfuricum dichloratum

List of remedy abbreviations

aethylicum = aethyl.
aethylium nitrosum = nit-s-d.
aethylum aceticum = aethyl-act.
aethylum nitricum = aethyl-n.
aethylum oxidum = aether

agar. — agaricus muscarius
agar-cit. — agaricus citrinus
agar-cpn. — agaricus campanulatus
agar-cps. — agaricus campestris
agar-em. — agaricus emeticus
agar-pa. — agaricus pantherinus
agar-ph. — agaricus phalloides
agar-pr. — agaricus procerus
agar-se. — agaricus semiglobatus
agar-st. — agaricus stercorarius
agaricus bulbosus = agar-ph.
agaricus laricis = bol-la.
agarin. — agaricinum
agav-a. — agave Americana
agav-t. — agave tequilana
agave rigida = agav-t.
agkistrodon contortrix = cench.
agkistrodon piscivorus = ancis-p.
agn. — agnus castus
agra. — agraphis nutans
agri. — agrimonia eupatoria
agro. — agrostema githago
agropyron repens = tritic.
agropyrum repens = tritic.
agrostemma githago = agro.
agrosti-a. — agrostis alba
agrosti-vg. — agrostis vulgaris
ail. — ailanthus glandulosa
ailanthus altissima = ail.
aka joanesia asoca = joan.
alarconia helenoides = wye.
alco. — alcoholus
ald. — aldehydum
alet. — aletris farinosa
alexandra senna = senn.
alf. — alfalfa
alis-p. — alisma plantago
alkekengi = physal-al.
all-c. — allium cepa
all-s. — allium sativum
allox. — alloxanum

allylsulfocarbamida = thiosin.
aln. — alnus rubra
alnus serrulata = aln.
aloe vera = aloe
aloe — aloe socotrina
alpha-tocopherolum = tocoph.
alpina officinarum = galan.
alpinia officinarum = galan.
alsidium helminthocorton = helm.
alsine media = stel.
alst. — alstonia constricta
alst-b. — alstonia boonei
alst-s. — alstonia scholaris
alth. — althaea officinalis
alting-e. — altingia excellsa
alum. — alumina
alum-p. — alumina phosphorica
alum-sil. — alumina silicata
alumen chronicum = kali-s-chr.
alumen crudum = alumn.
alumin. — aluminium metallicum
alumin-act. — aluminium aceticum
alumin-m. — aluminium muriaticum
alumin-p. — aluminium phosphoricum
alumin-sil. — aluminium silicicum
aluminii chloridum hexahydricum = alumin-m.
aluminium chloridum = alumin-m.
aluminium kalium sulphuricum = alumn.
aluminium oxide = alum.
aluminium silico-sulpho-calcite = slag
aluminum chloridum = alumin-m. .
alumn. — alumen
am-act. — ammonium aceticum
am-be. — ammonium benzoicum
am-br. — ammonium bromatum
am-c. — ammonium carbonicum
am-caust. — ammonium causticum
am-i. — ammonium iodatum
am-m. — ammonium muriaticum
am-n. — ammonium nitricum
am-p. — ammonium phosphoricum
am-pic. — ammonium picricum
am-t. — ammonium tartaricum
am-val. — ammonium valerianicum
am-van. — ammonium vanadinicum
amanita bulbosa = agar-ph.

List of remedy abbreviations

amanita muscaria = agar.

amanita phalloides = agar-ph.

amara = ign.

ambr. ambra grisea

ambra succinum = succ.

ambro. ambrosia artemisiaefolia

aminoaceticum acidum = glyco.

aminobenzene = anil.

aminobenzolum = anil.

aml-ns. amylenum nitrosum

amm-fml. ammonium formaldehydum

ammc. ammoniacum gummi

ammoniacum = ammc.

ammonii chloridum = am-m.

ammonium auricum = aur-fu.

ammonium chloratum = am-m.

ammonium chloridum = am-m.

ammonium hydratum = am-caust.

amn-l. amnii liquor

amor-r. amorphophallus riviere

amoracia = coch.

ampe-qu. ampelopsis quinquefolia

ampe-tr. ampelopsis trifoliata

amph. amphisbaena vermicularis

amphet-s. amphetaminum sulfuricum

amyg. amygdalus communis

amyg-p. amygdalus persica

amygdala amara = amyg.

amygdalae amarae aqua = amyg.

amygdalus communis amara = amyg.

amylam. amylaminum hydrochloricum

amylium nitricum = aml-ns.

amylium nitrosum = aml-ns.

amyloc-m. amylocainum muriaticum

anac. anacardium orientale

anac-oc. anacardium occidentale

anag. anagallis arvensis

anagy. anagyris foetida

anagyroides = cyt-l.

anamirta cocculus = cocc.

anan. anantherum muricatum

anas barbariae hepatinii et cardiae extractum = oscilloc.

ancis-p. ancistrodon piscivorus

ancistrodon contortrix = cench.

ancistrodon mokeson = cench.

andalusite rock = alum-sil.

anders. andersonia

andira araroba = chrysar.

andira inermis = geo.

andr. androsace lactea

androc. androctonus amoreuxii hebraeus

androctonus amurreuxi hebraeus = androc.

androctonus Australis = buth-a.

androg-p. andrographis paniculata

andromeda arborea = oxyd.

andropogon muraticus = anan.

andropogon muricatus = anan.

andropogon squarrosus = anan.

anemone hepatica = hepat.

anemone ludoviciana = puls-n.

anemone nuttaliana = puls-n.

anemone pratensis = puls.

anemone pulsatilla = puls.

anemps. anemopsis californica

anethum foeniculum = foen-an.

anethum vulgare = foen-an.

ang. angustura vera

ange. angelica atropurpurea

ange-s. angelicae sinensis

angelicae sinensis radix = ange-s.

ango. angophora lanceolata

anguillae serum = ser-ang.

angustura falsa = bruc.

angustura spuria falsa = bruc.

angustura spuria = bruc.

anh. anhalonium lewinii

anil. anilinum

anis. anisum stellatum

anisatum = anis.

ankistrodon contortrix mokeson = cench.

ankistrodon contortrix = cench.

anona triloba = asim.

ant-ar. antimonium arsenicosum

ant-c. antimonium crudum

ant-i. antimonium iodatum

ant-m. antimonium muriaticum

List of remedy abbreviations

ant-o.   antimonium oxydatum
ant-s-aur.   antimonium sulphuratum
    auratum
ant-s-r.   antimonium sulphuratum
    rubrum
ant-t.   antimonium tartaricum
antennaria dioica = gnaph.
anth.   anthemis nobilis
anthemis pyrethrum = pyre-p.
antho.   anthoxanthum odoratum
anthraci.   anthracinum
anthraco.   anthracokali
anthrakokali = anthraco.
anthraq.   anthraquinone
anthrokokali = anthraco.
antiaris toxicaria = upa-a.
antifebrinum = acetan.
antimonium arsenicicum = ant-ar.
antimonium chloridum = ant-m.
antimonium sulphuratum aureum = ant-s-aur.
antimonium sulphuratum nigrum = ant-c.
antip.   antipyrinum
antirrhinum linaria = lina.
ap-d.   apium dulce
ap-g.   apium graveolens
apat.   apatit
aphis   aphis chenopodii glauci
apiol.   apiolum
apisin.   apisinum
apis   apis mellifica
apium petroselinum = petros.
apium virus = apisin.
apoc.   apocynum cannabinum
apoc-a.   apocynum
    androsaemifolium
apom.   apomorphinum
    hydrochloricum
apom-m.   apomorphinum
    muriaticum
apomorphia = apom.
apomorphini hydrochloridum = apom-m.
append-xyz.   appendictitis nosode
    unknown species
aq-calc.   aqua calcarea
aq-mar.   aqua marina
aq-pet.   aqua petra
aq-sil.   aqua silicata

aqua calcis = aq-calc.
aqua regia = nit-m-ac.
aqua sanicula = sanic.
aqueous calendula = calen.
aqui.   aquilegia vulgaris
arag.   aragallus lamberti
aral.   aralia racemosa
aral-h.   aralia hispida
aralia ginseng = gins.
aralia quinquefolia = gins.
aran.   aranea diadema
aran-ix.   aranea ixobola
aran-sc.   aranea scinencia
aranea avicularia = mygal.
araneae tela = tela
aranearum tela = tela
araneus ixobolus Thorell = aran-ix.
araroba = chrysar.
arb.   arbutus andrachne
arbin.   arbutinum
arbor tristis = nyct.
arbutus uva ursi = uva
arctium lappa = lappa
arctium majus = lappa
arctostaphylos uva ursi = uva
arctostaphylos uva-ursi = uva
arec.   areca catechu
aren.   arenaria glabra
arg-cy.   argentum cyanatum
arg-i.   argentum iodatum
arg-met.   argentum metallicum
arg-mur.   argentum muriaticum
arg-n.   argentum nitricum
arg-o.   argentum oxydatum
arg-p.   argentum phosphoricum
arg-s.   argentum sulfuricum
arge.   argemone mexicana
arge-och.   argemone ochroleuca
argenti nitras = arg-n.
argentum chloratum = arg-mur.
argentum foliatum = arg-met.
argilla = alum.
arisaema atrorubens = arum-t.
arisaema triphyllum = arum-t.
arist-cl.   aristolochia clematitis
arist-m.   aristolochia milhomens

List of remedy abbreviations

aristolochia cymbifera = arist-m.	
aristolochia infesta = arist-cl.	
aristolochia serpentaria = serp.	
armoracia lapathifolia = coch.	
armoracia rusticana = coch.	
armoracia sativa = coch.	
arn.	arnica montana
ars.	arsenicum album
ars-br.	arsenicum bromatum
ars-h.	arsenicum hydrogenisatum
ars-i.	arsenicum iodatum
ars-met.	arsenicum metallicum
ars-n.	arsenicum nitricum
ars-s-f.	arsenicum sulphuratum flavum
ars-s-r.	arsenicum sulphuratum rubrum
arsenicum citrinum = ars-s-f.	
arsenicum rubrum = ars-s-r.	
arsenicum stibiatum = ant-ar.	
arsenicum tri-iodatum = ars-i.	
arsenicum tri-oxidum = ars.	
art-v.	artemisia vulgaris
artanthe elongata = mati.	
artemisia abrotanum = abrot.	
artemisia absinthium = absin.	
artemisia cina = cina	
artemisia contra = cina	
artemisia judaica = cina	
artemisia maritima = cina	
artemisia selengensis = art-v.	
arthr-u.	uratic arthritis nosode
arum seguinum = calad.	
arum-d.	arum dracontium
arum-dru.	arum dracunculus
arum-i.	arum italicum
arum-m.	arum maculatum
arum-t.	arum triphyllum
arund.	arundo mauritanica
arund-d.	arundo donax
asaf.	asa foetida
asagraea officinalis = sabad.	
asar.	asarum Europaeum
asar-c.	asarum canadense
asar-o.	asarum officinale

asarum rotundifolium = asar.	
asc-c.	asclepias cornuti
asc-i.	asclepias incarnata
asc-t.	asclepias tuberosa
ascar-l.	ascaris lumbricoides
ascaris vermicularis = enterob-v.	
asclepias decumbens = asc-t.	
asclepias gigantea = calo.	
asclepias syriaca = asc-c.	
asclepias vincetoxicum = vince.	
ashoka = joan.	
asim.	asimina triloba
aspar.	asparagus officinalis
asper.	asperula odorata
aspidin.	aspidospermium
aspidium filix mas = fil.	
aspidium panna = pann.	
aspidium = fil.	
aspidosperma quebracho = queb.	
aspidospermina = aspidin.	
aspirinum = acetyls-ac.	
assaku = hura	
astac.	astacus fluviatilis
aster.	asterias rubens
asteriacanthion rubens = aster.	
asthm-r.	asthma nosode Reckeweg
astra-e.	astragalus excapus
astra-m.	astragalus menziesii
astragalus mollissimus = astra-m.	
atha.	athamanta oreoselinum
atis.	atista indica
atis-r.	atista radix
atox.	atoxyl
atra-r.	atrax robustus
atri.	atriplex hortensis
atro.	atropinum-pur. + -s. (old abbr.)
atro-pur.	atropinum purum
atro-s.	atropinum sulphuricum
atropa bella-donna = bell.	
atropa belladona = bell.	
atropa mandragora = mand.	
atropini sulfas = atro-s.	
aur.	aurum metallicum
aur-ar.	aurum arsenicum
aur-br.	aurum bromatum

List of remedy abbreviations

aur-fu. — aurum fulminans
aur-i. — aurum iodatum
aur-m. — aurum muriaticum
aur-m-k. — aurum muriaticum kalinatum
aur-m-n. — aurum muriaticum natronatum
aur-n-f. — aurum natrum fluoricum
aur-p. — aurum phosphoricum
aur-s. — aurum sulphuratum
auran. — aurantii cortex
aurantiacum = ant-s-aur.
aurantii cortex = cit-v.
aurantium = cit-v.
aureum = ant-s-aur.
aurum arsenicicum = aur-ar.
aurum foliatum = aur.
aurum natrium chloratum = aur-m-n.
aven. — avena sativa
aviaire = tub-a.
avic. — avicularia
avocado = pers.
ayahuasca = banis-c.
ayhuasca = banis-c.
aza. — azadirachta indica
bac. — bacillinum Burnett
bac-t. — bacillinum testium
baccae juniperi = juni-c.
bacillus Calmette-Guérin = v-a-b.
bacillus clostridium botulinum = botul.
bacillus Friedländer = mucot.
bacillus leprae = lepr.
bacillus seven (Paterson) = bacls-7.
bacillus ten (Paterson) = bacls-10.
bacls-10. — bacillus 10 (Paterson)
bacls-7. — bacillus 7 (Paterson)
bacterium coli commune = coli.
bacterium coli = coli.
bacterium lactis aerogenes = mucot.
bad. — badiaga
bahia-pulver = chrysar.
baj. — = bry-la. = baja
bals-p. — balsamum peruvianum
bals-t. — balsamum tolutanum
balsamum copaivae siccum = cop.
balsamum copaivae = cop.

balsamum toluiferum = bals-t.
bamb-a. — bambusa arundinacea
bambusa vulgaris = bamb-a.
banana = musa
bananae flos = musa
banis-c. — banisteria caapi
banisteria quitensis = banis-c.
banisteriopsis caapi = banis-c.
bapt. — baptisia tinctoria
bapt-c. — baptisia confusa
baptisia confusa acetica = bapt-c.
bar-act. — baryta acetica
bar-c. — baryta carbonica
bar-i. — baryta iodata
bar-m. — baryta muriatica
bar-n. — baryta nitrica
bar-ox-suc. — baryta oxalsuccinata
bar-p. — baryta phosphorica
bar-s. — baryta sulphurica
barb. — barbae cyprini ova
barbiflora = orthos-s.
barbit. — barbital
barii sulphas = bar-s.
barium aceticum = bar-act.
barium carbonicum = bar-c.
barium chloratum = bar-m.
barium iodatum = bar-i.
barium nitricum = bar-n.
barium oxalsuccinicum = bar-ox-suc.
barium phosphoricum = bar-p.
barium sulfuricum = bar-s.
baros. — barosma crenulatum
barosma crenata = baros.
bart. — Bartfelder aqua
baryosma tongo = tong.
basaka = just.
basil. — basilicum
bcg = v-a-b.
bell. — belladonna
bell-p. — bellis perennis
ben. — benzinum
ben-d. — benzinum dinitricum
ben-n. — benzinum nitricum
benz-ac. — benzoicum acidum
benzenum = benzol.
benzo. — benzoin oderiferum

List of remedy abbreviations

benzol.	benzolum
benzq.	benzoquinonum
berb.	berberis vulgaris
berb-a.	berberis aquifolium
berbin.	berberinum
beryl.	beryllium metallicum
beta rapa = beta	
beta	beta vulgaris
beto.	betonica aquatica
betonica officinalis = stach.	
betonica stachys = stach.	
betu.	betula alba
betula pendula = betu.	
betula verrucosa = betu.	
bignonia caroba = jac-c.	
bignonia catalpa = catal.	
bignonia copaia = jac-c.	
bilinum = fel	
bism.	bismuthum-sn. + -o. (old abbr.)
bism-met.	bismuthum metallicum
bism-n.	bismuthum nitricum
bism-o.	bismuthum oxydatum
bism-sn.	bismuthum subnitricum
bit-ar.	bitis arietans arietans
bit-ga.	bitis gabonica
bitis arietans = bit-ar.	
bix.	bixa orellana
blatta-a.	blatta Americana
blatta-o.	blatta orientalis
blum-o.	blumea odorata
boerh-d.	boerhavia diffusa
boerhavia repens = boerh-d.	
bofareira = ric.	
bol-la.	boletus laricis
bol-lu.	boletus luridus
bol-s.	boletus satanas
bold.	boldo fragrans
boletus pinicola = polyp-p.	
bolus alba = alumin-sil.	
bomb-chr.	bombyx chrysorrhea
bomb-pr.	bombyx processionea
bombyx mori = bomb-chr.	
bomh.	bomhenia
bond.	Bondonneau aqua
bor-ac.	boricum acidum

bor-pur.	borium purum
bora-o.	borago officinalis
boracicum acidum = bor-ac.	
borx.	borax veneta
bos taurus bilis = fel	
both.	bothrops lanceolatus
both-a.	bothrops alternatus
both-ax.	bothrops atrox
bothrops jacara = both.	
bothrops urutu = both.	
botul.	botulinum
bougainvillea = bougv.	
bougmanica = dat-a.	
bougv.	bougenville
bounafa = ferul.	
bov.	bovista lycoperdon
bovista gigantea = bov.	
brach.	brachyglottis repens
brahea serrulata = sabal	
bran.	= acanth-mo. = branca ursina (old abbr.)
brass.	brassica napus oleifera (old abbr.)
brass-c.	brassica campestris
brass-n-o.	brassica napus oleifera
brass-o.	brassica oleracea
brassica alba = sin-a.	
brassica nigra = sin-n.	
brassica rapa = brass-c.	
brayera anthelmintica = kou.	
bro-r.	bromus ramosus
brom.	bromium
bromus racemosus = bro-r.	
bros-gau.	brosimum gaudichaudi
bruc.	brucea antidysenterica
brucel.	brucella melitensis
brucin.	brucinum
brugmansia candida = dat-a.	
brunfelsia hopeana = franc.	
brunfelsia uniflora = franc.	
bry.	bryonia alba
bryophyllum calycinum = kal.	
bryophyllum pinnatum = kal.	
bufo cinereus = bufo	
bufo sahytiensis Mure = bufo-s.	
bufo vulgaris = bufo	

List of remedy abbreviations

bufo-s.   bufo sahytiensis
bufonis saliva = bufo
bufo   bufo rana
bung-cd.   bungarus candidus
bung-fa.   bungarus fasciatus
bungarus facia = bung-fa.
buni-o.   bunias orientalis
bunium carvi = caru.
bursa pastoris = thlas.
but-ac.   butyricum acidum
buth-a.   buthus Australis
butyl chloralhydratum = crot-chlol.
bux.   buxus sempervirens
cac.   cacao
cact.   cactus grandiflorus
cactin-m.   cactinum mexicanum
cactus bonplandii = cere-b.
cactus opuntia = opun-v.
cactus selenicereus grandiflorus = cact.
cactus serpentinus = cere-s.
cadm-act.   cadmium aceticum
cadm-ar.   cadmium arsenicosum
cadm-bi.   cadmium bichromatum
cadm-br.   cadmium bromatum
cadm-calc-f.   cadmium calcarea fluoricum
cadm-chl.   cadmium chloratum
cadm-chr.   cadmium chromatum
cadm-f.   cadmium fluoratum
cadm-gl.   cadmium gluconicum
cadm-i.   cadmium iodatum
cadm-m.   cadmium muriaticum
cadm-met.   cadmium metallicum
cadm-n.   cadmium nitricum
cadm-o.   cadmium oxydatum
cadm-p.   cadmium phosphoricum
cadm-s.   cadmium sulphuratum
cadm-sel.   cadmium selenicosum
cael.   caela zacatechichi
caes-met.   caesium metallicum
caesal-b.   caesalpinia bonducella
caffeinum = coffin.
cahinca racemosa = cain.
cahinca = cain.
cain.   cainca
caj.   cajuputum
cal-bil.   calculus biliari

cal-ren.   calculus renalis
calabar = phys.
calad.   caladium seguinum
calag.   calaguala
calam.   calamus aromaticus
calc.   calcarea carbonica
calc-act.   calcarea acetica
calc-ar.   calcarea arsenicosa
calc-br.   calcarea bromata
calc-caust.   calcarea caustica
calc-chln.   calcarea chlorinata
calc-cn.   calcarea calcinata
calc-f.   calcarea fluorica
calc-hi.   calcarea hydriodica
calc-hp.   calcarea hypophosphorosa
calc-hs.   calcarea hyposulfurosa
calc-i.   calcarea iodata
calc-lac.   calcarea lactica
calc-ln.   calcarea lactica natronata
calc-lp.   calcarea lactophosphorica
calc-m.   calcarea muriatica
calc-n.   calcarea nitrica
calc-o.   calcarea oyxdata
calc-o-t.   calcarea ovi testae
calc-ox.   calcarea oxalica
calc-p.   calcarea phosphorica
calc-pic.   calcarea picrica
calc-s.   calcarea sulphurica
calc-sil.   calcarea silicata
calc-st-s.   calcarea stibiato-sulphurata
calcarea biliaris = cal-bil.
calcarea caustica segini = calc-caust.
calcarea fluorata = calc-f.
calcarea hypochlorata = calc-chln.
calcarea lactica phosphorica = calc-lp.
calcarea renalis praeparata = cal-ren.
calcarea renalis = cal-ren.
calcarea silicica = calc-sil.
calcarea sulphurata hahnemanni = hep.
calcarea sulphurata stibiata = calc-st-s.
calcii arsenias = calc-ar.
calcii bromidum = calc-br.
calcii carbonas = calc.
calcii chloridum = calc-caust.
calcii lactas = calc-lac.

List of remedy abbreviations

calcium aceticum = calc-act.
calcium arsenicosum = calc-ar.
calcium bromatum = calc-br.
calcium carbonicum = calc.
calcium causticum = calc-caust.
calcium chloratum = calc-m.
calcium chlorinatum = calc-chln.
calcium fluoricum = calc-f.
calcium hypophosphoricum = calc-hp.
calcium iodatum = calc-i.
calcium lacticum = calc-lac.
calcium ovi testae = calc-o-t.
calcium oxalicum = calc-ox.
calcium oxydatum = calc-o.
calcium phosphoricum = calc-p.
calcium picricum = calc-pic.
calcium silicatum = calc-sil.
calcium stibiato-sulphuratum = calc-st-s.
calcium sulphuricum = calc-s.
calculus urinae = cal-ren.

calen.	calendula officinalis
calendula cerate = calen.	
calli-h.	calliandra houstoni
callilaris = pin-c.	
calluna vulgaris = eric-vg.	
calo.	calotropis gigantea
calo-l.	calotropis lactum
calomel = merc-d.	
calth.	caltha palustris
camellia sinensis = thea	
campan-ra.	campanula rapunculus
camph.	camphora officinalis
camph-ac.	camphoricum acidum
camph-br.	camphora bromata
camph-mbr.	= camph-br. = camphora monobromata
camphora monobromata = camph-br.	
camphora racemica = camph.	
cancer astacus = astac.	
cancer fluviatilis = astac.	
cancerinum = carc.	
canch.	canchalagua
cand.	candida parapsilosis
candida albicans = moni.	
cann-i.	cannabis indica

cann-s.	cannabis sativa
cann-xyz.	cannabis unknown species
canna	canna angustifolia
canth.	cantharis vesicatoria
canthin.	cantharidinum
capp-crc.	capparis coriaccea
caps.	capsicum annuum
capsella bursa pastoris = thlas.	
capsella bursa-pastoris = thlas.	
car.	carissa schimperi
carb-ac.	carbolicum acidum
carb-an.	carbo animalis
carb-v.	carbo vegetabilis
carbamidum = urea-n.	
carbn.	carboneum
carbn-chl.	carboneum chloratum
carbn-h.	carboneum hydrogenisatum
carbn-o.	carboneum oxygenisatum
carbn-s.	carboneum sulphuratum
carbn-tm.	carboneum tetramuriaticum
carbo ligni = carb-v.	
carboneum tetrachloridum = carbn-tm.	
carc.	carcinosinum
carc-col-ad.	carcinosinum colon adeno
carc-st.	carcinosinum stomach
carc-st-ad.	carcinosinum stomach adeno
carc-st-sc.	carcinosinum stomach scirrhus
carcinosinum burnett = carc.	
carcinosinum foubister = carc.	
carcinosinum mammae scirrhus = scir.	
card-b.	carduus benedictus
card-m.	carduus marianus
cardios-h.	cardiospermum halicacabum
carl.	Carlsbad aqua
carli-a.	carlina acaulis
caroba = jac-c.	
carp-b.	carpinus betulus
carthamnus ceriferus = myric.	
caru.	carum carvi
carum aureum = ziz.	
cary.	carya alba

cas-s.	cascara sagrada
casc.	cascarilla
cascabela thevetia = thev.	
cascara = cas-s.	
cass.	cassada
cassia acutifolia = senn.	
cassia angustifolia = senn.	
cassia senna = senn.	
cassia sophora = cassia-s.	
cassia-f.	cassia fistula
cassia-s.	cassia sophera
castalia pudica = nymph.	
castanea sativa = castn-v.	
castanea vulgaris = castn-v.	
caste.	castella texana
castm.	castoreum canadense
castn-v.	castanea vesca
castor-eq.	castor equi
castoreum muscovitum = castm.	
castoreum sibericum = castm.	
castoreum sibinicum = castm.	
castoreum sibiricum = castm.	
catal.	catalpa bignonoides
catar.	cataria nepeta
catharanthus roseus = vinc-r.	
caul.	caulophyllum thalictroides
caust.	causticum
causticum hahnemanni = caust.	
Cayenne pepper = caps.	
cean.	ceanothus Americanus
cean-tr.	ceanothus thrysiflorus
ceanothus virginiana = cean.	
cecr.	cecropia mexicana
cedr.	cedron
celt.	celtis occidentalis
cem.	cement
cench.	cenchris contortrix
cenchris piscivorus = ancis-p.	
cent.	centaurea tagana
cent-cy.	centaurea cyanus
cent-u.	= centa-er. = centaurium umbellatum (old abbr.)
centaurium erythraea = canch.	
centaurium = canch.	
centella asiatica = hydrc.	

cepa vulgaris = all-c.	
cepa = all-c.	
ceph.	cephalanthus occidentalis
cephaelis ipecacuanha = ip.	
cephd-i.	cephalandra indica
cer-o.	cerium oxydatum
cer-ox.	cerium oxalicum
cer-s.	cerium sulfuricum
cerasus padus = prun-p.	
cerasus virginia = prun-v.	
ceratostigma willmottiana = cerstig-w.	
cerbera thevetia = thev.	
cerc-s.	cercis siliquastrum
cere-b.	cereus bonplandii
cere-s.	cereus serpentinus
cereus grandiflorus = cact.	
cerev-lg.	cerevisia lager
cerevisiae fermentum = tor.	
cerstig-w.	ceratostigma willmottigma
cerv.	cervus brasilicus
cervus brasilicus campestris = cerv.	
cesium metallicum = caes-met.	
ceto.	cetonia aurata
cetr.	cetraria islandica
cham.	chamomilla
chamae.	chamaedrys
chamaecyparis lawsonia = cupre-l.	
chamaelirium carolinianum = helon.	
chamaelirium luteum = helon.	
chamaelirium = helon.	
chamaemelum nobile = anth.	
chamaerops serrulata = sabal	
chamomilla recutita = cham.	
chamomilla romana = anth.	
chamomilla vulgaris = cham.	
chap.	chaparro amargoso
chaul.	chaulmoogra
cheir.	cheiranthus cheiri
chel.	chelidonium majus
chelin.	chelidoninum
chelo.	chelone glabra
chen-a.	chenopodium anthelminticum
chen-g.	chenopodium glaucum
chen-v.	chenopodium vulvaria

List of remedy abbreviations

chen-vg.	chenopodium vulgare
chenopodii glauci aphis = aphis	
chenopodium ambrosioides = chen-a.	
chenopodium olidum = chen-v.	
chicorium intybus = cich.	
chim.	chimaphila umbellata
chim-m.	chimaphila maculata
chin.	china officinalis
chin-b.	china boliviana
chin-su.	cinchona succirubra
chinchonae cortex = chin.	
chinin-ar.	chininum arsenicosum
chinin-brh.	chininum bromhydricum
chinin-fcit.	chininum ferri citricum
chinin-hcy.	chininum hydrocyanicum
chinin-m.	chininum muriaticum
chinin-pur.	chininum purum
chinin-s.	chininum sulphuricum
chinin-sal.	chininum salicylicum
chinini hydrochloridum = chinin-m.	
chinini sulfas = chinin-s.	
chiococca densifolia = cain.	
chiococca racemosa = cain.	
chion.	chionanthus virginica
chionanthus Americana = chion.	
chionanthus latifolia = chion.	
chir-fl.	chironex fleckeri
chlf.	chloroformium
chlol.	chloralum hydratum
chlor.	chlorum
chloram.	chloramphenicolum
chlorinum = chlor.	
chlornitrosum acidum = nit-m-ac.	
chloroformum = chlf.	
chloromycetinum = chloram.	
chlorpr.	chlorpromazinum
cho.	cholas terrapina
choc.	chocolate
chol.	cholesterinum
cholesterolum = chol.	
cholin.	cholinum
chondodendron tomentosa = pareir.	
chondodendron tormentosum = pareir.	
chopn.	chopheenee
chr-ac.	chromicum acidum
chr-met.	chromium metallicum

chr-o.	chromium oxydatum
chr-s.	chromium sulphuricum
chromium kali sulphuratum = kali-s-chr.	
chromium kaliumsulfuricum = kali-s-chr.	
chrys-ac.	chrysophanicum acidum
chrysan.	chrysanthemum leucanthemum
chrysanthemum vulgare = tanac.	
chrysanthenum parthenium = pyre-p.	
chrysar.	chrysarobinum
chrysol.	chrysolite
cic.	cicuta virosa
cic-m.	cicuta maculata
cich.	cichorium intybus
cimic.	cimicifuga racemosa
cimx.	cimex lectularius
cina	cina maritima
cinch.	cinchoninum sulphuricum
cinchona boliviana = chin-b.	
cinchona calisaya = chin-b.	
cinchona officinalis = chin.	
cinchona pubescens = chin-su.	
cinchona regia = chin.	
cine.	cineraria maritima
cinnamomi cortex = cinnm.	
cinnamomum camphora = camph.	
cinnamomum ceylancium = cinnm.	
cinnamonum verum = cinnm.	
cinnb.	cinnabaris
cinnm.	cinnamomum zeylanicum
cinnmd-c.	cinnamodendron corticosum
cisplat.	cisplatina
cist.	cistus canadensis
cistus vulgaris = cist.	
cit-ac.	citricum acidum
cit-d.	citrus decumana
cit-l.	citrus limonum
cit-v.	citrus vulgaris
citrullus colocynthis = coloc.	
citrullus lanatus = cuc-c.	
citrus aurantium = cit-v.	
citrus canadensis = cist.	
cladon.	cladonia pyxidata
claviceps purpurea = sec.	
clem.	clematis erecta

List of remedy abbreviations

clem-vit. clematis vitalba
clematis recta = clem.
clerod-g. clerodendron glabrum
clomip. clomipramine
clostridium botulinum = botul.
cloth. = bit-ar. = clotho arietans
(old abbr.)
clotho arietans = bit-ar.
cnic-ar. cnicus arvensis
cnicus benedictus = card-b.
cob. cobaltum metallicum
cob-act. cobaltum aceticum
cob-m. cobaltum muriaticum
cob-n. cobaltum nitricum
cobaltum chloratum = cob-m.
cobaltum chloridum = cob-m.
cobra corallinus = elaps
coc-c. coccus cacti
cocain. cocainum hydrochloricum
cocaini hydrochloricum = cocain.
cocainum muriaticum = cocain.
coca coca
cocc. cocculus indicus
cocc-s. coccinella septempunctata
cocculus platyphylla = pareir.
coch. cochlearia armoracia
coch-o. cochlearia officinalis
cochlearia armoracea = coch.
cochlearia pyrenaica = coch-o.
cochlearia rusticana = coch.
cod. codeinum
cod-p. codeinum phosphoricum
coenz-a. coenzyme A
coenz-q. coenzyme Q
coff. coffea cruda
coff-t. coffea tosta
coffea arabica = coff.
coffin. coffeinum
cola acuminata = kola
cola nitida = kola
cola vera = kola
colch. colchicum autumnale
colchin. colchicinum
coleus-a. coleus aromaticus
coli. colibacillinum
coll. collinsonia canadensis

collod. collodion
coloc. colocynthis
colocin. colocynthinum
colocynthis citrullus = coloc.
colos. colostrum
colubrina = nux-v.
columbine = aqui.
com. comocladia dentata
combr-r. combretum raimbaultii
con. conium maculatum
conch. conchiolinum
conchae praeparatae = calc.
condurango = cund.
congo-r. congo red
conin. coniinum
conin-br. coniinum bromatum
coninum = conin.
conv. convallaria majalis
convo-a. convolvulus arvensis
convo-d. convolvulus duartinus
convo-s. convolvulus stans
convolvulus purga = jal.
convolvulus purpureus = ipom-p.
convolvulus scammonia = scam.
convolvulus turpenthum = oper.
conyza canadensis = erig.
cop. copaiva officinalis
copahu = cop.
copaiba = cop.
copaifera langdorfii = cop.
copaifera officinalis = cop.
coqueluchinum = pert.
cor-r. corallium rubrum
cordelistris syphilitica = jac-c.
corh. corallorhiza odontorhiza
cori-m. coriaria myrtifolia
cori-r. coriaria ruscifolia
corn. cornus circinata
corn-a. cornus alternifolia
corn-f. cornus florida
corn-s. cornus sericea
coron-v. coronilla varia
corpus luteum = lutin.
cortico. corticotropinum
cortiso. cortisonum
cortisoni acetas = cortiso.

List of remedy abbreviations

cory.	corydalis formosa
cory-c.	corydalis cava
corydalis canadensis = cory.	
corynanthe yohimbe = yohim.	
cot.	cotyledon umbilicus
cotinus coggygria = rhus-c.	
coto	coto
coumarinum = cumin.	
coxs.	coxsackie virus nosode
crat.	crataegus oxyacantha
crataegus laevigata = crat.	
crataegus monogyna = crat.	
creat.	creatinum
cresolum = kres.	
cresylolum = kres.	
croc.	crocus sativus
crocus stigmates = croc.	
crot-c.	crotalus cascavella
crot-chlol.	croton chloralum
crot-h.	crotalus horridus
crot-t.	croton tiglium
croton cascarilla = casc.	
croton chloralhydratum = crot-chlol.	
croton eluteria = casc.	
cryp.	cryptopinum
cub.	cubeba officinalis
cuc-c.	cucurbita citrullus
cuc-p.	cucurbita pepo
cucum-m.	cucumis melo
cucumis colocynthis = coloc.	
culx.	culex musca
cumin.	cumarinum
cund.	cundurango
cunila pulegioides = hedeo.	
cuph.	cuphea viscosissima
cuphea petiolata = cuph.	
cupr.	cuprum metallicum
cupr-act.	cuprum aceticum
cupr-am-s.	cuprum ammoniae sulphuricum
cupr-ar.	cuprum arsenicosum
cupr-c.	cuprum carbonicum
cupr-cy.	cuprum cyanatum
cupr-m.	cuprum muriaticum
cupr-n.	cuprum nitricum
cupr-o.	cuprum oxydatum nigrum

cupr-ox.	cuprum oxalicum
cupr-s.	cuprum sulphuricum
cupre-au.	cupressus Australis
cupre-l.	cupressus lawsoniana
cupri sulfas anhydricus = cupr-s.	
cur.	curare
curc.	= curc-x. = curcuma javanensis (old abbr.)
cuscus = anan.	
cusparia febrifuga = ang.	
cyanhydricum acidum = hydr-ac.	
cycl.	cyclamen Europaeum
cyclamen purpurascens = cycl.	
cyclop.	cyclophosphamide
cyclosp.	cyclosporinum
cyd.	cydonia vulgaris
cymin.	cymarinum
cyn-d.	cynodon dactylon
cyna.	cynara scolymus
cynanchum = vince.	
cypr.	cypripedium pubescens
cystisus laburnum = cyt-l.	
cyt-l.	cytisus laburnum
cytin.	cytisinum
cytisus scoparius = saroth.	
daboia russellii = vip-d.	
daboia = vip-d.	
dactylopius coccus = coc-c.	
dam.	damiana
damiana aphrodisiaca = dam.	
daph.	daphne indica
daphne mezereum = mez.	
daphne odora = daph.	
daphne odorata = daph.	
dat-a.	datura arborea
dat-f.	datura ferox
dat-m.	datura metel
dat-s.	datura sanguinea
datin.	daturinum
datura stramonium = stram.	
del.	delphinus amazonicus
delphin.	delphininum staphysagria
delphinium staphysagria = staph.	
dema.	dematium petraeum
dendr-pol.	dendroaspis polylepsis
denys = tub-d.	

List of remedy abbreviations

deoxyribonucleicum acidum = des-ac.

der.   derris pinnata

derris elliptica = der.

des-ac.   desoxyribonucleicum
                              acidum

dextrum lacticum acidum = sarcol-ac.

di-ammonii phospas = am-p.

diabolus metallorum = stann.

diadema aranea = aran.

dicentra canadensis = cory.

dicentra formosa = cory.

dicha.   dichapetalum

dict.   dictamnus albus

dictamnus = orig-d.

dictamus fraxinella = dict.

dieffenbachia seguinum = calad.

dig.   digitalis purpurea

digin.   digitalinum

digitalis purpureae folium = dig.

digox.   digitoxinum

dikalii carbonas = kali-c.

dikalii phosphas = kali-p.

dikalii sulphas = kali-s.

dinatrii phosphas dodecahydricus = nat-p.

dios.   dioscorea villosa

dioscorea paniculata = dios.

diosm.   diosma lincaris

diosma crenata = baros.

dip.   dipodium punctatum

diph.   diphtherinum

diph-t-tpt.   diphthero-tetano-typho-pa
                              ratyphoidicum

diphthericum = diph.

diphthericum-tetanicum-typho-parathyphoidicum =
diph-t-tpt.

diphtox.   diphtherotoxinum

dipterix odorata = tong.

dirc.   dirca palustris

distemp-vc.   distemperinum vaccinum

dna = des-ac.

dol.   dolichos pruriens

dor.   doryphora decemlineata

dorema ammoniacum = ammc.

doryphora leptinotarsa = dor.

draconitum foetidum = ictod.

dracunculus vulgaris = arum-dru.

dros.   drosera rotundifolia

drymis winteri = cinnmd-c.

dryopteris filix mas = fil.

dryopteris filix-mas = fil.

dt-tab. = diph-t-tpt.

DTTAB = diph-t-tpt.

dub.   duboisinum + dubo-m.
                              (old abbr.)

dubo-h.   duboisia hopwoodi

dubo-m.   duboisia myoporoides

duboin.   duboisinum

duboisinum sulphatum = duboin.

dulc.   dulcamara

durb.   durbital

dys. co. (bach) = dys.

dys.   bacillus dysenteriae
                              (Bach)

dysenteriae (bach) = dys.

dysenteriae compound (bach) = dys.

eaux   Eaux Bonnes aqua

eberth.   eberthinum

ecballium elaterium = elat.

echi.   echinacea angustifolia

echi-p.   echinacea purpurea

echiichthys vipera = trach-v.

echis carinatus = vip-a-c.

echit.   echites suberecta

eel serum = ser-ang.

either = aether

elae.   elaeis guineensis

elaps   elaps corallinus

elat.   elaterium

elaterium officinarum = elat.

elec.   electricitas

electricitas frictionale = elec.

electro-magnetismus = m-ambo.

elem.   = guat. = elemuy gauteria
                              (old abbr.)

elymus repens = tritic.

elytrigia repens = tritic.

emb-r.   embelia ribes

emblc.   embelica officinalis

emeticus = ant-t.

emetin.   emetinum

endymion nutans = agra.

enterob-v.   enterobius vermicularis

List of remedy abbreviations

enteroc.   enterococcinum
enterotoxinum = enteroc.
eos.   eosinum
ephe.   ephedra vulgaris
ephedrini hydrochloridum = ephin-m.
ephin-m.   ephedrinum muriatium
epig.   epigea repens
epigaea repens = epig.
epih.   epihysterinum
epil.   epilobium palustre
epinephrinum = adren.
epiph.   epiphegus virginiana
epiphegus Americanus = epiph.
epiphysinum = pineal.
epiphysis cerebri = pineal.
equis-a.   equisetum arvense
equis-h.   equisetum hyemale
eran.   eranthis hymnalis
erech.   erechthites hieracifolia
ergot.   ergotinum
eric-vg.   erica vulgaris
erig.   erigeron canadense
erinus lobelia = lob-e.
erio.   eriodictyon californicum
eriodyction californicum = erio.
eriodyction glutinosum = erio.
erod.   erodium cicutarium
eruca alba = sin-a.
ery-a.   eryngium aquaticum
ery-m.   eryngium maritimum
eryt-j.   erythrophlaeum judiciale
eryth.   erythrinus
erythraea centaurium = canch.
erythraea chilensis = canch.
erythrina corallodendron = pisc.
erythroxylon coca = coca
esch.   eschscholtzia californica
escherichia coli = coli.
escoba amargo = parth.
esin.   eserinum
esin-sal.   eserinum salicylicum
esp-g.   espeletia grandiflora
esponjilla = luf-op.
estrone = foll.
etherum = aether
ethylene-ethenyl-diamine = lysd.

ethylicum aceticum = aethyl-act.
ethylicum nitricum = aethyl-n.
ethylicum sulfuricum dichloratum = aethyl-s-d.
ethylicum = aethyl.
eucal.   eucalyptus globulus
eucal-r.   eucalyptus rostrata
eucalypti aetheroleum = ol-eucal.
eucalypti folium = eucal.
eucol.   eucalyptolum
eug.   eugenia jambos
eugenia cheken = myrt-ch.
eugenia jambolana = syzyg.
eugenia vulgaris = eug.
euginia chequen = myrt-ch.
euon.   euonymus europaeus
euon-a.   euonymus atropurpurea
euonin.   euonyminum
euonymus Europaea = euon.
euonymus vulgaris = euon.
eup-a.   eupatorium aromaticum
eup-c.   eupatorium cannabinum
eup-per.   eupatorium perfoliatum
eup-pur.   eupatorium purpureum
eupatorium aya-pana = eup-a.
eupatorium satureiaefolium = gua.
eupatorium triplinerve = eup-a.
eupatorium verticullatum = eup-pur.
euph.   euphorbium officinarum
euph-a.   euphorbia amygdaloides
euph-c.   euphorbia corollata
euph-cy.   euphorbia cyparissias
euph-he.   euphorbia heterodoxa
euph-hy.   euphorbia hypericifolia
euph-ip.   euphorbia ipecacuanhae
euph-l.   euphorbia lathyris
euph-m.   euphorbia marginata
euph-pe.   euphorbia peplus
euph-pi.   euphorbia pilulifera
euph-po.   euphorbia polycarpa
euph-pr.   euphorbia prostata
euph-re.   = euph. = euphorbia
    resinifera (old abbr.)
euphorbia sylvatica = euph-a.
euphr.   euphrasia officinalis
euphrasia rostkoviana = euphr.
eupi.   eupionum

List of remedy abbreviations

euryangium sumbul = sumb.
euscorpius italicus = scor.
euspongia officinalis = spong.
evonymus atropurpureus = euon-a.
evonymus Europeus = euon.
evonymus vulgaris = euon.
exogonium purga = jal.

eys.	eysenhardtia polystachia
fab.	fabiana imbricata
faec.	bacillus Faecalis (Bach)

faecalis (bach) = faec.

fago.	fagopyrum esculentum
fagu.	fagus sylvatica
falco-pe.	falcon peregrinus disciplinatus

farfara = tus-fa.
felix domestica lac = lac-f.

fel	fel tauri
ferr.	ferrum metallicum
ferr-act.	ferrum aceticum
ferr-ar.	ferrum arsenicosum
ferr-br.	ferrum bromatum
ferr-c.	ferrum carbonicum
ferr-cit.	ferrum citricum
ferr-cy.	ferrum cyanatum
ferr-i.	ferrum iodatum
ferr-lac.	ferrum lacticum
ferr-m.	ferrum muriaticum
ferr-ma.	ferrum magneticum
ferr-n.	ferrum nitricum
ferr-ox.	ferrum oxalicum
ferr-p.	ferrum phosphoricum
ferr-p-h.	ferrum phosphoricum hydricum
ferr-pern.	ferrum pernitricum
ferr-pic.	ferrum picricum
ferr-prox.	ferrum protoxalatum
ferr-py.	ferrum pyrophosphoricum
ferr-r.	ferrum reductum
ferr-s.	ferrum sulphuricum
ferr-t.	ferrum tartaricum
ferr-val.	ferrum valerianicum

ferrum arsenicicum = ferr-ar.
ferrum chloratum = ferr-m.
ferrum sulfas = ferr-s.

| ferul. | = ferul-gl. = ferula glauca (old abbr.) |

| ferul-ga. | ferula galbanifera |

ferula asa foetida = asaf.
ferula communis = ferul.
ferula moschata = sumb.
ferula narthex = asaf.
ferula scorodosma = asaf.
ferula sumbul = sumb.

fic-c.	ficus carica
fic-r.	ficus religiosa
fic-v.	ficus venosa

ficaria ranunculoides = ran-fi.
ficaria verna = ran-fi.
ficus indica = opun-f.
ficus opuntia = opun-f.
fiel di piedra = flor-p.

| fil. | filix mas |

filipendula ulmaria = spirae.

| fl-ac. | fluoricum acidum |
| flav. | flavus |

flaveinum = lutin.

| flf. | fluoroformium |
| flor-p. | flor de piedra |

flos solis = helia.

| foen. | foeniculum sativum |
| foen-an. | foeniculum anethum |

foeniculum aquaticum = phel.
foeniculum vulgare = foen-an.

foll.	folliculinum
form.	formica rufa
form-ac.	formicicum acidum
formal.	formalinum

formaldehydi solutio = formal.

| frag. | fragaria vesca |

fragaria elatior = frag.

| fram. | framboesinum |
| franc. | franciscea uniflora |

franciscaea uniflora = franc.
frangula = rham-f.
frangulae cortex = rham-f.

franz.	Franzensbad aqua
frax.	fraxinus Americana
frax-e.	fraxinus excelsior
friedr.	Friedrichshaller aqua
fruc-m-s.	fructi mixtus sucus

fructus phytolaccae = phyt-b.

| fuc. | fucus vesiculosus |

List of remedy abbreviations

fuch.   fuchsinum
fuchsin = fuch.
fuli.   fuligo ligni
fum.   fumaria officinalis
fuma-ac.   fumaricum acidum
funiculus umbilicalis suis = suis-chord-umb.
gad.   gadus morrhua
gaert.   bacillus Gaertner (Bach)
gaertner (bach) = gaert.
gal-ac.   gallicum acidum
gal-met.   gallium metallicum
gala.   galanthus nivalis
galan.   galanga
galeg.   galega officinalis
galeoc-c-h.   galeocerdo cuvier hepar
gali.   galium aparine
galin.   galinsoga parviflora
galipea cusparia = ang.
galipea officinalis = ang.
galium odoratum = asper.
gallinae stomachi tunica interior = ing.
galph.   galphimia glauca
galv.   galvanismus
gamb.   gambogia
garcinia hanburyi = gamb.
garcinia morella = gamb.
garcinia sp. = gamb.
gardenalum = phenob.
garlic = all-s.
gast.   Gastein aqua
gaul.   gaultheria procumbens
gaulteriae aetherolum = gaul.
gaultheria humilis = gaul.
gaultheria repens = gaul.
gelin.   gelatinum
gels.   gelsemium sempervirens
gelsemium nitidum = gels.
genist.   genista tinctoria
genista scoparia = saroth.
gent-am.   gentiana amarella
gent-c.   gentiana cruciata
gent-l.   gentiana lutea
gent-q.   gentiana quinquefolia
gentiana quinqueflora = gent-q.
geo.   geoffroya vermifuga
geoffroya inermis = geo.

ger.   geranium maculatum
geranium pusillum = ger.
germ-met.   germanium metallicum
get.   Gettysburg aqua
geum   geum rivale
gink-b.   ginkgo biloba
gins.   ginseng quinquefolium
glanderinum = hippoz.
glandula parathyroidea = parathyr.
glandula parotis = parot.
glandula pinealis = pineal.
glandula suprarenalis = suprar.
glandula thymus = thym-gl.
glandula thyreoidea = thyr.
glech.   glechoma hederacea
glinicum = med.
glon.   glonoinum
gluca.   glucagon
glucagonum = gluca.
glucinium metallicum = beryl.
glyc.   glycerinum
glycinum = glyco.
glyco.   glycocollum
glycosmis pentaphylla = atis.
glycyr-g.   glycyrrhiza glabra
glycyrrhiza glabra linn. = glycyr-g.
glynicum = med.
gnaph.   gnaphalium polycephalum
gnaphalium dioicum = gnaph.
golondrina = euph-po.
gonococcinum = med.
gonolubus cundurango = cund.
gonotox.   gonotoxinum
goss.   gossypium herbaceum
gran.   granatum
granit-m.   granitum murvey
granite murvey = granit-m.
graph.   graphites
graphites naturalis = graph.
grat.   gratiola officinalis
grin.   grindelia robusta
gua.   guaco
guaiacum officinale = guaj.
guaj.   guajacum officinale
guajol.   guajacolum
guako = gua.

List of remedy abbreviations

guan.   guano Australis
guao = com.
guar.   guarana
guaraninum = coffin.
guare.   guarea trichiloides
guarea guidonia = guare.
guat.   guatteria gaumeri
guilandina dioica = gymno.
guips.   guipsinum
gummi guttae = gamb.
gummi gutti = gamb.
gunp.   gunpowder
gymne.   gymnema sylvestre
gymno.   gymnocladus canadensis
gymnocladus dioicus = gymno.
gymnocladus distica = gymno.
gynocardia odorata = chaul.
gyrotheca tinctoria = lachn.
haem.   haematoxylon
                                     campechianum
haff.   haffkine
hagenia abyssinica = kou.
haliae-lc.   haliaeetus leucocephalus
haliaethus leukocapitus = haliae-lc.
hall   Hall aqua
halo.   haloperidolum
ham.   hamamelis virginiana
hamamelis virginica = ham.
harp.   harpagophytum
                                     procumbens
harpagophyti radix = harp.
hecla   Hecla lava
hed.   hedera helix
hedeo.   hedeoma pulegioides
hedy.   hedysarum ildefonsianum
hekla lava = hecla
heli-n.   helianthemum
                                     nummularium
helia.   helianthus annuus
helianthemum canadense = cist.
helianthus vulgare = helia.
helic-p.   helicobacter pylori
helin.   heloninum
helio.   heliotropium peruvianum
helios = sol
hell.   helleborus niger

hell-f.   helleborus foetidus
hell-o.   helleborus orientalis
hell-v.   helleborus viridis
helm.   helminthochortos
helo.   heloderma-h. + -s. (old
                                     abbr.)
helo-h.   heloderma horridum
helo-s.   heloderma suspectum
helon.   helonias dioica
helonias viridis = verat-v.
helx.   helix tosta
hep.   hepar sulphur
hepar sulphuris calcareum = hep.
hepar sulphuris kalinum = kali-sula.
hepar sulphuris = hep.
hepat.   hepatica triloba
hepatica nobilis = hepat.
hera.   heracleum sphondylium
heracleum branca = hera.
heuch.   heuchera Americana
hier-p.   hieracium pilosella
hip-ac.   hippuricum acidum
hipp.   hippomanes
hippomane mancinella = manc.
hippoz.   hippozaeninum
hir.   hirudo medicinalis
hirudo officinalis = hir.
hist.   histaminum
hist-m.   histaminum muriaticum
histamini dihydrochloridum = hist-m.
histaminum hydrochloricum = hist-m.
histrix prehensilis = sphing.
histrix subspinosum = sphing.
hoang-nan = strych-g.
hoit.   hoitzia coccinea
holarrhena antidysenterica = kurch.
holothuria physalis = physala-p.
hom-xyz.   homarus unknown species
home.   homeria collina
hoorali = cur.
hott-p.   hottonia palustris
humulus lupulus = lup.
hura-c.   hura crepitans
hura   hura brasiliensis
hydr.   hydrastis canadensis
hydr-ac.   hydrocyanicum acidum

116

List of remedy abbreviations

hydrang.   hydrangea arborescens
hydrangea frutescens = hydrang.
hydrargyri bichloridum = merc-c.
hydrargyri bijodidum = merc-i-r.
hydrargyri cyanidum = merc-cy.
hydrargyri oxydum rubrum = merc-pr-r.
hydrargyri oxydum subsulphuricum = merc-sul.
hydrargyri subchloridum mite = merc-d.
hydrargyrum bichloratum = merc-c.
hydrargyrum bicyanatum = merc-cy.
hydrargyrum bijodatum rubrum = merc-i-r.
hydrargyrum depuratum = merc.
hydrargyrum oxydulatum nitricum crystallisatum = merc-n.
hydrargyrum stibiato-sulfuratum = aethi-a.
hydrargyrum stibiatosulfuratum = aethi-a.
hydrargyrum sulfuratum = aethi-m.
hydrargyrum sulphuratum nigrum = aethi-m.
hydratum = am-caust.
hydrc.   hydrocotyle asiatica
hydrin-m.   hydrastinum muriaticum
hydrin-s.   hydrastinum sulphuricum
hydrinin-m.   hydrastininum muriaticum
hydro-v.   hydrophyllum virginicum
hydrobr-ac.   hydrobromicum acidum
hydrochl-ac.   hydrochloridum acidum
hydrochloricum = amylam.
hydrocort.   hydrocortisone
hydrofluoricum acidum = fl-ac.
hydrog.   hydrogenium
hydroph.   hydrophis cyanocinctus
hydrophobinum = lyss.
hydrophylium virginianum = hydro-v.
hydroq.   hydroquinone
hygroph-s.   hygrophilia sphinosa
hygrophila spinosa = hygroph-s.
hymos.   hymosa
hyos.   hyoscyamus niger
hyosciamus niger = hyos.
hyoscinum bromhydricum = scopin-hbr.
hyoscyami folium = hyos.
hyoscyaminum hydrobromatum = hyosin-hbr.
hyosin.   hyosciaminum-s. + -hbr.
                           (old abbr.)
hyosin-hbr.   hyosciaminum
                           hydrobromatum

hyper.   hypericum perforatum
hypo.   hypophyllum sanguineum
hypophysinum = pituin.
hypophysis anterior = pitu-a.
hypophysis cerebri = pitu-gl.
hypophysis glandula = pitu-gl.
hypophysis posterior = pitu-p.
hypoth.   hypothalamus
hypothalamus of the ox = hypoth.
hyss-o.   hyssopus officinalis
iber.   iberis amara
ichth.   ichthyolum
ichthyolammonium = ichth.
ichthyotoxinum = ser-ang.
ictod.   ictodes foetida
Iecoris aselli oleum = ol-j.
ign.   ignatia amara
ignis-alc.   ignis alcoholis
ikshugandha = trib.
ilex cassine = ilx-c.
Ilex opaca = ilx-a.
ilex paraguaiensis = mate
ilex paraguariensis = mate
ille.   illecebrum verticillatum
illicium anisatum = anis.
illicium stellatum = anis.
illicium verum = anis.
ilx-a.   ilex aquifolium
ilx-c.   ilex casseine
ilx-v.   ilex vomitoria
immunoserum diphthericum = diphtox.
imp.   imperatoria ostruthium
impa-g.   impatiens glandulifera
impatiens roylei = impa-g.
imperatoria peucedanum = imp.
ind.   indium metallicum
indg.   indigo tinctoria
indgf-a.   indigofera atriceps
indigofera tinctoria = indg.
indol.   indolum
influ.   influenzinum
influenzinum vaccinus = influ.
ing.   ingluvin
ins.   insulinum
inul.   inula helenium
iod.   iodium

117

List of remedy abbreviations

iod-h.   iodium hydrogenisatum
iodium purum = iod.
iodof.   iodoformium
iodoformum = iodof.
iodothyrinum = thyroid.
ip.   ipecacuanha
ipeca = ip.
ipom-p.   ipomoea purpurea
ipomea purga = jal.
ipomea turpenthum = oper.
ipomoea bona-nox = convo-d.
ipomoea hirsutula = ipom-p.
ipomoea stans = convo-s.
irid-m.   iridium muriaticum
irid-met.   iridium metallicum
iridinum = irisin.
iridium chloride = irid-m.
iris minor = iris-t.
iris-fa.   iris factissima
iris-fl.   iris florentina
iris-foe.   iris foetidissima
iris-g.   iris germanica
iris-t.   iris tenax
irisin.   irisinum
iris   iris versicolor
itu   itu
jab.   jaborandi
jac-c.   jacaranda caroba
jac-g.   jacaranda gualandai
jacaranda braziliensis = jac-c.
jacaranda procera = jac-c.
jacea = viol-t.
jal.   jalapa
jambos eugenia = eug.
jambosa vulgaris = eug.
janosia = joan.
jararaca = both.
jararacussu = both.
jasm.   jasminum officinale
jatr-c.   jatropha curcas
jatr-g.   jatropha gossypifolia
jatr-u.   jatropha urens
jatropha manihot = cass.
jenosia ashoka = joan.
jequirity = abr.
joan.   joanesia asoca

jodium = iod.
jonosia asoka = joan.
jug-c.   juglans cinerea
jug-r.   juglans regia
jugin.   juglandinum
juglans cathartica = jug-c.
junc-e.   juncus effusus
juncus communis = junc-e.
juni-c.   juniperus communis
juni-v.   juniperus virginiana
juniperus sabina = sabin.
juniperus virginianus = juni-v.
just.   justicia adhatoda
just-r.   justicia rubrum
justicia cydoniifolia = just.
justicia paniculata = androg-p.
kal.   kalanchoe pinnatum
kalag.   kalagua
kali hydriodicum = kali-i.
kali hydriodium = kali-i.
kali hydroiodicum = kali-i.
kali silicatum = kali-sil.
kali-act.   kalium aceticum
kali-ar.   kalium arsenicosum
kali-bi.   kalium bichromicum
kali-bit.   kalium bitartaricum
kali-br.   kalium bromatum
kali-c.   kalium carbonicum
kali-chl.   kalium chloricum
kali-chls.   kalium chlorosum
kali-chr.   kalium chromicum
kali-cit.   kalium citricum
kali-cy.   kalium cyanatum
kali-f.   kalium fluoratum
kali-fcy.   kalium ferrocyanatum
kali-hox.   kalium hydroxydum
kali-hp.   kalium hypophosphoricum
kali-i.   kalium iodatum
kali-l.   kalium lacticum
kali-m.   kalium muriaticum
kali-n.   kalium nitricum
kali-o.   kalium oxydatum
kali-ox.   kalium oxalicum
kali-p.   kalium phosphoricum
kali-perm.   kalium permanganatum
kali-pic.   kalium picricum

List of remedy abbreviations

kali-s.   kalium sulphuricum
kali-s-chr.   kalium sulphuricum chromicum
kali-sal.   kalium salicylicum
kali-sil.   kalium silicicum
kali-sula.   kalium sulphuratum
kali-sulo.   kalium sulphurosum
kali-t.   kalium tartaricum
kali-tcy.   kalium thiocyanatum
kali-tel.   kalium telluricum
kali-x.   kalium xanthogenicum
kalii acetas = kali-act.
kalii antimoniotartras = ant-t.
kalii bichromas = kali-bi.
kalii bromidum = kali-br.
kalii chloridum = kali-m.
kalii chromas = kali-chr.
kalii citras = kali-cit.
kalii dihyrogenphosphas = kali-p.
kalii iodidum = kali-i.
kalii nitras = kali-n.
kalii permangas = kali-perm.
kalium chromicum sulphuricum = kali-s-chr.
kalium hypermanganicum = kali-perm.
kalium iodicum = kali-i.
kalium manganicum = kali-perm.
kalium stibyltartaricum = ant-t.
kalm.   kalmia latifolia
kam.   kamala
kaol.   kaolinum
kaolinit = kaol.
kaolinum ponderosum = alumin-sil.
kaolinum ponderosum = kaol.
kara   karaka
karlsbad aqua = carl.
karw-h.   karwinskia humboldtiana
katipo = lat-k.
kava-kava = pip-m.
kerose.   kerosenum
keroso.   kerosolenum
ketogl-ac.   ketoglutaricum acidum
kinkeliba = combr-r.
kino australiense = ango.
kino   kino pterocarpi
kiss.   Kissingen aqua
Klebsiella pneumoniae = mucot.

kobra = naja
kola   kola
koso = kou.
kou.   kousso
krameria triandra = rat.
kreos.   kreosotum
kres.   kresolum
kurch.   kurchi
laburnum anagyroides = cyt-l.
lac defloratum = lac-d.
lac delphinum = lac-del.
lac equie = lac-e.
lac leonis = lac-leo.
lac vaccini flos = lac-v-f.
lac-ac.   lacticum acidum
lac-c.   lac caninum
lac-cp.   lac caprinum
lac-d.   lac vaccinum defloratum
lac-del.   lac delphinum
lac-e.   lac equinum
lac-f.   lac felinum
lac-h.   lac humanum
lac-leo.   lac leoninum
lac-loxod-a.   lac loxodonta Africana
lac-lup.   lac lupinum
lac-mat.   lac maternum
lac-v.   lac vaccinum
lac-v-c.   lac vaccinum coagulatum
lac-v-f.   lac vaccinum flos
lacer.   lacerta agilis
lach.   lachesis muta
lachesis alternatus = both-a.
lachesis lanceolatus = both.
lachn.   lachnanthes tinctoria
lact.   lactuca virosa (old abbr.)
lact-sa.   lactuca sativa
lact-v.   lactuca virosa
lacticum acidum dextrum = sarcol-ac.
lactis acidum = lac-ac.
lactis vaccini flos = lac-v-f.
lactuca silvestris = lact-v.
Lager beer = cerev-lg.
lam.   lamium album
lang.   langebrucken aqua
lap-a.   lapis albus
lap-la.   lapis lazuli

List of remedy abbreviations

lapa.   lapathum acutum
lapathum sylvestre = lapa.
lapis granites murvey = granit-m.
lapis renalis = cal-ren.
lappa major = lappa
lappa officinalis = lappa
lappa tomentosa = lappa
lappa   lappa arctium
laps.   lapsana communis
lar-d.   larix decidua
laricifomes officinalis = bol-la.
lasidora cubana = mygal.
lat-h.   latrodectus haseltii
lat-k.   latrodectus katipo
lat-m.   latrodectus mactans
lath.   lathyrus sativus
lathyrus cicera = lath.
lathyrus odoratus = lath.
latrodectus curassavicus = ther.
latrodectus mactans hasselti = lat-h.
laur.   laurocerasus
laurus benzoin = benzo.
laurus camphora = camph.
laurus sassafras = sass.
laurustinus = vib-t.
lava heclae = hecla
lava scoriae = hecla
lavand-a.   lavandula angustifolia
lavandula officinalis = lavand-a.
lavandula vera = lavand-a.
lavandulae aetheroleum = ol-lav.
lec.   lecithinum
led.   ledum palustre
lem-m.   lemna minor
leon.   leonurus cardiaca
leontice thalictroides = caul.
lepi.   lepidium bonariense
lepr.   leprominium
lept.   leptandra virginica
leptilon canadense = erig.
leptos-ih.   leptospira ictero-hemorrhagica
lesp-c.   lespedeza capitata
lesp-s.   lespedeza sieboldii
lespedeza thunbergii = lesp-s.
leucanthemum parthenium = pyre-p.

leucanthemum vulgare = chrysan.
leucas-a.   leucas aspera
lev.   Levico aqua
levist.   levisticum officinale
levo.   levomepromazinum
liat.   liatris spicata
lichen islandicus = cetr.
lignum nephriticum = eys.
lignum vitae = guaj.
lil-s.   lilium superbum
lil-t.   lilium tigrinum
lilium lancifolium = lil-t.
lim.   limulus cyclops
limen-b-c.   limenitis bredowii californica
limx.   = arion = limex ater (old abbr.)
lina.   linaria vulgaris
lindera benzoin = benzo.
lingusticum levisticum = levist.
lini semen = linu-u.
linu-c.   linum catharticum
linu-u.   linum usitatissimum
linum cartharticum = linu-c.
lip.   lippia mexicana
lipp.   Lippspringe aqua
liquor ammoni caustici = am-caust.
lir-o.   liriosma ovata
lister.   listeriosis nosode
lith-be.   lithium benzoicum
lith-br.   lithium bromatum
lith-c.   lithium carbonicum
lith-chl.   lithium chloricum
lith-f.   lithium fluoratum
lith-lac.   lithium lacticum
lith-m.   lithium muriaticum
lith-sal.   lithium salicylicum
lithii benzoas = lith-be.
lithii carbonas = lith-c.
lithospermum virginicum = onos.
lob.   lobelia inflata
lob-a.   lobelia acetum
lob-c.   lobelia cardinalis
lob-d.   lobelia dortmanna
lob-e.   lobelia erinus
lob-p.   lobelia purpurascens
lob-s.   lobelia syphilitica

List of remedy abbreviations

lobaria pulmonaria = stict.

lobelia coerulea = lob-s.

lobelia glandulosa = lob-s.

lobelia siphilitica = lob-s.

lobin.   lobelinum

lol.   lolium temulentum

loleum temulentum = lol.

lon-c.   lonicera caprifolium

lon-p.   lonicera periclymenum

lon-x.   lonicera xylosteum

lonicera ochroleuca = lon-x.

lophophora williamsii = anh.

lophophytum leandri = flor-p.

lophophytum mirabile = flor-p.

lophophytum spectabile = flor-p.

loxo-parr.   loxosceles parrami

loxo-recl.   loxosceles reclusa

loxosceles reclusus = loxo-recl.

luesinum = syph.

lueticum = syph.

luf-act.   luffa actangula

luf-am.   luffa amara

luf-b.   luffa bindal

luf-op.   luffa operculata

luminal = phenob.

luna   luna

lup.   lupulus humulus

lupin.   lupulinum

lutin.   luteinum

lyc.   lycopodium clavatum

lychnis githago = agro.

lycoperdon bovista = bov.

lycopus aqauticus = lycps-eu.

lycosa fasciiventris = tarent.

lycosa tarentula = tarent.

lycpr.   lycopersicon esculentum

lycps-eu.   lycopus Europaeus

lycps-v.   lycopus virginicus

lys.   lysinum

lysd.   lysidinum

lyss.   lyssinum

lythrum petiolatum = cuph.

lytta vesicatoria = canth.

m-ambo.   magnetis poli ambo

m-arct.   magnetis polus arcticus

m-aust.   magnetis polus Australis

macro.   macrotinum

macrotys racemosa = cimic.

macroz.   macrozamia spiralis

madar = calo.

madura album = calo.

mag-act.   magnesium aceticum

mag-art.   magnesium artificialis

mag-bcit.   magnesium borocitricum

mag-c.   magnesium carbonicum

mag-f.   magnesium fluoratum

mag-i.   magnesium iodatum

mag-lac.   magnesium lacticum

mag-m.   magnesium muriaticum

mag-met.   magnesium metallicum

mag-n.   magnesium nitricum

mag-o.   magnesium oxydatum

mag-p.   magnesium phosphoricum

mag-s.   magnesium sulphuricum

mag-sil.   magnesium silicatum

magenta = fuch.

magistery of bismuth = bism-sn.

magn-gl.   magnolia glauca

magn-gr.   magnolia grandiflora

magnes artificialis = m-ambo.

magnesia = mag-o.

magnesii chloridum hexahydricum = mag-m.

magnesii oxydum = mag-o.

magnesii subcarbonas levis = mag-c.

magnesii sulfas = mag-s.

magnesium calcinatum = mag-o.

mahonia aquifolium = berb-a.

maias-l.   maiasaura lapidea

majeptilum = thiop.

mal-ac.   malicum acidum

malachite = cupr-c.

maland.   malandrinum

malar.   malaria nosode

malatox.   malariatoxinum

malleinum = hippoz.

mallotus philippinensis = kam.

malosma laurina = rhus-l.

malus sylvestris = malus-c.

malus-c.   malus communis

mamm.   glandula mammalis

mamma glandula = mamm.

manaca = franc.

List of remedy abbreviations

manc.	mancinella
mand.	mandragora officinarum
mang.	manganum-act. + -c. (old abbr.)
mang-act.	manganum aceticum
mang-c.	manganum carbonicum
mang-coll.	manganum colloidale
mang-i.	manganum iodatum
mang-m.	manganum muriaticum
mang-met.	manganum metallicum
mang-o.	manganum oxydatum
mang-p.	manganum phosphoricum
mang-s.	manganum sulphuricum

mangana sulfas = mang-s.

manganum dioxydum = mang-o.

manganum oxydatum nativum = mang-o.

manganum peroxydum = mang-o.

mangi.	mangifera indica

manihot utilissima = cass.

manioc = cass.

mapato = rat.

marigoldin = calen.

marr.	= marr-vg. = marrubium album (old abbr.)
marr-vg.	marrubium vulgare

marrubium album = marr-vg.

marsdenia cundurango = cund.

marum verum = teucr.

mastoid.	mastoiditis nosode

mater perlarum = conch.

mate	ilex mate
mati.	matico

matricaria chamomilla = cham.

matricaria recutita = cham.

matth.	matthiola graeca

mauritanica = arund-d.

mec.	meconinum
med.	medorrhinum

medicago sativa = alf.

medul-o.	medulla oblongata
medul-os-si.	medulla ossis suis
medul-spi.	medulla spinalis
medus.	medusa
mel-c-s.	mel cum sale
mela.	melastoma Ackermanni

melaleuca leucodendron = caj.

meli.	melilotus officinalis
meli-a.	melilotus alba
meli-xyz.	melilotus off. + -a.

melia azadirachta indica = aza.

melia azadirachta = aza.

melia grandiflora = guare.

melis.	melissa officinalis
melit.	melitagrinum

melitococcinum = brucel.

melitotoxinum = brucel.

meloe vesicatoris = canth.

meningoc.	meningococcinum
menis.	menispermum canadense

menispermum cocculus = cocc.

menth.	mentha piperita
menth-pu.	mentha pulegium
menth-v.	mentha viridis
mentho.	mentholum
meny.	menyanthes trifoliata
meph.	mephitis putorius

mephitis americana = meph.

mephitis mephitica = meph.

merc.	mercurius solubilis
merc-act.	mercurius aceticus
merc-aur.	mercurius auratus
merc-br.	mercurius bromatus
merc-c.	mercurius corrosivus
merc-cy.	mercurius cyanatus
merc-d.	mercurius dulcis
merc-i-f.	mercurius iodatus flavus
merc-i-r.	mercurius iodatus ruber
merc-k-i.	mercurius biniodatus cum kali iodatum
merc-meth.	mercurius methylenus
merc-n.	mercurius nitricus
merc-ns.	mercurius nitrosus
merc-p.	mercurius phosphoricus
merc-pn.	mercurius proto-nitricus
merc-pr-a.	mercurius praecipitatus albus
merc-pr-r.	mercurius praecipitatus ruber
merc-s-cy.	mercurius sulphocyanatus
merc-sul.	mercurius sulphuricus
merc-tn.	mercurius tannicus

mercenaria mercenaria = ven-m.

mercs-n.	mercuresceinum natricum

List of remedy abbreviations

mercurius bi-iodatus = merc-i-r.

mercurius biniodatus = merc-i-r.

mercurius cum kali = aethi-m.

mercurius et kali iodatus = merc-k-i.

mercurius nitricus oxydulatus = merc-ns.

mercurius oxydatulus niger = merc.

mercurius oxydatus = merc-pr-r.

mercurius proto-iodatus = merc-i-f.

mercurius protoiodatus = merc-i-f.

mercurius solubilis hahnemanni = merc.

mercurius sublimatus corrosivus = merc-c.

mercurius sublimatus = merc-c.

mercurius sulphuratus niger = aethi-m.

mercurius sulphuratus ruber = cinnb.

merl.	mercurialis perennis

metallum album = ars.

metallum iodatum = ars-i.

meth-ae-ae.	methylium aethyloaethereum
meth-bchl.	methylenum bichloratum
meth-sal.	methylium salicylicum
methan.	methanol
methyl.	methylenum coeruleum

methylene blue = methyl.

methylenum trichloratum = chlf.

methylenum trichloride = chlf.

methylglycoxalidine = lysd.

methys.	methysergidum

metrosideros costatus = ango.

mez.	mezereum
mica	mica
micr.	micromeria douglasii

micrococcus catarrhalis = mucot.

micrococcus melitensis = brucel.

micrococcus tetragenius = mucot.

microphyllus pennatifolius = jab.

micrurus corallinus = elaps

micrurus fulvius = elaps

mikania guaco = gua.

mill.	millefolium

millipedes = onis.

mim-h.	mimosa humilis
mim-p.	mimosa pudica
miml-g.	mimulus guttatus
miss.	Mississquoi aqua

mit.	mitchella repens
moly-met.	molybdenium metallicum

molybdaenum metallicum = moly-met.

mom-b.	momordica balsamica
mom-ch.	momordica charantia

momordica balsamina = mom-b.

momordica elaterium = elat.

moni.	= cand-al. = monilia albicans (old abbr.)
mono.	monotropa uniflora
mons.	monsonia ovata
morb.	morbillinum
morg.	bacillus Morgan (Bach)
morg-g.	bacillus Morgan-Gaertner (Paterson)
morg-p.	bacillus Morgan pure (Paterson)

morgan (bach) = morg.

morgan pure (paterson) = morg-p.

morgan-gaertner (paterson) = morg-g.

morph.	morphinum and salts (old abbr.)
morph-act.	morphinum aceticum
morph-m.	morphinum muriaticum
morph-s.	morphinum sulphuricum

morphini hydrochloridum = morph-m.

morphini sulfas = morph-s.

mosch.	moschus

moschus moschiferus = mosch.

ms.	multiple sclerosis nosode
muc-u.	mucuna urens
mucoc.	mucococcinum

mucocatarrhalis = mucot.

mucor-a-p.	mucor cum aspergillus cum penicillinum
mucor	mucor mucedo
mucot.	mucotoxinum

mucuna pruriens = dol.

mudar = calo.

mur-ac.	muriaticum acidum
muru.	murure leite
murx.	murex purpurea
musa	musa sapientum
muscin.	muscarinum

mustela foetida = meph.

mygal.	mygale lasiodora

mygale avicularia = mygal.

List of remedy abbreviations

myos-a.   myosotis arvensis
myos-s.   myosotis symphytifolia
myosotis avicularia = myos-a.
myosotis intermedia = myos-a.
myric.   myrica cerifera
myris.   myristica sebifera
myristica fragrans = nux-m.
myristica officinalis = nux-m.
myrmexin = form.
myrobalanum chebula = term-c.
myrocylon peruvianum = bals-p.
myrospermum pereirae = bals-p.
myroxylon pereira = bals-p.
myroxylon peruvianum = bals-p.
myrt-c.   myrtus communis
myrt-ch.   myrtus cheken
myrtillus = vacc-m.
myrtus jambos = eug.
myrtus pimenta = pime.
myxoedema parotitis = ourl.
nabal.   nabalus serpentarius
nabulus albus = nabal.
naja   naja tripudians
nalox.   naloxon
naloxone = nalox.
napellus = acon.
napht.   naphtha
naphthoq.   naphthoquinone
naphtin.   naphthalinum
narc-po.   narcissus poeticus
narc-ps.   narcissus pseudonarcissus
narcin.   narceinum
narcot.   narcotinum
narcot-m.   narcotinum muriaticum
narz.   Narzan aqua
nast.   = nast-o. = nasturtium aquaticum (old abbr.)
nast-o.   nasturtium officinale
nasturtium aquaticum = nast-o.
nat-act.   natrium aceticum
nat-ae-s.   natrium aethylosulphuricum
nat-ar.   natrium arsenicosum
nat-bic.   natrium bicarbonicum
nat-br.   natrium bromatum
nat-c.   natrium carbonicum

nat-cac.   = nat-c. = natrium cacodylicum
nat-caust.   natrium causticum
nat-ch.   natrium choleinicum
nat-chl.   natrium chloricum
nat-f.   natrium fluoratum
nat-hchls.   natrium hypochlorosum
nat-hp.   natrium hypophosphorum
nat-hsulo.   natrium hyposulphurosum
nat-i.   natrium iodatum
nat-lac.   natrium lacticum
nat-m.   natrium muriaticum
nat-n.   natrium nitricum
nat-ns.   natrium nitrosum
nat-ox-act.   natrium oxalaceticum
nat-p.   natrium phosphoricum
nat-pyru.   natrium pyruvicum
nat-s.   natrium sulphuricum
nat-s-c.   natrium sulphocarbolicum
nat-sal.   natrium salicylicum
nat-sel.   natrium selenicum
nat-sil.   natrium silicicum
nat-sil-f.   natrium silicofluoricum
nat-sula.   natrium sulphuratum
nat-sulo.   natrium sulphurosum
nat-taur.   natrium taurocholicum
nat-tel.   natrium telluricum
nat-tmcy.   natrium thiosinaminum cyanatum
nat-uric.   natrium uricum
natrii acetas = nat-act.
natrii bromidum = nat-br.
natrii carbonas monohydricus = nat-c.
natrii chloridum = nat-m.
natrii fluoridum = nat-f.
natrii hydroxydum = nat-caust.
natrii hypophosphis = nat-hp.
natrii iodidum = nat-i.
natrii lactatis solutio = nat-lac.
natrii nitras = nat-n.
natrii nitris = nat-ns.
natrii phosphas = nat-p.
natrii salicylas = nat-sal.
natrii sulfas anhydricus = nat-s.
natrium arsenicicum = nat-ar.
natrium biboracicum = borx.

List of remedy abbreviations

natrium biboratum = borx.

natrium cacodylicum = nat-c.

natrium chloratum = nat-m.

natrium silicatum = nat-sil.

natrium sulphorinicum = nat-ae-s.

natrium tetraboracicum = borx.

natrium tetrachloroauratum = aur-m-n.

nectrin.   nectrianinum

neg.   negundium Americanum

negundo aceroides = neg.

negundo Americanum = neg.

neisseria flava = flav.

neon   neon

nep.   nepenthes distillatoria

nepet.   = catar. = nepeta cataria

nerium odorum = olnd.

nerium oleander = olnd.

neurohypophysis = pitu-p.

nicc.   niccolum-met. + -c. (old
                                 abbr.)

nicc-br.   niccolum bromidum

nicc-c.   niccolum carbonicum

nicc-met.   niccolum metallicum

nicc-s.   niccolum sulphuricum

niccolum bromatum = nicc-br.

nicot.   nicotinum

nicotiana tabacum = tab.

nid.   nidus edulis

nig-s.   nigella sativa

nit-ac.   nitricum acidum

nit-m-ac.   nitromuriaticum acidum

nit-s-d.   nitri spiritus dulcis

nitri acidum = nit-ac.

nitro-o.   nitrogenium oxygenatum

nitrob.   nitrobenzolum

nitrobenzenum = nitrob.

nitrogenii oxidum = nitro-o.

nitrogenum oxygenatum = nitro-o.

nitroglycerinum = glon.

nitroso-muriaticum acidum = nit-m-ac.

nitrum = kali-n.

nuph.   nuphar luteum

nux colae = kola

nux juglans = jug-r.

nux-a.   nux absurda

nux-m.   nux moschata

nux-v.   nux vomica

nyct.   nyctanthes arbor tristis

nymph.   nymphaea odorata

nymphaea lutea = nuph.

nymphea odorata = nymph.

oci.   ocimum canum

oci-car.   ocimum caryophyllatum

oci-g.   ocimum gratissimum

oci-sa.   ocimum sanctum

ocimum basilicum = basil.

oena.   oenanthe crocata

oenanthe aquaticum = phel.

oenanthe phellandrium = phel.

oeno.   oenothera biennis

oest.   oestrus cameli

oestronum = foll.

officinalis polyporus = bol-la.

oidium albicans = moni.

okou.   okoubaka aubrevillei

ol-an.   oleum animale aethereum

ol-car.   oleum caryophyllatum

ol-eucal.   oleum eucalyptus

ol-j.   oleum jecoris aselli

ol-lav.   oleum lavandulae

ol-myr.   oleum myristicae

ol-sant.   oleum santali

ol-suc.   oleum succinum

olden-h.   oldenlandia herbacea

oleum animae aetherum dippeli = ol-an.

oleum cajuputi = caj.

oleum carvi = caru.

oleum chaulmoogra = chaul.

oleum cornu cervi = ol-an.

oleum dippeli = ol-an.

oleum elaeis = elae.

oleum jecoris morrhuae = ol-j.

oleum morrhuae = ol-j.

oleum petrae = petr.

oleum ricini = ric.

oleum ricinus = ric.

oleum sussini non rectificatum = ol-suc.

oleum terebinthinae = ter.

oleum wittnebianum = caj.

olib-sac.   olibanum sacrum

olnd.   oleander

onis.   oniscus asellus

List of remedy abbreviations

onon.	ononis spinosa
ononis arvensis = onon.	
onop.	onopordon acanthium
onos.	onosmodium virginianum
onosmodium virginicum = onos.	
oophorinum = ov.	
oorari = cur.	
op.	opium
oper.	operculina turpenthum
operculina turpethum = oper.	
opianyl = mec.	
opium crudum = op.	
opl.	oplia farinosa
opun-a.	opuntia aciculata
opun-f.	opuntia ficus-indica
opun-s.	opuntia spina alba
opun-v.	= opun-f. = opuntia vulgaris (old abbr.)
opun-xyz.	opun-s. + opun-f.
orch.	orchitinum
oreo.	oreodaphne californica
orex-tann.	orexinum tannaticum
orig.	origanum majorana
orig-d.	origanum dictamnus
orig-v.	origanum vulgare
origanum hortensis = orig.	
origanum majorana = orig.	
orni.	ornithogalum umbellatum
ornithogalum nutans = agra.	
orobanche virginiana = epiph.	
orot-ac.	oroticum acidum
orteaga = eys.	
orthos-s.	orthosiphon stamineus
orthosiphonis folium = orthos-s.	
oscilloc.	oscillococcinum
osm.	osmium met. + -ac. (old abbr.)
osm-ac.	osmicum acidum
osm-met.	osmium metallicum
osm-o.	osmium oxydatum
osmium tetroxidum = osm-o.	
ost.	ostrya virginica
osteo-a.	osteo-arthriticum
osteo-mye.	osteomyelitis nosode
osteo-mye-scl.	osteomyelosclerosis nosode
ostrea edulis = calc.	

otit-m-xyz.	otitis media nosode unknown species
ouabin.	ouabainum
ourl.	ourlianum
ov.	ovininum
ova tosta = ovi-p.	
oval buchu = baros.	
ovar.	ovaries
ovi gallinae testa = calc-o-t.	
ovi testa = calc-o-t.	
ovi-p.	ovi gallinae pellicula
ox-ac.	oxalicum acidum
oxal-a.	oxalis acetosella
oxeod.	= oreo. = oxeodaphne (old abbr.)
oxyd.	oxydendron arboreum
oxyg.	oxygenium
oxyt.	oxytropis lamberti
oxyte-chl.	oxytetracycline chlorhydrate
oxytrophis = oxyt.	
oxyuris vermicularis = enterob-v.	
ozone	ozonum
p-benzq.	parabenzoquinonum
padus avium = prun-p.	
paeon.	paeonia officinalis
paico = chen-a.	
pakur = fic-r.	
pall.	palladium metallicum
palo.	paloondo
pambotano = calli-h.	
pambt.	pambotano
pana.	panacea arvensis
panax ginseng = gins.	
panax quinquefolia = gins.	
pancr.	pancreatinum
pancreatis pulvis = pancr.	
pann.	panna
pap-r.	papaver rhoeas
papaver somniferum = op.	
papaver vulgaris = pap-r.	
papaya vulgaris = asim.	
papin.	papaverinum
par.	paris quadrifolia
para-benzoquinonum = p-benzq.	
paraf.	paraffinum

126

List of remedy abbreviations

paraffinum liquidum = paraf.

paraph.   paraphenylendiaminum

parat.   paratyphoidinum

parat-b.   paratyphoidinum B

parathormonum = parathyr.

parathyr.   parathyreoidinum

parathyreoid glands = parathyr.

paratyphoidinum a = parat.

pareir.   pareira brava

pariet.   parietaria officinalis

paro-i.   paronychia illecebrum

parot.   parotidinum

parotitis nosode = parot.

parth.   parthenium hysterophorus

parthenium hysterophorus lynn = parth.

parthenocissus = ampe-qu.

passi.   passiflora incarnata

past.   pastinaca sativa

paull.   paullinia pinnata

paullinia sorbilis = guar.

pausinystalia yohimba = yohim.

pect.   pecten jacobaeus

ped.   pediculus capitis

pedclr.   pedicularis canadensis

pelarg.   pelargonium reniforme

pelias berus = vip.

pellin.   pelletierinum

pen.   penthorum sedoides

penic.   penicillinum

peps.   pepsinum

pepsini pulvis = peps.

perh.   perhexilinum

perh-mal.   perhexilinum maleatum

peri.   periploca graeca

periproc.   periproctitic abscess nosode

perlarum mater = conch.

pers.   persea Americana

persea gratissima = pers.

persica amygdalus = amyg-p.

persica vulgaris = amyg-p.

persicaria acris = polyg-h.

persicaria urens = polyg-pe.

pert.   pertussinum

pert-vc.   pertussis vaccinus

pest.   pestinum

petasites fragrans = tus-fr.

petasites hybridus = tus-p.

petasites officinalis = tus-p.

petasites vulgaris = tus-p.

peti.   petiveria tetandra

peti-a.   petiveria alliacea

petr.   petroleum

petros.   petroselinum sativum

petroselinum crispum = petros.

petroselinum hortense = petros.

peucedanum oreoselo = atha.

peucedanum ostruthium = imp.

peumus boldo = bold.

pexid = perh-mal.

peyotl = anh.

ph-ac.   phosphoricum acidum

phal.   phallus impudicus

pharbitis purpurea = ipom-p.

phase.   phaseolus nanus

phase-vg.   phaseolus vulgaris

phase-xyz.   phase.+ phase-vg.

phel.   phellandrium aquaticum

phenac.   phenacetinum

phenob.   phenobarbitalum

phenol = carb-ac.

phenolum = carb-ac.

phenylaethylimalonylureum = phenob.

phle.   phleum pratense

phlor.   phlorizinum

phos.   phosphorus

phos-h.   phosphorus hydrogenatus

phos-pchl.   = phos-m. = phosphorus pentachloratus

phosphorus muriaticus = phos-pchl.

phyllitis scolopendrium = scolo-v.

phylloquinone = hydroq.

phys.   physostigma venenosum

physal-al.   physalis alkekengi

physala-p.   physalia pelagica

physalia arethusa = physala-p.

physalia caravella = physala-p.

physalia physalis = physala-p.

physalia utriculus = physala-p.

physostigminum = esin.

phyt.   phytolacca decandra

phyt-b.   phytolacca berry

List of remedy abbreviations

phytolacca tetandra = peti.

pic-ac.   picricum acidum

picea mariana = abies-n.

picea nigra = abies-n.

pichi-pichi = fab.

picro.   picrotoxinum

picro-ac.   picrotoxinum acidum

picronitricum acidum = pic-ac.

pili-pili = caps.

pilo.   pilocarpinum + salts (old
                                       abbr.)

pilo-m.   pilocarpinum muriaticum

pilocarpini hydrochloridum = pilo-m.

pilocarpus jaborandi = jab.

pilocarpus microphyllus = jab.

pilocarpus pennatifolius = jab.

pilosella = hier-p.

pime.   pimenta officinalis

pimp.   pimpinella saxifraga

pimpinella alba = pimp.

pimpinella major = pimp.

pin-c.   pinus cupressus

pin-l.   pinus lambertiana

pin-s.   pinus silvestris

pineal.   pinealis

pinus canadensis = abies-c.

pinus murrayana = pin-s.

pinus sylvestris = pin-s.

pip-m.   piper methysticum

pip-n.   piper nigrum

pipe.   piperazinum

piper angustifolium elongatum = mati.

piper angustifolium = mati.

piper cubeba = cub.

piper elongatum = mati.

pisc.   piscidia erythrina

pitu.   pituitaria posterior (old
                                       abbr.)

pitu-a.   pituitaria anterior

pitu-gl.   pituitaria glandula

pitu-p.   pituitaria posterior

pituin.   = pitu-gl. = pituitrinum

pituitaria cerebri = pitu-gl.

pituitarium anteriorum = pitu-a.

pituitarium posteriorum = pitu-p.

piturinum = dubo-h.

pix   pix liquida

plac.   placenta humana

plan.   plantago major

plan-mi.   plantago minor

planifolia = vanil.

plantago aquatica = alis-p.

plat.   platinum metallicum

plat-m.   platinum muriaticum

plat-m-n.   platinum muriaticum
                                       natronatum

platan. old = platan-oc. + -or. = platan.

platan.   platan-oc. + -or. (old
                                       abbr.)

platan-oc.   platanus occidentalis

platan-or.   platanus orientalis

platanus acerifolia = platan-or.

platina = plat.

platinum chloratum = plat-m.

plb.   plumbum metallicum

plb-act.   plumbum aceticum

plb-c.   plumbum carbonicum

plb-chr.   plumbum chromicum

plb-i.   plumbum iodatum

plb-m.   plumbum muriaticum

plb-o.   plumbum oxydatum

plb-p.   plumbum phosphoricum

plb-tae.   plumbum tetra-aethylicum

plb-xyz.   plumbum met. + -act. +
                                       -c.

plect.   plectranthus fruticosus

plumbg.   plumbago littoralis

plumbii acetas = plb-act.

plut-n.   plutonium nitricum

pneu.   pneumococcinum

pneumococcus = pneu.

podo.   podophyllum peltatum

podoin.   podophyllinum

polio   polio

poll.   pollantinum

pollen = poll.

polyg-a.   polygonum aviculare

polyg-h.   polygonum
                                       hydropiperoides

polyg-pe.   polygonum persicaria

polyg-s.   polygonum sagittatum

polyg-xyz.   polygonum h. + -pe. + ?

polygala senega = seneg.

List of remedy abbreviations

polygonum acre = polyg-h.
polygonum fagopyrum = fago.
polygonum hydropiper = polyg-pe.
polygonum punctatum = polyg-h.

polym.	polymnia uvedalia
polyp-p.	polyporus pinicola

polypodium calaguala = calag.
polypodium leucotomos = calag.
polyporus officinalis = bol-la.

polys.	polystyrenum
polytr.	polytrichum juniperinum
polytr-c.	polytrichum commune
pop.	populus tremuloides
pop-c-t.	populus balsamifera trichocarpa
pop-cand.	populus candicans

populus alba = pop-cand.
populus balsamifera = pop-cand.
populus tremula = pop.

positr.	positronium
pot-a.	potentilla anserina
pot-e.	potentilla erecta

potamobius astacus = astac.
potassium xantate = kali-x.
potentilla recta = pot-e.
potentilla tormentilla = pot-e.
pothos foetidus = ictod.
prenanthes serpentaria = nabal.

prim-f.	primula farinosa
prim-o.	primula obconica
prim-v.	primula veris
prim-vl.	primula vulgaris

primula obconca = prim-o.
primula officinalis = prim-v.
primulae veris radix = prim-v.

prin.	prinos verticillatus

prionurus Australis = buth-a.

prop.	propylaminum
prost.	prostate gland
prot.	bacillus Proteus (Bach)

proteus (bach) = prot.
proteus mirabilis = prot.
proteus vulgaris = prot.

protg.	protargol
prots-m.	= prot. = proteus mirabilis
prun.	prunus spinosa

prun-cf.	prunus cerasifera
prun-p.	prunus padus
prun-v.	prunus virginiana
prune.	prunella vulgaris

prunus dulcis var. amara = amyg.
prunus laurocerasus = laur.
psalliota bispora = agar-cps.
psalliota hortensis = agar-cps.
pseudognaphalium obtusifolium = gnaph.

pseuts-m.	pseudotsuga menziesii
psil.	psilocybe caerulescens
psor.	psorinum
psoral.	psoralea bituminosa

psoricum = psor.
psychotria ipecacuanha = ip.
psychotria viridis = banis-c.

ptel.	ptelea trifoliata

pterocarpus erinaceus = kino
pterocarpus marsupium = kino
ptetrocarpus santalinus = santal.

pull-g.	pullus gallinaceus
pulm-a.	pulmo anaphylacticus
pulm-v.	vulpes pulmo

pulmo vulpis = pulm-v.

puls.	pulsatilla pratensis
puls-n.	pulsatilla nuttaliana

pulsatilla nigricans = puls.

pulx.	pulex irritans

punica granatum = gran.

pycnop-sa.	pycnoporus sanguineus
pyrar.	pyrarara
pyre-p.	pyrethrum parthenium
pyrog.	pyrogenium

pyrola umbellata = chim.
pyrus malus = malus-c.

pyrus	pyrus Americana
quas.	quassia amara
queb.	quebracho
querc.	quercus
querc-r.	quercus robur
querc-r-g-s.	quercus robur glandium spiritus

quercus fructus = querc.
quercus pedunculata = querc-r.
quercus sessilifera = querc-r.

quill.	quillaya saponaria

List of remedy abbreviations

quillaya smegmaderma = quill.

quinhydr.	quinhydrone
quinid.	quinidinum
rad-br.	radium bromatum
rad-met.	radium metallicum

Rademacher's solution = zinc-act.

radix angelicae sinensis = ange-s.

raja-s.	rajania subsamarata
ran-a.	ranunculus acris
ran-b.	ranunculus bulbosus
ran-fi.	ranunculus ficaria
ran-fl.	ranunculus flammula
ran-g.	ranunculus glacialis
ran-r.	ranunculus repens
ran-s.	ranunculus sceleratus

rana bufo = bufo

raph.	raphanus sativus
rat.	ratanhia peruviana

ratanhiae peruvianae radix = rat.

rauvolfia serpentina = rauw.

rauw.	rauwolfia serpentina

realgar = ars-s-r.

rein.	Reinerz aqua
ren.	kidneys
res.	resorcinum
reser.	reserpinum

resina cimifugae = macro.

resina itu = itu

resina piceae = abies-n.

retin-ac.	retinoicum acidum
rham-cal.	rhamnus californica
rham-cath.	rhamnus cathartica
rham-f.	rhamnus frangula

rhamni purshianae cortex = cas-s.

rhamnus purshiana = cas-s.

rheum officinale = rheum

rheum	rheum palmatum
rhod.	rhododendron chrysanthum

rhodallinum = thiosin.

rhodi.	rhodium metallicum
rhodi-o-n.	rhodium oxydatum nitricum

rhus canadensis = rhus-a.

rhus radicans = rhus-t.

rhus vernix = rhus-v.

rhus-a.	rhus aromatica
rhus-c.	rhus cotinus
rhus-d.	rhus diversiloba
rhus-g.	rhus glabra
rhus-l.	rhus laurina
rhus-r.	rhus radicans
rhus-t.	rhus toxicodendron
rhus-v.	rhus venenata
rib-ac.	ribonucleicum acidum
ribes-n.	ribes nigrum
ric.	ricinus communis

rna = rib-ac.

rob.	robinia pseudacacia

rorippa nasturtium aquaticum = nast-o.

ros-ca.	rosa canina
ros-d.	rosa damascena
rosm.	rosmarinus officinalis
rub-t.	rubia tinctorum
rubella	rubella nosode

rubia tinctoria = rub-t.

rubu.	rubus villosus

rudbeckia angustifolia = echi.

rudbeckia purpurea = echi-p.

ruizia fragrans = bold.

rumex obtusifolius = lapa.

rumx.	rumex crispus
rumx-ab.	rumex abyssinicus
rumx-act.	rumex acetosa
rumx-p.	rumex patientia
rusc-a.	ruscus aculeatus
russ.	russula foetens

russula emetica = agar-em.

ruta	ruta graveolens
sabad.	sabadilla
sabal	sabal serrulata
sabb.	sabbatia angularis
sabin.	sabina
sacch.	saccharum officinale
sacch-a.	saccharum album
sacch-l.	saccharum lactis

saccharomyces cerevisiae = tor.

saccharomyces ceru = tor.

saccharum raffinatum = sacch-a.

sal amarum = mag-s.

sal glauberi = nat-s.

sal-ac.	salicylicum acidum
sal-al.	salix alba

List of remedy abbreviations

sal-l.   salix lasiolepis
sal-mar.   sal marinum
sal-mo.   salix mollissima
sal-n.   salix nigra
sal-p.   salix purpurea
salam.   salamandra maculata
salamandra maculosa = salam.
salicylate of soda = nat-sal.
salin.   salicinum
salisburia adiantifolia = gink-b.
salix nigricans = sal-p.
salix vitellina = sal-l.
salmonella parathyphoidea = parat.
salmonella schotmullieri = parat-b.
salmonella typhi = eberth.
salol.   salolum
salv.   salvia officinalis
salviae officinalis folium = salv.
sam-ox.   samarium oxalicum
samars.   samarskite
samb.   sambucus nigra
samb-c.   sambucus canadensis
sambuci nigrae flos = samb.
sang.   sanguinaria canadensis
sangin-act.   sanguinarinum aceticum
sangin-n.   sanguinarinum nitricum
sangin-t.   sanguinarinum tartaricum
sanguis-s.   sanguis soricis
sanguiso.   sanguisorba officinalis
sanguisuga officinalis = hir.
sanic.   sanicula aqua
santa.   santalum album
santal.   santalinus
santalum = ol-sant.
santin.   santoninum
sapin.   saponinum
sapium sylvaticum = still.
sapo.   saponaria officinalis
saraca indica = joan.
sarcol-ac.   sarcolacticum acidum
saroth.   sarothamnus scoparius
sarr.   sarracenia purpurea
sars.   sarsaparilla officinalis
sass.   sassafras officinalis
saur.   saururus cernuus
saxi.   saxifraga granulata

saxon.   saxonitum
scam.   scammonium
scand-met.   scandium metallicum
scarl.   scarlatinum
scarlatininum = scarl.
schin.   schinus molle
schoenocaulon officinale = sabad.
scilla maritima = squil.
scilla-non-scripta = agra.
scir.   scirrhinum
scler.   scleranthus annuus
scol.   scolopendra morsitans
scolo-v.   scolopendrium vulgare
scolopendrium officinale = scolo-v.
scop.   scopolia carniolica
scopin-hbr.   scopolaminum
    bromhydricum
scopla.   scopola
scopolaminum hydrobromidum = scopin-hbr.
scor.   scorpio Europaeus
scorodosma foetida = asaf.
scorpio Australis = buth-a.
scorpionida = scor.
scroph-n.   scrophularia nodosa
scroph-xyz.   scroph-m. + scroph-n.
scut.   scutellaria laterifolia
scutellaria lateriflora = scut.
sec.   secale cornutum
secret.   secretinum
sed-ac.   sedum acre
sed-r.   sedum repens
sed-t.   sedum telephium
sedi.   sedinha
sedum alpestre = sed-r.
sedum purpureum = sed-t.
sel.   selenium metallicum
sela.   selaginella apus
selaginella = sela.
selenicereus grandiflorus = cact.
selenicereus spinulosus = cact.
sem-t.   semen tiglii
semecarpus anacardium = anac.
semen contra = cina
semp.   sempervivum tectorum
senebiera pinnatifida = lepi.
senec.   senecio aureus

senec-fu.	senecio fuschii
senec-j.	senecio jacobaea
senecio cineraria = cine.	
senecio gragglis = senec.	
seneg.	senega
senn.	senna
sennae folium = senn.	
sep.	sepia officinalis
sepia succus = sep.	
sepsinum = pyrog.	
septi.	septicaeminum
seq-s.	sequoia sempervirens
ser-a-c.	serum anti colibacillum
ser-ang.	serum anguillae
ser-febr-s.	serum febris suis
serenoa repens = sabal	
serenoa serrulata = sabal	
serot-cs.	serotoninum creatininum
	sulfuricum
serp.	serpentaria aristolochia
serratula tinctoria = liat.	
seven (Paterson) = bacls-7.	
shigella dysenteriae = dys.	
sieg.	siegesbeckia orientalis
sil.	silicea terra
sil-mar.	silica marina
silphium laciniatum = silphu.	
silpho.	silphion cyrenaicum
silphu.	silphium lacinatum
silybum marianum = card-m.	
sima.	simaruba amara
simaba cedron = cedr.	
simaruba cedron = cedr.	
simaruba ferroginea = cedr.	
simaruba officinalis = cedr.	
sin-a.	sinapis alba
sin-n.	sinapis nigra
sisy.	sisyrinchium galaxoides
sium	sium latifolium
skat.	skatolum
skook.	Skookum Chuck aqua
slag	slag silica
smilax offinialis = sars.	
smilax sarsaparilla = sars.	
smilcin.	smilacinum
smyrnium aureum = ziz.	

sol-a.	solanum arrebenta
sol-crl.	solanum carolinense
sol-mm.	solanum mammosum
sol-ni.	solanum nigrum
sol-o.	solanum oleraceum
sol-ps.	solanum pseudocapsicum
sol-t.	solanum tuberosum
sol-t-ae.	solanum tuberosum
	aegrotans
sol-x.	solanum xanthocarpum
solalinum = solin.	
solania = solin.	
solanum dulcamara = dulc.	
solanum lycopersicum = lycpr.	
solanum oleaceum = sol-o.	
solanum vesicarium = physal-al.	
solid.	solidago virgaurea
solidago virga avrea = solid.	
solin.	solaninum pur. + -act.
	(old abbr.)
solin-act.	solaninum aceticum
solin-pur.	solaninum purum
sol	sol
sorb-a.	sorbus aucuparia
sorbus Americana = pyrus	
spartin.	sparteinum
spartin-s.	sparteinum sulfuricum
spartini sulfas = spartin-s.	
spartium scoparium = saroth.	
sperminum = orch.	
sphaerococcus helminthochortos = helm.	
sphing.	sphingurus martini
spig.	spigelia anthelmia
spig-m.	spigelia marylandica
spigelia anthelmintica = spig.	
spiggurus martini = sphing.	
spir-aeth-c.	spiritus aetheris
	compositus
spir-n-d.	= nit-s-d. = spiritus nitri
	dulcis (old abbr.)
spira.	spiranthes autumnalis
spirae.	spiraea ulmaria
spiritus aetheris nitrosi = nit-s-d.	
spiritus dulcis nitri = nit-s-d.	
spiritus glandium quercus robur = querc-r-g-s.	
spiritus nitrico-aethereus = nit-s-d.	

List of remedy abbreviations

spong.	spongia tosta
spongia fluvialitis = bad.	
spongia officinalis = spong.	
spongilla fluvialitis = bad.	
squil.	squilla maritima
stach.	stachys betonica
stachys officinalis = stach.	
stann.	stannum metallicum
stann-i.	stannum iodatum
stann-m.	stannum muriaticum
staph.	staphisagria
staphycoc.	staphylococcinum
staphylocinum = staphycoc.	
staphysagria = staph.	
staphytox.	staphylotoxinum
stel.	stellaria media
sterculia acuminata = kola	
stibio-kali tartaricum = ant-t.	
stibium arsenicosum = ant-ar.	
stibium chloridum = ant-m.	
stibium crudum = ant-c.	
stibium iodatum = ant-i.	
stibium muriaticum = ant-m.	
stibium oxydatum = ant-o.	
stibium sulfuratum aurantiacum = ant-s-aur.	
stibium sulfuratum nigrum = ant-c.	
stibium sulfuratum rubrum = ant-s-r.	
stibium sulphuratum auratum = ant-s-aur.	
stibium tartaricum = ant-t.	
stict.	sticta pulmonaria
stigm.	stigmata maydis
still.	stillingia silvatica
stizolobium pruriens = dol.	
stovaine = amyloc-m.	
stram.	stramonium
strept-ent.	bacillus strepto-enterococcus
streptoc.	streptococcinum unknown species
streptococcus haemolyticus = streptoc.	
streptococcus pyogenes = streptoc.	
streptococcus scarlatinae = streptoc.	
streptococcus viridans = streptoc.	
streptom.	streptomycinum
streptom-s.	streptomycinum sulphatum

stront-br.	strontium bromatum
stront-c.	strontium carbonicum
stront-i.	strontium iodatum
stront-met.	strontium metallicum
stront-n.	strontium nitricum
stroph-h.	strophanthus hispidus
stroph-s.	strophanthus sarmentosus
stroph-xyz.	strophanthus species unknown
stry.	strychninum purum
stry-af-cit.	strychninum citricum cum ammonioferri-citricum
stry-ar.	strychninum arsenicosum
stry-n.	strychninum nitricum
stry-p.	strychninum phosphoricum
stry-s.	strychninum sulphuricum
stry-val.	strychninum valerianicum
stry-xyz.	strychinum unknown type
strych-g.	strychnos gaultheriana
strychnini et ferri citras = stry-af-cit.	
strychnos ignatiae = ign.	
strychnos nux vomica = nux-v.	
strychnos nux-vomica = nux-v.	
strychnos tieut = upa.	
succ.	succinimidum
succ-ac.	succinicum acidum
succ-xyz.	succ. + succ-ac. + ol-suc.
suis-chord-umb.	suis (chorda umbilicalis)
suis-cu.	cutis suis
sul-ac.	sulphuricum acidum
sul-ac-ar.	sulphuricum acidum aromaticum
sul-h.	sulphur hydrogenisatum
sul-i.	sulphur iodatum
sul-ter.	sulphur terebinthinatum
sulfa.	sulfanilamidum
sulfag.	sulfaguanidinum
sulfon.	sulfonalum
sulfonam.	sulfonamidum
sulfur = sulph.	
sulo-ac.	sulphurosum acidum
sulph.	sulphur
sulphur lotum = sulph.	
sulphur sublimatum = sulph.	
sulphuricum aromaticum acidum = sul-ac-ar.	
sumb.	sumbulus moschatus

List of remedy abbreviations

sumbul ferula = sumb.

suprar.   suprarenalis

suprarenalis glandula = suprar.

surukuku = lach.

syc.   bacillus Sycoccus
                             (Paterson)

sycoccus (paterson) = syc.

sycoccus bacillus (paterson) = syc.

sycotic co. (paterson) = syc.

sycotic compound (paterson) = syc.

sym-r.   symphoricarpus
                             racemosus

symph.   symphytum officinale

symphoricarpos albus = sym-r.

symphoricarpus rivularis = sym-r.

symplocarpus foetidum = ictod.

syph.   syphilinum

syriaca = asc-c.

syzyg.   syzygium jambolanum

syzygium cumini = syzyg.

syzygium jambos = eug.

tab.   tabacum

tam.   tamus communis

tamrnd.   tamarindus indica

tanac.   tanacetum vulgare

tang.   tanghinia venenifera

tann-ac.   tannicum acidum

tanninum = tann-ac.

taraktogenos kurzii = chaul.

taraktogenos = chaul.

tarantula cubensis = tarent-c.

tarantula hispanica = tarent.

tarax.   taraxacum officinale

taraxacum dens leonis = tarax.

tarent.   tarentula hispanica

tarent-c.   tarentula cubensis

tart-ac.   tartaricum acidum

tartarus depuratus = kali-bit.

tartarus emeticus = ant-t.

tartarus stibiatus = ant-t.

tax.   taxus baccata

tax-br.   taxus brevifolia

tela aranearum = tela

tela   teła araneae

teleamethylthioninum chloridum = methyl.

tell.   tellurium metallicum

ten (Paterson) = bacls-10.

tep.   Teplitz aqua

ter.   terebinthinae oleum

teramycin = oxyte-chl.

tere-ch.   terebinthina chios

terebe.   terebenum

term-a.   terminalia arjuna

term-c.   terminalia chebula

terp-h.   terpini hydras

terra silicea = sil.

test.   testosterone base

testa praeparata = calc-o-t.

testis   testicles

tet.   tetradymitum

tetox.   tetanotoxinum

tetrabromfluoresceinum = eos.

tetrac.   tetracyclinum

tetramethylaminum = prop.

teucr.   teucrium marum verum

teucr-s.   teucrium scorodonia

teucrium chamaedrys = chamae.

thal.   thallium met. + -act. (old
                             abbr.)

thal-act.   thallium aceticum

thal-met.   thallium metallicum

thal-s.   thallium sulphuricum

thala.   thalamus

thap-g.   thapsia garganica

thaspium aureum = ziz.

thea sinensis = thea

thea   thea chinensis

thebaicum = op.

thebin.   thebainum

thein.   theinum

theobroma cacao = cac.

ther.   theridion curassavicum

thev.   thevetia nerifolia

thiop.   thioproperazinum

thiosin.   thiosinaminum

thlas.   thlaspi bursa pastoris

thrombidium = trom.

thryallis glauca = galph.

thuj.   thuja occidentalis

thuj-l.   thuja lobii

thym-gl.   thymi glandulae
                             extractum

thymoidinum = thym-gl.

List of remedy abbreviations

thymol.	thymolum
thymonucleicum acidum = des-ac.	
thymu.	thymus serpyllum
thymul.	thymulinum
thymus = thym-gl.	
thyr.	thyreoidinum
thyreostimulinum = thyreotr.	
thyreotr.	thyreotropinum
thyroid = thyr.	
thyroidinum = thyr.	
thyroiod.	thyro-iodinum
thyroiodinum = thyroiod.	
til.	tilia Europaea
tilia cordata = til.	
tilia silvestris = til.	
tinas.	tinospora cordifolia
tinctura sine kali = caust.	
tip.	tipida aqua
titan.	titanium metallicum
titan-xyz.	titan-g. + titan-n.
tocoph.	tocopherolum
toluiferum = bals-t.	
tonca = tong.	
tong.	tongo odorata
tor.	torula cerevisiae
tormentilla erecta = pot-e.	
tox-th.	= acok-op. = toxicophlaea thunbergii (old abbr.)
toxi.	= ancis-p. = toxicophis pugnax (old abbr.)
toxicodendron diversilobum = rhus-d.	
toxicodendron quercifolium vernix = rhus-t.	
toxicodendron radicans = rhus-t.	
toxicodendron vernixa = rhus-v.	
toxicophloea thunbergi = tox-th.	
toxo-g.	toxoplasma gondii
toxoplasmosis nosode = toxo-g.	
toxoplasms gondi = toxo-g.	
trach.	trachinus draco
trach-v.	trachinus vipera
trach-xyz.	trach. + trach-v.
trad.	tradescantia diuretica
triat.	triatoma
triatema = triat.	
trib.	tribulus terrestris
trich.	trichosanthes amara

trichom.	trichomonas vaginalis
trichosanthes dioica = trich.	
trif-p.	trifolium pratense
trif-r.	trifolium repens
trifolium album = trif-r.	
trifolium fibrinum = meny.	
trigonocephalus contortrix = cench.	
trigonocephalus lachesis = lach.	
trigonocephalus piscivorus = ancis-p.	
tril-c.	trillium cernuum
tril-p.	trillium pendulum
trillium erectum = tril-p.	
trim.	trimeresurus wagleri
trimethylaminum = prop.	
trimethylxanthin = coffin.	
trinit.	trinitrotoluenum
trinitrophenolum = pic-ac.	
trion.	trional
trios.	triosteum perfoliatum
tritic.	triticum repens
tritic-vg.	triticum vulgare
triticum aestivum = tritic-vg.	
trom.	trombidium muscae domesticae
trop.	tropaeolum majus
trychs.	trychosanthes
tsuga canadensis = abies-c.	
tub.	tuberculinum bovinum Kent
tub-a.	tuberculinum avis
tub-d.	tuberculinum Denys
tub-k.	tuberculinum Koch
tub-m.	tuberculinum Marmoreck
tub-r.	tuberculinum residuum Koch
tub-ro.	tuberculinum Rosenbach
tub-sp.	tuberculinum Spengler
tuberculini aviarii derivatum = tub-a.	
tuberculini bovini derivatum = tub.	
tuberculinum aviaire = tub-a.	
tuberculinum pristinum = tub-k.	
tung-met.	tungstenium metallicum
turnera aphrodisiaca = dam.	
turnera diffusa = dam.	
turpethum minerale = merc-sul.	
tus-fa.	tussilago farfara

List of remedy abbreviations

tus-fr.	tussilago fragrans
tus-p.	tussilago petasites
tyl-i.	tylophora indica
typh.	typha latifolia
typhobacillinum = eberth.	
typhoidinum = eberth.	
ulm-c.	ulmus campestris
ulm-pra.	ulmus procera
ulx-eu.	ulex Europaeus
umbellularia californica = oreo.	
umbilicus pendulinus = cot.	
uncar-tom.	uncaria tomentosa
upa.	upas tieuté
upa-a.	upas antiaris
ur-ac.	uricum acidum
uragoga ipecacuanha = ip.	
uran-m.	uranium muriaticum
uran-met.	uranium metallicum
uran-n.	uranium nitricum
urea-n.	urea nitrica
urea	urea pura
urginea maritima = squil.	
urin.	urinum
urine = urin.	
urotrop.	urotropinum
urt-c.	urtica crenulata
urt-g.	urtica gigas
urt-u.	urtica urens
usn.	usnea barbata
ust.	ustilago maydis
uva	uva ursi
uza.	uzara
v-a-b.	vaccin atténué bilié
vac.	vaccininum
vacc-m.	vaccinium myrtillus
Vaccin of Haffkine = pest.	
vaccinotoxinum = vac.	
vaccinum influenzae inactivatum = influ.	
valer.	valeriana officinalis
valerianae radix = valer.	
vanad.	vanadium metallicum
vanil.	vanilla aromatica
vanilla planifolia = vanil.	
varech = fuc.	
vario.	variolinum
ven-m.	venus mercenaria
verat.	veratrum album

verat-n.	veratrum nigrum
verat-v.	veratrum viride
veratrum luteum = helon.	
verb.	verbascum thapsus
verbe-h.	verbena hastata
verbe-o.	verbena officinalis
verbe-u.	verbena urticaefolia
verin.	veratrinum
vern-a.	vernonia anthelmintica
vero-o.	veronica officinalis
veronal = barbit.	
veronastricum virginicum = lept.	
veronica virginica = lept.	
verr.	verrucinum
vesi.	vesicaria communis
vesp.	vespa crabro
vesp-xyz.	vespa crabro + vespul-m.
+vespul-vg.	
vespul-vg.	vespula vulgaris
vetiver = anan.	
vetiveria zizanioides = anan.	
vib.	viburnum opulus
vib-od.	viburnum oderatissinum
vib-p.	viburnum prunifolium
vib-t.	viburnum tinus
viburnum oderiferum = vib-od.	
vichy-g.	Vichy aqua Grande Grille
vichy-h.	Vichy aqua Hôpital
vinc.	vinca minor
vinc-ma.	vinca major
vinc-r.	vinca rosea
vince.	vincetoxicum officinale
viol-o.	viola odorata
viol-t.	viola tricolor
vip.	vipera berus
vip-a.	vipera aspis
vip-a-c.	vipera acontica carinata
vip-d.	vipera daboia
vip-l-f.	vipera lachesis fel
vip-t.	= vip. = vipera torva (old abbr.)
vipera communis = vip.	
vipera redi = vip-a.	
vipera russelli = vip-d.	
virola sebifera = myric.	
virus poliomyelitis = polio	
visc.	viscum album

List of remedy abbreviations

vit.	vitex trifolia	zinc.	zincum metallicum
vit-b-x.	vitamin b1+b2+b6+b12	zinc-act.	zincum aceticum
vitamin e = tocoph.		zinc-ar.	zincum arsenicosum
vitamin-d	vit d2 and/or vit d3	zinc-br.	zincum bromatum
vitex agnus castus = agn.		zinc-c.	zincum carbonicum
vitex agnus-castus = agn.		zinc-chl.	zincum chloricum
vitis alba = bry.		zinc-chr.	zincum chromicum
vitis quinquefolia = ampe-qu.		zinc-cy.	zincum cyanatum
vitis rubra = ampe-qu.		zinc-fcy.	zincum ferrocyanatum
vitis-v.	vitis vinifera	zinc-i.	zincum iodatum
vitr-an.	vitrum antimonii	zinc-m.	zincum muriaticum
vitr-cor.	vitrum coroni	zinc-o.	zincum oxydatum
voes.	Voeslau aqua	zinc-ox.	zincum oxalicum
wies.	Wiesbaden aqua	zinc-p.	zincum phosphoricum (old abbr.)
wigardia californica = erio.			
wildb.	Wildbad aqua	zinc-phic.	zincum phosphoricum
wist-s.	wisteria sinensis	zinc-pic.	zincum picricum
wood alcohol = methan.		zinc-s.	zincum sulphuricum
woorali = cur.		zinc-val.	zincum valerianicum
woorara = cur.		zinci oxidum = zinc-o.	
wrightia antidysenterica = kurch.		zinci sulphas = zinc-s.	
wrightia tincto = kurch.		zincum chromatum = zinc-chr.	
wye.	wyethia helenoides	zincum isovalerianicum = zinc-val.	
wyethia = wye.		zing.	zingiber officinale
x-ray	x-ray	zingiber = zing.	
xan.	xanthoxylum fraxineum	ziz.	zizia aurea
xanrhi.	xanthorrhiza apifolia		
xanrhoe.	xanthorrhoea arborea		
xanth.	xanthium spinosum		
xanthoxylum Americanum = xan.			
xero.	xerophyllum asphodeloides		
xiphosura = lim.			
yaupon = ilx-v.			
yerba buena = micr.			
yerba mansa = anemps.			
yerba santa = erio.			
yers.	serum yersiniae		
Yersin = yers.			
yohim.	yohimbinum		
yohimbehe = yohim.			
yuc.	yucca filamentosa		
zanthoxylum fraxineum = xan.			
zea mais = stigm.			
zea putrefatto = zea-i.			
zea-i.	zea italica		

List of remedy abbreviations

Index of words

A

abandoned *[Mind]* **1**
abashed *[Mind]* **1**
abdomen *[Coug]* 1137, *[Drea]* 1675
abdominal *[Resp]* 1113
abducted *[Extr]* 1351
ability *[Mind]* **1**
abortion *[Mind]* 15, 20, 38, 45, 65, 82, 101, 104,
    144, 169, 188, *[Mout]* 638, *[Abdo]* 869, *[Rect]* 935,
    [Blad] 960, *[Fema]* **1043**, 1043, 1050, 1051, 1053,
    1058, 1061, 1063, 1064, 1068, 1069, 1070, 1071,
    1077, 1090, 1091, *[Resp]* 1121, *[Coug]* 1151,
    1156, *[Ches]* 1230, *[Back]* 1284, 1347, *[Extr]*
    1496, *[Slee]* 1672, *[Drea]* **1675**, *[Chil]* 1702, *[Feve]*
    1719, *[Gene]* 1800, 1801, 1818, 1840, 1870, 1954,
    1965
abraded *[Extr]* 1351
abrasion *[Eye]* **389**
abroad *[Mind]* **1**
abrupt *[Mind]* **1**, 195
abscess *[Vert]* 233, *[Head]* 239, *[Ear]* **461**, *[Nose]*
    505, *[Face]* 545, *[Mout]* 605, 605, 614, 635, 656,
    [Teet] **661**, *[Thro]* 683, *[Exte]* **715**, *[Abdo]* **803**,
    [Rect] 897, 937, *[Kidn]* **973**, *[Pros]* **981**, *[Uret]* **985**,
    [Male] **1013**, *[Fema]* **1044**, *[Ches]* **1177**, 1177,
    1195, 1197, 1219, 1263, *[Back]* **1269**, *[Extr]* **1351**,
    1367, *[Skin]* 1771, *[Gene]* 1845
abscesses *[Eye]* **389**, *[Skin]* 1747, *[Gene]* 1797
absences *[Mind]* **1**, *[Gene]* 1798
absent *[Abdo]* **803**, *[Male]* **1013**, *[Back]* **1269**, *[Chil]*
    1702, *[Pers]* 1737
absent father *[Mind]* **1**
absent mother *[Mind]* **1**
absentminded *[Mind]* **1**
absorbed *[Mind]* **1**
absorption *[Gene]* 1798
abstract thinking *[Mind]* **2**
abstraction of mind *[Mind]* **2**
absurd *[Mind]* **2**, *[Drea]* 1675
abused *[Mind]* **2**, *[Drea]* 1675
abused sexually *[Drea]* 1675
abusing *[Drea]* 1675
abusive *[Mind]* **2**
abyss *[Drea]* 1675
acanthosis *[Skin]* 1747
acarophobia *[Mind]* **2**
accelerated *[Resp]* 1113

accident-prone *[Mind]* **2**
accidents *[Drea]* 1675
accommodation *[Visi]* **443**
accompanied by *[Vert]* 226, *[Coug]* 1137, *[Drea]*
    1675, *[Chil]* **1702**, *[Feve]* **1719**, *[Pers]* 1737
accumulation *[Gene]* 1798
accusations *[Drea]* 1675
acetonemia *[Stom]* **723**, *[Gene]* 1798
acetonuria *[Urin]* **999**
acid *[Urin]* **999**
acidity *[Teet]* **661**, *[Stom]* **723**
acidosis *[Gene]* 1798
acids *[Coug]* **1138**, *[Chil]* **1702**
acne *[Mind]* 182, *[Ear]* 465, *[Hear]* 504, *[Nose]* 527,
    [Face] 560, 561, *[Stom]* 790, *[Fema]* 1066, *[Ches]*
    1188, 1189, *[Back]* 1274, *[Extr]* 1385, 1395, *[Skin]*
    1755, *[Gene]* 1830, 1837
aconite *[Gene]* 1798
acquaintances *[Drea]* 1675
acrid *[Eye]* 394, 435, *[Nose]* 509, 513, 521, 530,
    534, *[Face]* 561, 567, 570, 601, *[Mout]* 629, 640,
    648, *[Thro]* 711, *[Stom]* 738, 796, *[Rect]* 913, 922,
    933, *[Stoo]* **939**, 944, *[Uret]* 985, 990, *[Urin]* **999**,
    1006, *[Male]* 1025, *[Fema]* 1053, 1055, 1057,
    1058, 1060, 1064, 1068, *[Resp]* 1115, *[Coug]*
    1138, *[Expe]* **1169**, 1170, *[Ches]* 1256, *[Extr]*
    1391, 1398, *[Pers]* **1737**, *[Skin]* 1747, 1773, *[Gene]*
    1797, 1814, 1832, 1869, 1890
acridity *[Face]* **545**, *[Stom]* **723**, *[Gene]* 1798
acrocyanosis *[Extr]* 1351
acromegaly *[Extr]* 1351, *[Gene]* 1798
acromion *[Extr]* 1408, 1539, 1588
acrophobia *[Mind]* **2**
actinomycosis *[Skin]* 1747, *[Gene]* 1879
action *[Mind]* **2**
actions *[Mind]* **2**
active *[Drea]* 1675
activity *[Mind]* **2**, *[Gene]* 1798
actors *[Drea]* 1675
acute *[Visi]* **443**, *[Hear]* **501**
acute diseases *[Pers]* 1737
acuteness *[Mind]* **3**
adams-stokes *[Ches]* **1177**
adaptability *[Mind]* **3**
addison's *[Kidn]* **973**
adenitis *[Gene]* 1799
adenoids *[Hear]* 502, *[Nose]* **505**, *[Thro]* **683**, 712,
    [Resp] 1133, *[Gene]* **1799**

Index of words

adenopathy *[Gene]* **1799**

adhere *[Teet]* **661**, *[Male]* **1013**

adherent *[Back]* **1269**, *[Skin]* **1747**

adheres *[Mout]* **605**, *[Coug]* **1138**

adhesion *[Head]* **239**, *[Face]* **545**, *[Stom]* **723**, *[Abdo]* **803**, *[Extr]* **1351**

adhesions *[Eye]* **389**, *[Ear]* **461**, *[Fema]* **1044**, *[Ches]* **1177**, *[Gene]* **1799**

adhesive *[Thro]* **683**

adiposogenital dystrophy *[Gene]* **1799**

admonition *[Mind]* **3**, 3, 219

adrenal glands *[Gene]* **1979**

adulterous *[Mind]* **3**

adventurous *[Mind]* **3**, *[Drea]* **1675**

adynamic fever *[Feve]* **1719**

aerials *[Drea]* **1675**

aerophagia *[Stom]* **723**

affability *[Mind]* **3**

affectation *[Mind]* **3**

affected *[Mind]* **3**, *[Slee]* **1641**, *[Chil]* **1702**, *[Feve]* **1719**, *[Pers]* **1737**

affecting *[Drea]* **1675**

affection *[Mind]* **3**

affectionate *[Mind]* **3**, *[Drea]* **1675**

affections *[Ches]* **1177**

afraid *[Mind]* **3**

afternoon *[Vert]* **225**, *[Coug]* **1136**, *[Expe]* **1169**, *[Chil]* **1700**, *[Feve]* **1718**, *[Pers]* **1735**, *[Gene]* **1794**

afterpains *[Head]* **292**, *[Abdo]* **862**, *[Fema]* **1044**, 1071, *[Back]* 1330, *[Extr]* **1490**, *[Gene]* 1840

agalactia *[Ches]* **1177**

agg *[Expe]* **1169**

agglutinated *[Eye]* **389**

agglutination *[Ear]* **461**, *[Nose]* **505**, *[Uret]* **985**, *[Gene]* **1799**

aggravates *[Coug]* **1138**, *[Pers]* **1737**

aggression *[Mind]* **3**

agility *[Mind]* **3**, *[Extr]* **1351**, *[Gene]* **1799**

agitation *[Mind]* **3**, *[Coug]* **1138**

agony *[Mind]* **3**

agoraphobia *[Mind]* **3**

agranulocytosis *[Gene]* **1799**, 1879

agreeable *[Drea]* **1675**

ague *[Gene]* **1799**

aichmophobia *[Mind]* **3**

aids *[Gene]* **1799**

ailments *[Gene]* **1799**

ailments from *[Mind]* **3**

ailurophobia *[Mind]* **7**

air *[Mind]* **7**, *[Head]* **239**, *[Eye]* **389**, *[Ear]* **461**, *[Face]* **545**, *[Mout]* **605**, *[Teet]* **661**, *[Exte]* **715**, *[Blad]* **951**, *[Uret]* **985**, *[Fema]* **1044**, *[Lary]* **1093**, *[Expe]* **1169**, *[Ches]* **1177**, *[Extr]* **1351**, *[Drea]* **1675**, *[Chil]* **1703**, *[Skin]* **1747**, *[Gene]* **1799**

air ; in open *[Resp]* **1113**

air agg *[Vert]* **227**, *[Head]* **239**, *[Coug]* **1138**, *[Back]* **1269**

air attacks *[Drea]* **1675**

air hunger *[Gene]* **1799**

air; draft of *[Chil]* **1703**, *[Gene]* **1799**

air; in open *[Vert]* **227**, *[Nose]* **505**, *[Stom]* **723**, *[Coug]* **1138**, *[Expe]* **1169**, *[Ches]* **1177**, *[Chil]* **1703**, *[Feve]* **1719**, *[Pers]* **1737**, *[Gene]* **1799**

air; open *[Gene]* **1800**

airplane *[Stom]* **723**, *[Gene]* **1800**

airplanes *[Drea]* **1675**

akinesia *[Gene]* **1800**

alarms *[Drea]* **1675**

albuminous *[Stoo]* **939**, *[Urin]* **999**, *[Expe]* **1169**

albuminuria *[Urin]* **999**, *[Gene]* **1800**

alcohol *[Mind]* **7**, *[Coug]* **1138**, *[Chil]* **1703**

alcoholic *[Vert]* **227**, *[Gene]* **1800**

alcoholics *[Vert]* **227**

alcoholism *[Mind]* **7**, *[Gene]* **1800**

alert *[Mind]* **7**

algophobia *[Mind]* **7**

alienated *[Mind]* **7**

alive *[Head]* **239**, *[Ear]* **461**, *[Teet]* **661**, *[Thro]* **683**, *[Exte]* **715**, *[Stom]* **723**, *[Abdo]* **803**, *[Ches]* **1177**, *[Extr]* **1351**, *[Skin]* **1747**, *[Gene]* **1800**

alkaline *[Urin]* **999**

allergic *[Coug]* **1138**, *[Gene]* **1800**

allergy *[Skin]* **1747**

alone *[Mind]* **7**, *[Drea]* **1675**

aloof *[Mind]* **7**

alopecia *[Head]* **239**, *[Skin]* **1747**, *[Gene]* **1800**

altered *[Urin]* **1000**

alternating *[Mind]* **7**, *[Coug]* **1138**, *[Expe]* **1169**, *[Ches]* **1177**, *[Drea]* **1675**, *[Feve]* **1719**, *[Pers]* **1737**, *[Gene]* **1801**

alternating sides *[Pers]* **1735**

alternating with *[Vert]* **227**, *[Chil]* **1703**

altitude *[Gene]* **1801**

aluminium *[Gene]* **1801**

alzheimer's disease *[Gene]* **1801**

amathophobia *[Mind]* **7**

Index of words

amativeness *[Mind]* **7**

amaurosis *[Eye]* **389**, *[Visi]* **443**

amaxophobia *[Mind]* **7**

ambition *[Mind]* **7**

amblyopia *[Eye]* **389**, *[Visi]* **443**

amebiasis *[Gene]* **1801**

amel *[Expe]* **1169**

ameliorates *[Pers]* **1737**

amenorrhea *[Fema]* **1044**

amnesia *[Mind]* **8**, 22, 96

amorous *[Mind]* **8**, *[Drea]* **1675**

amputated *[Extr]* **1351**

amputation *[Drea]* **1676**

amusement *[Mind]* **8**

amyotrophic lateral sclerosis *[Gene]* **1801**

anal fixation *[Mind]* **8**

analgesia *[Extr]* **1351**, *[Gene]* **1801**

analgesics *[Kidn]* **973**, *[Gene]* **1801**

analytical thinking *[Mind]* **8**

anaphylaxis *[Gene]* **1801**

anarchist *[Mind]* **8**

anasarca *[Gene]* **1801**

androphobia *[Mind]* **8**

anemia *[Vert]* 226, 227, *[Head]* **239**, 276, *[Eye]* **389**, *[Hear]* **504**, *[Nose]* 521, *[Face]* 555, 574, *[Stom]* 791, *[Abdo]* 818, 894, 896, *[Rect]* 898, *[Blad]* 960, 965, *[Urin]* 1004, *[Male]* 1014, *[Fema]* 1043, 1045, 1054, 1068, *[Resp]* 1121, *[Ches]* 1251, 1264, *[Back]* **1269**, *[Slee]* 1654, *[Feve]* 1726, *[Pers]* 1742, *[Gene]* **1801**, 1810, 1833, 1837, 1840, 1844, 1886, 1897, 1966, 1968

anemic *[Face]* **545**

anemophobia *[Mind]* **8**

anesthesia *[Mind]* 95, *[Thro]* **683**, *[Lary]* **1093**, *[Resp]* 1116, *[Ches]* 1192, *[Extr]* **1351**, *[Skin]* 1747, *[Gene]* **1802**, 1818, 1937

aneurysm *[Abdo]* **803**, 885, *[Ches]* **1177**, *[Gene]* **1802**

anger *[Mind]* **8**, *[Vert]* **227**, *[Head]* **239**, *[Abdo]* **803**, *[Coug]* **1138**, *[Drea]* **1676**, *[Chil]* **1703**, *[Feve]* **1720**, *[Pers]* **1737**

angina *[Thro]* **683**, *[Ches]* **1177**

angioma *[Face]* **545**, *[Skin]* 1755, *[Gene]* 1807, 1955

angiophobia *[Mind]* **11**

anguish *[Mind]* **11**

anhidrosis *[Skin]* **1747**

animal *[Mind]* 50, 140, *[Head]* 280, 288, *[Stom]* 754, 798, *[Gene]* 1810, 1837, 1846, 1870

animals *[Mind]* **12**, 12, 42, 50, 51, 57, 58, 70, 73, 88, 101, 104, 107, 149, 205, 206, *[Visi]* 444, *[Nose]* 529, *[Abdo]* 896, *[Drea]* **1676**, 1676, 1677, 1684, 1691, 1696, *[Gene]* 1978

animated *[Mind]* **12**

animation *[Mind]* **12**

animus possession *[Mind]* **12**

ankle-drop *[Extr]* **1351**

ankles *[Extr]* **1632**

ankylosing *[Back]* **1269**

ankylosis *[Back]* **1269**, *[Extr]* **1351**

annoyed *[Mind]* **12**

annoying *[Drea]* **1676**

annual *[Chil]* **1703**

anorexia mentalis *[Mind]* **12**

anorexia nervosa *[Mind]* **12**

anosmia *[Nose]* **505**

anosognosia *[Mind]* 130

another person *[Drea]* **1676**

anoxia *[Head]* **239**

answering *[Mind]* **12**

antagonism *[Mind]* **13**

anterior *[Chil]* **1703**

anthrax *[Extr]* **1351**, *[Skin]* 1755

anthropophobia *[Mind]* **13**, 101, 110

antibiotics *[Gene]* **1802**

anticipating *[Chil]* **1703**, *[Feve]* **1720**

anticipation *[Mind]* **13**

antics *[Mind]* **14**

antipyretics *[Gene]* **1802**

antisocial *[Mind]* **14**

antitragus *[Ear]* 466, 469, 490, 496

ants *[Skin]* **1747**

anus *[Rect]* **937**

anxiety *[Mind]* **14**, *[Vert]* **227**, *[Head]* **239**, *[Thro]* **683**, *[Stom]* **723**, *[Abdo]* **803**, *[Ches]* **1177**, *[Extr]* **1351**, *[Chil]* **1703**, *[Pers]* **1737**, *[Gene]* **1802**

anxious *[Eye]* **389**, *[Resp]* 1113, *[Slee]* **1641**, *[Drea]* **1676**, *[Feve]* **1720**

aorta *[Abdo]* 833, 885, *[Ches]* **1177**, 1195, 1219, 1258, 1266

aortic *[Ches]* **1178**

apathy *[Mind]* **22**

ape *[Drea]* **1677**

aphasia *[Mind]* **22**, 152, *[Mout]* 638, *[Extr]* **1436**, *[Gene]* 1918

aphrodisiac *[Male]* **1013**, *[Fema]* **1044**

Index of words

aphthae *[Mind]* 189, *[Eye]* 393, *[Nose]* **505**, *[Face]* **545**, *[Mout]* **605**, 605, 609, 642, 645, 647, *[Thro]* **683**, 686, *[Male]* **1013**, *[Fema]* **1044**, 1051, *[Ches]* **1178**, 1257, *[Feve]* 1732, *[Skin]* 1771, *[Gene]* **1802**, 1955

aphthous *[Rect]* 897

aplomb *[Mind]* 22

apnea *[Resp]* 1113

apoplectic *[Mind]* 33, 45, 202, *[Eye]* 404, *[Drea]* 1680, *[Gene]* 1820

apoplexy *[Mind]* 22, 51, 101, 133, 163, 213, *[Head]* **239**, 246, 256, 282, 346, 372, *[Eye]* **389**, 440, *[Hear]* 504, *[Face]* 549, 551, 555, *[Mout]* 642, 643, 646, *[Stom]* 786, *[Extr]* 1579, 1581, 1582, 1631, *[Slee]* 1641, 1643, 1650, 1655, 1661, *[Gene]* **1802**, 1818, 1844, 1872, 1918, 1919, 1928, 1929, 1930, 1958, 1966

appearance *[Mind]* **22**, *[Face]* **545**, *[Gene]* **1803**

appearing suddenly *[Gene]* **1803**

appendicitis *[Abdo]* **803**

appetite *[Stom]* **723**

applauded *[Drea]* **1677**

apple *[Thro]* **683**

appreciation *[Mind]* 22

apprehension *[Stom]* **728**, *[Abdo]* **803**, *[Blad]* **951**, *[Coug]* **1138**, *[Ches]* **1179**

apprehensions *[Mind]* 22

approach *[Visi]* **443**

approached *[Mind]* 22

approval *[Mind]* 22

apyrexia *[Feve]* **1720**

aquaphobia *[Mind]* 22

arachnophobia *[Mind]* 22

arching *[Back]* **1269**

arcus senilis *[Eye]* **389**

ardent *[Mind]* 22

arguing *[Mind]* 22

argumentative *[Mind]* 22

arm *[Drea]* **1677**

armies *[Drea]* **1677**

armor *[Drea]* **1677**

arms *[Coug]* **1139**, *[Extr]* **1632**

arms away from the body *[Gene]* **1803**

arrested *[Resp]* **1113**, *[Drea]* **1677**

arrhythmia *[Ches]* **1179**

arrogance *[Mind]* **22**

arrows *[Drea]* **1677**

arsenic *[Chil]* **1703**

arsenical *[Coug]* **1139**, *[Gene]* **1803**

art *[Mind]* 22

arteries *[Head]* 264, 277, 311, 375, *[Eye]* 432, *[Ear]* 495, *[Abdo]* 885, *[Ches]* 1177, 1257, *[Gene]* 1805, 1817, 1874, 1896, 1924, 1949

arteriosclerosis *[Ches]* **1179**, 1264, *[Gene]* **1803**, 1830

arteriosclerotic *[Mind]* 153, *[Vert]* **227**, *[Ches]* 1265

arthralgia *[Gene]* **1803**

arthritic *[Extr]* **1351**

arthritis *[Extr]* **1352**, *[Gene]* **1803**

arthritis deformans *[Extr]* **1352**

arthrosis *[Extr]* **1352**

artistic *[Mind]* 22

ascarides *[Rect]* 921, *[Fema]* **1044**, *[Skin]* 1769

ascending *[Vert]* **228**, *[Head]* **239**, *[Fema]* **1044**, *[Resp]* **1114**, *[Drea]* **1677**, *[Chil]* **1703**, *[Feve]* **1720**, *[Pers]* **1737**, *[Gene]* **1803**

ascending stairs *[Coug]* **1139**

ascetic *[Mind]* 22

ascites *[Mout]* 619, *[Abdo]* **803**, 804, 812, 817, 894, *[Ches]* 1264, *[Gene]* 1966

ash-colored *[Stoo]* **939**, *[Expe]* **1169**

asking *[Mind]* 22

asleep *[Head]* **239**, *[Mout]* **606**, *[Male]* **1013**, *[Back]* **1269**, *[Extr]* **1352**, *[Slee]* **1641**, *[Skin]* **1747**

asphyxia *[Mind]* 33, 213, *[Resp]* **1114**, *[Gene]* **1803**, 1829

aspirin *[Gene]* **1803**

aspiring *[Drea]* **1677**

assemblies *[Drea]* **1677**

assertive *[Mind]* 22

assimilation *[Gene]* **1803**

assurance *[Mind]* 22

asthenopia *[Head]* 276, *[Eye]* **389**, *[Visi]* **443**

asthma *[Mind]* 16, 144, 145, 177, 222, *[Head]* 276, 279, *[Nose]* 526, 540, *[Face]* 550, 555, 601, *[Mout]* 629, 635, 642, *[Thro]* 699, *[Stom]* 723, 733, 736, 746, 750, 756, 757, 782, 792, 794, *[Rect]* 904, *[Fema]* 1067, *[Lary]* 1105, *[Resp]* 1117, *[Ches]* 1187, 1188, 1189, *[Extr]* 1382, 1389, 1398, 1497, *[Pers]* 1742, *[Skin]* 1755, 1765, 1769, *[Gene]* 1809, 1834, 1840, 1844, 1864, 1871, 1965

asthmatic *[Resp]* **1114**, *[Coug]* **1139**

asthmatic bronchitis *[Ches]* **1179**

astigmatism *[Eye]* **390**, *[Visi]* **443**, 456

astonished *[Mind]* 22

astraphobia *[Mind]* 22

Index of words

astray *[Drea]* **1677**
astringent *[Mout]* **606**, *[Thro]* **683**
ataxia *[Extr]* **1352**
atelectasis *[Ches]* **1179**
atheroma *[Gene]* **1803**
athetosis *[Extr]* **1352**
athlete's *[Extr]* **1352**
atony *[Stom]* **728**, *[Blad]* **951**, *[Fema]* **1044**
atrophy *[Head]* **239**, *[Eye]* **390**, *[Nose]* **505**, *[Mout]* **606**, *[Stom]* **728**, *[Abdo]* **803**, *[Kidn]* **973**, *[Male]* **1013**, *[Fema]* **1044**, *[Ches]* **1179**, *[Back]* **1269**, *[Extr]* **1352**, *[Skin]* **1747**, *[Gene]* **1803**
attached *[Mind]* **22**
attack *[Mind]* **23**
attacked *[Drea]* **1677**
attended *[Mind]* **23**
attention *[Mind]* **23**
attention deficit hyperactive disorder *[Mind]* **23**
attention seeking *[Mind]* **23**
attitudes *[Mind]* **23**
audacity *[Mind]* **23**
aura *[Fema]* **1044**
aura epileptica *[Stom]* **728**
autism *[Mind]* **23**
autoimmune *[Gene]* **1803**
automatic *[Mind]* **23**, 118, 207, 214, *[Extr]* 1428, 1429
automatism *[Mind]* **23**
autophobia *[Mind]* **23**
autophony *[Hear]* **501**
autopsies *[Drea]* **1677**
autumn *[Coug]* **1139**, *[Chil]* **1703**, *[Gene]* **1803**
autumnal *[Chil]* **1703**, *[Feve]* **1720**
avarice *[Mind]* **23**
aversion *[Mind]* **23**, *[Stom]* **728**, *[Male]* **1013**, *[Fema]* **1044**
aviator's disease *[Gene]* **1803**
awake *[Slee]* **1641**, *[Pers]* **1737**
awakening *[Mind]* **24**
aware *[Slee]* **1641**
awareness *[Mind]* **24**, *[Ches]* **1179**
away *[Drea]* **1677**
awe *[Mind]* **24**
awkward *[Mind]* **24**, 118, 124, 196, 211, *[Extr]* 1429, 1623
awkwardness *[Extr]* **1352**
axilla *[Ches]* **1264**

B

back *[Vert]* **228**, *[Drea]* **1677**
backache *[Back]* **1269**
backwardness *[Mind]* **24**
backwards in time *[Drea]* **1677**
bad *[Slee]* **1641**
bad mood *[Mind]* **24**
bad news *[Mind]* **24**, *[Vert]* **228**
bad parts *[Mind]* **24**
bad temper *[Mind]* **24**
baffled *[Drea]* **1677**
balance *[Mind]* **24**
balanced *[Stom]* **728**
balancing *[Vert]* **228**, *[Head]* **239**
balanitis *[Male]* **1013**
bald *[Ear]* **461**
baldness *[Head]* **239**, 346, 385
ball *[Head]* **239**, *[Thro]* **683**, *[Stom]* **728**, *[Abdo]* **803**, *[Rect]* **897**, *[Blad]* **951**, *[Pros]* **981**, *[Uret]* **985**, *[Fema]* **1044**, *[Lary]* **1093**, *[Expe]* **1169**, *[Ches]* **1179**, *[Gene]* **1803**
ballism *[Extr]* **1352**
balls *[Visi]* **443**, *[Stoo]* **939**, *[Expe]* **1169**, *[Extr]* **1352**, *[Drea]* **1677**
band *[Mind]* **78**, *[Head]* **239**, 247, 248, 280, 297, 317, 319, 321, 339, 351, 367, *[Eye]* **390**, *[Nose]* 542, *[Mout]* 615, *[Abdo]* **803**, 807, 850, *[Blad]* **951**, *[Fema]* **1046**, *[Ches]* **1179**, 1184, 1185, *[Back]* **1269**, 1273, *[Extr]* **1365**, 1542, *[Slee]* **1672**, *[Gene]* **1803**, 1817, 1818
bandaged *[Extr]* **1352**
bandaging *[Head]* **250**, 280, 316, 336, *[Stom]* **767**, *[Abdo]* **803**, *[Back]* **1318**, 1333, *[Extr]* **1353**, 1490, *[Gene]* **1803**
banquet *[Drea]* **1677**
bar *[Stom]* **728**, *[Ches]* **1179**, *[Back]* **1269**, 1289
barber's itch *[Face]* **545**
bargaining *[Mind]* **24**
barking *[Mind]* **24**, 45, 144, *[Stom]* **736**, *[Lary]* **1106**, *[Coug]* **1139**, 1149
bartholin's c *[Fema]* **1044**
baseball *[Drea]* **1677**
basedow *[Exte]* **716**
basedow's *[Gene]* **1804**
bashful *[Mind]* **24**
basic *[Mind]* **24**
basphobia *[Mind]* **24**

Index of words

bath *[Skin]* **1747**

bathing *[Mind]* **24**, *[Vert]* **228**, *[Head]* **239**, *[Eye]* **390**, *[Coug]* **1139**, *[Drea]* **1677**, *[Chil]* **1703**, *[Gene]* **1804**

bats *[Drea]* **1677**

batter *[Expe]* **1169**

battles *[Mind]* **24**, *[Drea]* **1677**

beard *[Face]* **545**

bearing *[Abdo]* **803**, *[Male]* **1013**

bearing down *[Gene]* **1804**

beaten *[Ches]* **1179**, *[Drea]* **1677**

beating *[Mind]* **24**

beautiful *[Mind]* **24**

bed *[Mind]* **24**, *[Vert]* **228**, *[Coug]* **1139**, *[Expe]* **1169**, *[Drea]* **1677**, *[Chil]* **1703**, *[Feve]* **1720**, *[Pers]* **1737**

bedsores *[Extr]* **1353**, *[Skin]* **1747**

bed-wetting *[Blad]* **951**

beer *[Mind]* 16, **25**, 37, 38, 90, 96, 201, *[Vert]* **228**, *[Head]* 257, 261, 280, 281, 377, *[Eye]* 412, *[Nose]* 529, 538, *[Mout]* 641, 650, 652, 653, 654, 655, 656, *[Teet]* **661**, 669, *[Thro]* 709, *[Stom]* 725, 732, 736, 740, 746, 748, 751, 753, 757, 759, 767, 786, 792, *[Abdo]* 810, 830, 833, *[Rect]* 905, 917, *[Blad]* 958, *[Urin]* 1001, *[Male]* 1037, *[Resp]* 1122, *[Coug]* **1139**, 1143, *[Ches]* 1247, 1252, *[Back]* 1312, *[Extr]* 1589, *[Slee]* 1642, 1646, 1655, 1661, *[Chil]* 1702, *[Feve]* 1719, **1720**, *[Gene]* 1803, 1846, 1847, 1867, 1895, 1966

bees *[Drea]* **1677**, *[Skin]* **1747**

beetles *[Drea]* **1677**

beggars *[Drea]* **1677**

begging *[Mind]* **25**

beginning *[Vert]* **228**, *[Chil]* **1703**

behavior problems *[Mind]* **25**

belching *[Stom]* **728**

belladonna *[Gene]* **1804**

bellowing *[Mind]* **25**

bell's palsy *[Face]* **545**

bellyache *[Abdo]* **803**

belonephobia *[Mind]* **25**

bemoaning *[Mind]* **25**

bending *[Vert]* **228**, *[Head]* **239**, *[Stom]* **728**, *[Male]* **1013**, *[Fema]* **1044**, *[Lary]* **1093**, *[Resp]* **1119**, *[Coug]* **1139**, *[Ches]* **1179**, *[Back]* **1269**, *[Extr]* **1353**, *[Gene]* **1804**

bending double *[Coug]* **1139**

bending head backward *[Eye]* **390**

benevolence *[Mind]* **25**

bent *[Extr]* **1353**, *[Gene]* **1805**

benumbed *[Mind]* **25**

bereavement *[Mind]* **25**

berger' *[Extr]* **1353**

berger's disease *[Kidn]* **973**

beriberi *[Gene]* **1805**

beside oneself *[Mind]* **25**

besnier-boeck-schaumann *[Gene]* **1805**

betrayed *[Drea]* **1677**

bewildered *[Mind]* **25**

biceps *[Extr]* **1377**, **1422**, **1565**, **1582**, **1597**, **1608**, 1619

bicycle *[Drea]* **1677**

bifida *[Back]* **1269**

bile *[Urin]* **1000**

biliary colic *[Abdo]* **803**

bilious *[Mind]* **25**, *[Stoo]* **939**, *[Expe]* **1169**, *[Feve]* **1720**

binding *[Head]* **240**

binding up *[Gene]* **1805**

birds *[Mind]* 52, 102, *[Ear]* 479, *[Drea]* **1677**

birth *[Fema]* **1044**

birthmarks *[Face]* **545**

bites *[Skin]* **1747**, *[Gene]* **1805**

biting *[Mind]* **25**, *[Face]* **545**, *[Mout]* **606**, *[Teet]* **661**, *[Thro]* **683**, *[Urin]* **1000**, *[Extr]* **1353**, *[Skin]* **1747**, *[Gene]* **1805**

bitten *[Drea]* **1677**, *[Skin]* **1747**

bitter *[Mind]* 122, 183, 185, 220, *[Head]* 277, *[Nose]* 514, 529, *[Mout]* 608, 640, 648, 649, 650, 651, 652, 655, *[Thro]* 694, 696, 710, *[Stom]* **728**, 739, 740, 741, 742, 743, 756, 786, 797, 799, *[Expe]* 1169, 1174, *[Ches]* 1200, *[Pers]* 1740, *[Gene]* 1832, 1847, 1848, 1849, 1941

black *[Mind]* **26**, *[Nose]* **505**, *[Thro]* **683**, *[Rect]* **897**, *[Stoo]* **939**

black spots *[Visi]* **443**

blackish *[Expe]* **1169**

blackness *[Gene]* **1805**

blackout *[Mind]* **26**

blackwater *[Feve]* **1720**

bladder *[Skin]* **1747**

blames *[Mind]* **26**

blank *[Mind]* **26**

blanket *[Coug]* **1139**

blasphemy *[Mind]* **26**

Index of words

bleeding *[Eye]* **390**, *[Ear]* **461**, *[Nose]* **505**, *[Face]* **545**, *[Mout]* **606**, *[Teet]* **661**, *[Abdo]* **803**, *[Rect]* **897**, *[Male]* **1013**, *[Fema]* **1044**, *[Ches]* **1179**, *[Gene]* **1805**

blennorrhea *[Male]* **1013**

blepharitis *[Eye]* **390**

blepharospasm *[Eye]* **390**

blind *[Drea]* **1677**

blindness *[Mind]* **26**, *[Eye]* **390**, *[Visi]* **443**

blinking *[Eye]* **390**

blissful *[Mind]* **26**

blistered *[Thro]* **683**

blisters *[Eye]* **390**, 397, *[Ear]* **465**, *[Nose]* **505**, *[Face]* 561, 568, 569, *[Mout]* **607**, *[Fema]* 1054, *[Ches]* 1188, 1189, *[Extr]* 1385, 1387, 1388, 1391, 1392, 1395, 1396, 1398, 1603, 1620, 1621, *[Drea]* **1677**, 1677, *[Skin]* 1748, 1755

bloated *[Eye]* **390**, *[Face]* **545**, *[Abdo]* **803**

bloating *[Back]* **1269**

blocked *[Face]* **545**

blond *[Gene]* **1805**

blood *[Mind]* **26**, *[Nose]* **505**, *[Face]* **602**, *[Thro]* **683**, *[Coug]* **1139**, *[Back]* **1269**, *[Extr]* **1353**, *[Drea]* **1677**, *[Feve]* **1720**, *[Skin]* **1747**, *[Gene]* **1979**

blood boils *[Face]* 561, *[Back]* 1274, *[Extr]* 1392, 1394, 1395, *[Skin]* 1756

blood circulation *[Extr]* **1632**, *[Gene]* **1805**

blood pressure *[Gene]* **1805**

blood vessels *[Head]* **240**, *[Gene]* **1805**

bloodshot *[Eye]* **390**

bloody *[Stoo]* **939**, *[Urin]* **1000**, *[Expe]* **1169**, *[Pers]* **1737**

blotches *[Head]* 251, *[Eye]* 398, *[Ear]* 465, 466, *[Face]* 555, 561, *[Mout]* **607**, 610, *[Thro]* **683**, *[Exte]* 715, *[Abdo]* 809, 813, *[Rect]* 912, *[Male]* 1020, 1021, *[Fema]* **1044**, *[Ches]* 1187, 1188, 1189, *[Back]* 1274, *[Extr]* **1353**, 1377, 1378, 1379, 1380, 1381, 1382, 1385, 1387, 1388, 1389, 1391, · 1392, 1393, 1394, 1395, 1396, 1397, 1398, *[Skin]* **1747**, 1755, 1765

blow *[Ear]* **461**, *[Face]* **545**, *[Teet]* **661**, *[Back]* **1269**

blowing *[Mind]* **26**, *[Eye]* **390**, *[Ear]* **461**, *[Mout]* **607**, *[Lary]* **1093**, *[Resp]* **1119**, *[Extr]* **1353**

blowing the nose *[Head]* **240**, *[Eye]* **390**, *[Ear]* **461**, *[Nose]* **505**, *[Ches]* **1179**, *[Back]* **1269**, *[Gene]* **1805**

blowing the nose agg *[Vert]* **228**

blows *[Eye]* **390**, *[Stom]* **728**, *[Gene]* **1805**

blueness *[Eye]* **390**, *[Male]* **1013**

bluish *[Stoo]* **940**, *[Expe]* **1171**, *[Back]* **1269**

blunt *[Mind]* **26**, *[Teet]* **661**

blunted *[Mind]* **26**

blurred *[Visi]* **443**

blushing *[Mind]* **26**

board *[Head]* **240**, *[Ear]* **461**, *[Back]* **1269**

boars *[Drea]* **1677**

boaster *[Mind]* **26**

boasting *[Drea]* **1677**

boat *[Drea]* **1677**

body *[Head]* **240**, *[Ear]* **461**, *[Drea]* **1677**, *[Feve]* **1720**, *[Skin]* **1747**

body; parts of *[Drea]* **1677**

boiling *[Head]* **240**, *[Abdo]* **803**, *[Ches]* **1179**, *[Gene]* **1805**

boils *[Head]* 251, *[Eye]* **390**, 397, 398, *[Ear]* 465, 466, 467, *[Nose]* **505**, *[Face]* 561, 597, *[Mout]* **607**, *[Exte]* 715, *[Abdo]* 813, *[Rect]* **897**, 905, 912, *[Male]* 1019, 1020, *[Fema]* 1048, *[Ches]* **1179**, 1188, 1189, 1219, *[Back]* **1269**, 1274, *[Extr]* 1385, 1386, 1387, 1388, 1389, 1390, 1391, 1392, 1393, 1394, 1395, 1396, 1397, 1398, *[Drea]* **1677**, *[Skin]* 1756, 1785, 1789, *[Gene]* 1830, 1870

boisterous *[Mind]* **26**

boldness *[Mind]* **26**

bone *[Thro]* **683**

bones *[Nose]* **543**, *[Gene]* **1979**

borborygmus *[Abdo]* **804**

bored *[Mind]* **26**

boredom *[Mind]* **26**

bores *[Head]* **240**

boring *[Head]* **240**, *[Ear]* **461**, *[Nose]* **505**, *[Gene]* **1805**

borreliosis *[Gene]* **1805**

borrowing *[Mind]* **26**

bossy *[Mind]* **26**

bound *[Extr]* **1353**, *[Drea]* **1678**

boundaries *[Mind]* **26**

boys *[Mind]* 88, 103, 114, 131, 154, 165, 185, *[Hear]* 504, *[Nose]* 522, *[Mout]* 618, *[Blad]* 961, 965, *[Coug]* 1144, *[Ches]* 1200, *[Drea]* 1689, *[Gene]* 1837, 1950

braggart *[Mind]* **26**

brain *[Head]* **384**

brain fag *[Mind]* **26**

brandy *[Coug]* **1139**

bran-like *[Skin]* **1747**

brassy *[Coug]* **1139**

Index of words

bread *[Vert]* **228**, *[Thro]* **683**, *[Coug]* **1139**

break *[Extr]* **1353**

breakfast *[Vert]* **228**, *[Stoo]* **940**, *[Coug]* **1139**, *[Expe]* **1171**, *[Chil]* **1704**, *[Feve]* **1720**, *[Pers]* **1737**, *[Gene]* **1805**

breaking *[Mind]* **26**, *[Teet]* **661**

breath *[Ear]* **461**, *[Mout]* **607**, *[Coug]* **1139**

breathing *[Vert]* **228**, *[Head]* **240**, *[Stom]* **728**, *[Abdo]* **804**, *[Resp]* **1119**, *[Coug]* **1139**, *[Ches]* **1179**, *[Back]* **1269**, *[Extr]* **1353**, *[Gene]* **1805**

breathless *[Resp]* **1119**

bregma *[Head]* **385**

brick-dust *[Urin]* **1000**, *[Expe]* **1171**

bridge *[Drea]* **1678**

bright *[Mind]* **26**, *[Visi]* **443**, *[Coug]* **1140**, *[Gene]* **1806**

bright colored *[Stoo]* **940**

bright's disease *[Gene]* **1806**

brilliant *[Eye]* **390**

brittle *[Head]* **240**, *[Extr]* **1353**

brittle bones *[Gene]* **1806**

broad *[Nose]* **505**, *[Face]* **545**

broad tongue *[Mout]* **607**

bromides *[Gene]* **1806**

bronchial *[Coug]* **1140**

bronchiectasis *[Ches]* **1179**, 1194

bronchitis *[Ches]* **1179**

bronchorrhea *[Ches]* **1179**

brontophobia *[Mind]* **26**

brooding *[Mind]* **26**

brotherhood *[Mind]* **26**

brown *[Stoo]* **940**, *[Back]* **1269**

brownish *[Expe]* **1171**

brown-séguard *[Gene]* **1806**

brucellosis *[Gene]* **1806**

bruised *[Gene]* **1806**

bruised p *[Skin]* **1747**

bruises *[Back]* **1269**, *[Gene]* **1806**

bruising *[Drea]* **1678**

brunet *[Gene]* **1806**

brunette *[Gene]* **1806**

brushing *[Teet]* **661**, *[Coug]* **1140**

brushing teeth *[Gene]* **1806**

brusque *[Mind]* **26**

brutality *[Mind]* **27**

bruxism *[Mout]* **607**, *[Teet]* **661**

bubble *[Ches]* **1179**

bubbles *[Rect]* **897**

bubbling *[Head]* **240**, *[Nose]* **505**, *[Face]* **545**, *[Thro]* **683**, *[Stom]* **728**, *[Abdo]* **804**, *[Kidn]* **973**, *[Uret]* **985**, *[Male]* **1013**, *[Fema]* **1044**, *[Ches]* **1179**, *[Back]* **1269**, *[Extr]* **1353**, *[Skin]* **1747**, *[Gene]* **1806**

bubo *[Abdo]* **804**

bubonic *[Gene]* **1806**

bubonic- *[Feve]* **1720**

buccal cavity *[Mout]* **659**

buffoonery *[Mind]* **27**

bugs *[Drea]* **1678**, *[Skin]* **1747**

buildings *[Drea]* **1678**

bulbar *[Gene]* **1806**

bulging *[Head]* **240**

bulimia *[Mind]* **27**

bull *[Drea]* **1678**

bullying *[Drea]* **1678**

bunions *[Extr]* **1353**

buoyancy *[Mind]* **27**

buried *[Drea]* **1678**

burned *[Expe]* **1171**, *[Drea]* **1678**

burning *[Urin]* **1000**, *[Coug]* **1140**, *[Expe]* **1171**, *[Drea]* **1678**, *[Feve]* **1720**, *[Pers]* **1737**, *[Skin]* **1747**, *[Gene]* **1806**

burns *[Mind]* **102**, *[Eye]* **401**, *[Mout]* **607**, 609, 627, *[Rect]* **906**, *[Extr]* **1358**, *[Drea]* **1678**, *[Skin]* **1748**, 1750, *[Gene]* **1806**, 1806, 1819, 1953, 1978

burnt *[Nose]* **516**, 529, *[Face]* **545**, 581, *[Mout]* 607, 614, 626, 627, 629, 630, 631, 632, 633, 635, 636, 637, 651, 652, *[Thro]* 700, 707, *[Stom]* 739, *[Stoo]* 943, 945, *[Urin]* 1006, 1008, *[Male]* 1033, *[Fema]* 1056, *[Expe]* 1173, 1174, *[Back]* 1299, *[Extr]* 1452, 1557, *[Drea]* 1677, 1678, *[Pers]* 1740, *[Skin]* 1752, 1787, *[Gene]* 1849, 1898

burnt easily *[Skin]* **1748**

burrowing *[Gene]* **1806**

bursae *[Extr]* **1354**, *[Gene]* **1806**

burst *[Skin]* **1748**

business *[Mind]* 1, 2, 4, 9, 16, **27**, 27, 28, 45, 46, 54, 71, 83, 87, 90, 93, 99, 102, 106, 115, 122, 130, 133, 138, 146, 147, 150, 153, 161, 163, 169, 183, 196, 206, 207, 209, 211, *[Head]* 269, 317, *[Slee]* 1644, 1662, 1666, 1670, 1671, *[Drea]* 1676, **1678**, 1678, 1695

businessmen *[Mind]* **27**

busy *[Mind]* **27**, *[Drea]* **1678**

buzzing *[Ches]* **1179**, *[Back]* **1269**, *[Extr]* **1354**

Index of words

C

cachectic *[Face]* **545**
cachexia *[Gene]* **1806**
cadaveric *[Stoo]* 945
caged *[Gene]* **1806**
calcareous *[Ear]* **461**, *[Thro]* **683**, *[Expe]* **1171**, *[Back]* **1269**
calcification *[Back]* **1269**
calcium *[Stoo]* **940**, *[Urin]* **1000**
calculating *[Mind]* **27**, *[Drea]* **1678**
calculi *[Abdo]* **804**, *[Blad]* **951**, 960, *[Kidn]* **973**, 975, *[Urin]* 1009
calf *[Mind]* 46, *[Abdo]* 865, *[Rect]* 908, *[Extr]* 1353, 1362, 1371, 1381, 1450, 1465, 1494, 1508, 1547, 1599, 1624, *[Slee]* 1664, *[Gene]* 1820, 1948
calling out *[Drea]* **1678**
callosities *[Extr]* **1354**
callous *[Skin]* **1748**
calmness *[Mind]* **27**
calumniate *[Mind]* **27**
camphor *[Gene]* **1806**
cancer *[Mind]* 54, 57, 102, 105, 183, *[Head]* **240**, *[Eye]* **390**, *[Nose]* **505**, 529, *[Face]* **545**, *[Mout]* 606, **607**, 607, 612, 629, *[Thro]* **683**, *[Exte]* 716, *[Stom]* 724, **728**, 749, 768, 792, 797, 798, *[Abdo]* **804**, 831, *[Rect]* **897**, 899, 902, 906, 924, *[Blad]* **951**, *[Kidn]* **973**, *[Pros]* **981**, 981, 982, *[Male]* **1013**, 1040, *[Fema]* **1044**, 1056, 1067, 1068, 1069, 1072, 1082, *[Lary]* **1093**, 1107, *[Resp]* 1116, 1122, *[Ches]* **1179**, 1194, 1195, 1199, 1208, 1216, 1230, 1231, 1261, 1263, 1264, 1265, *[Back]* **1269**, 1296, *[Extr]* **1354**, 1414, 1538, *[Drea]* **1678**, *[Skin]* **1748**, *[Gene]* 1806, 1807, 1832, 1844, 1869, 1870, 1966, 1970, 1978, 1980
cancerous *[Ear]* **461**, *[Face]* 602, *[Abdo]* 822, *[Pros]* 983, *[Fema]* 1050, 1069, 1091, *[Ches]* 1180, 1263, *[Skin]* 1785, *[Gene]* **1806**, 1837, 1873, 1895, 1899
cancrum *[Mout]* **607**
candida albicans *[Mout]* **607**
canines *[Teet]* **681**
canker *[Mout]* **607**
cannonading *[Drea]* **1678**
cantharis *[Gene]* **1808**
canthi *[Eye]* **439**
capillaries *[Gene]* **1808**
capillary *[Ches]* **1180**
capriciousness *[Mind]* **27**

captivating *[Mind]* **27**
car exhaust *[Gene]* **1808**
carbon *[Coug]* **1140**
carbuncle *[Uret]* **985**
carbuncles *[Head]* 251, *[Face]* **546**, 562, *[Back]* **1269**, *[Extr]* **1354**, *[Gene]* 1830
cardiac *[Mind]* 11, 96, 138, 177, *[Head]* 282, *[Thro]* 684, 695, 711, 712, *[Exte]* 721, *[Stom]* 731, 732, 777, 780, *[Kidn]* 974, *[Resp]* 1116, *[Coug]* **1140**, 1150, 1162, *[Ches]* 1187, 1201, *[Extr]* 1598, *[Gene]* 1834, 1840
cardialgia *[Stom]* **729**, *[Ches]* **1180**
cardiomegaly *[Ches]* **1180**
cardiophobia *[Mind]* **27**
carefree *[Mind]* **27**
carefulness *[Mind]* **27**
careless *[Mind]* **28**
cares *[Mind]* **28**, *[Drea]* **1678**
caressed *[Mind]* **28**
caressing *[Mind]* **28**
caries *[Head]* **240**, *[Eye]* 404, *[Ear]* **461**, 463, *[Nose]* 505, *[Face]* **546**, 581, *[Mout]* **607**, 629, *[Teet]* **661**, *[Ches]* **1180**, *[Back]* **1269**, *[Extr]* **1354**, 1354, 1400, 1496, *[Pers]* **1742**, *[Gene]* **1808**, 1908
carotids *[Mind]* 46, *[Head]* 278, *[Exte]* 720
carousal *[Mind]* **28**
carousing *[Drea]* **1678**
carpal tunnel syndrome *[Extr]* **1354**
carphologia *[Mind]* **28**, 118, 119
carried *[Mind]* **28**, *[Gene]* **1808**
carrying *[Mind]* **28**, *[Vert]* **228**, *[Stom]* **729**, *[Gene]* **1808**
cars *[Mind]* **28**
carsickness *[Gene]* **1808**
cartilages *[Ches]* **1264**, *[Gene]* **1808**
cartilaginous *[Blad]* **951**, *[Uret]* **985**
caruncle *[Uret]* **985**
caseous *[Thro]* **683**
casting off *[Mind]* **28**
casts *[Urin]* **1000**, *[Expe]* **1171**
casualties *[Drea]* **1678**
catalepsy *[Mind]* **28**, 102, 152, 173, *[Eye]* 441, *[Male]* 1033, *[Extr]* **1354**, *[Slee]* 1642, *[Gene]* **1808**
cataract *[Eye]* **390**, 391, 409, *[Visi]* 452
catarrh *[Eye]* 391, *[Ear]* **461**, *[Nose]* **505**, *[Thro]* **683**, *[Stom]* **729**, *[Abdo]* **804**, *[Rect]* **897**, *[Blad]* **951**, *[Kidn]* **973**, *[Uret]* **985**, *[Fema]* **1044**, *[Lary]* **1093**, *[Ches]* **1180**, *[Gene]* **1808**

Index of words

catarrhal *[Pros]* 981, *[Coug]* 1140, *[Feve]* 1721

catatonia *[Mind]* 28

catching *[Resp]* 1119

catheter *[Feve]* 1721

catheterism *[Gene]* 1808

catnaps *[Slee]* 1641

catoptrophobia *[Mind]* 28

cats *[Mind]* 28, *[Drea]* 1678

cauda equina *[Back]* 1269

cauliflower *[Rect]* 897

cauterizing *[Drea]* 1678

cautery *[Gene]* 1808

cautious *[Mind]* 28

cavities *[Ches]* 1180

ceases *[Ches]* 1180

cecum *[Abdo]* 893

celibacy *[Male]* 1013, *[Fema]* 1044, *[Gene]* 1808

cellar *[Mind]* 54, *[Drea]* 1678

cellars *[Coug]* 1140, *[Ches]* 1180, *[Gene]* 1808

cellulitis *[Eye]* 404, *[Fema]* 1050, 1051, *[Back]* 1278, *[Extr]* 1602, *[Feve]* 1729, 1732, *[Gene]* 1808, 1873

cemetery *[Drea]* 1678

censorious *[Mind]* 28

centered *[Mind]* 29

cephalhematoma *[Head]* 240

cerebellar *[Head]* 240

cerebral *[Mind]* 29, *[Head]* 240, *[Gene]* 1808

cerebral hemorrhage *[Head]* 240

cerebrospinal *[Feve]* 1721

cerebrovascular accident *[Head]* 240

cerumen *[Ear]* 461

cervical region *[Back]* 1348

cervicitis *[Fema]* 1044

chafed *[Face]* 546, *[Extr]* 1354

chagrin *[Mind]* 29, *[Vert]* 228, *[Coug]* 1140

chalazae *[Eye]* 391

chalk *[Head]* 251, *[Nose]* 529, 539, *[Face]* 558, *[Mout]* 617, *[Stoo]* 949, *[Urin]* 1001, 1003, 1005, 1008, *[Expe]* 1174, *[Skin]* 1772, *[Gene]* 1848, 1854, 1977

chalky *[Stoo]* 940

chancre *[Uret]* 985, *[Gene]* 1808

change *[Mind]* 29, *[Gene]* 1808

changeable *[Mind]* 29, *[Stoo]* 940

changing *[Visi]* 443, *[Drea]* 1678, *[Chil]* 1704, *[Feve]* 1721

changing mood *[Mind]* 29

chaotic *[Mind]* 29

chapped *[Nose]* 506, *[Face]* 546, *[Extr]* 1354

chapping *[Skin]* 1748

character *[Mind]* 29

charming *[Mind]* 29

chased *[Drea]* 1678

chasing *[Mind]* 29, *[Drea]* 1678

chattering *[Teet]* 661

checking *[Mind]* 29

cheek *[Drea]* 1678

cheerful *[Mind]* 29, *[Drea]* 1678

cheese *[Expe]* 1171

cheesy *[Ear]* 463, *[Mout]* 617, 629, 651, *[Thro]* 683, 683, *[Stom]* 798, *[Stoo]* 944, *[Blad]* 964, *[Uret]* 986, *[Urin]* 1005, 1008, *[Male]* 1041, *[Fema]* 1044, *[Ches]* 1200, *[Pers]* 1740, *[Skin]* 1785

cheloid *[Gene]* 1955

chemical *[Gene]* 1809

chemosis *[Eye]* 391

chemotherapy *[Gene]* 1809

chest *[Drea]* 1678

chewing *[Head]* 240, *[Ear]* 461, *[Face]* 546, *[Mout]* 607, *[Back]* 1269, *[Gene]* 1809

cheyne-stokes *[Mind]* 213, *[Resp]* 1119, *[Gene]* 1805, 1809

chicken breast *[Ches]* 1180

chickenpox *[Coug]* 1140

chilblains *[Ear]* 461, *[Face]* 546, *[Extr]* 1354, *[Skin]* 1748

childbed *[Mind]* 31, *[Fema]* 1045, *[Gene]* 1809

childbirth *[Fema]* 1045

childish *[Mind]* 31

children *[Mind]* 1, 2, 3, 4, 5, 6, 9, 10, 11, 12, 14, 15, 16, 22, 23, 24, 25, 27, 28, 29, 31, 31, 34, 35, 36, 37, 38, 40, 41, 42, 43, 48, 50, 54, 60, 81, 83, 85, 86, 87, 88, 90, 92, 93, 94, 95, 96, 97, 98, 101, 102, 103, 105, 106, 110, 111, 112, 113, 114, 115, 116, 118, 119, 121, 122, 123, 124, 126, 127, 128, 129, 130, 132, 135, 136, 137, 138, 139, 140, 141, 142, 143, 144, 145, 146, 148, 149, 150, 151, 152, 153, 156, 157, 159, 160, 161, 163, 165, 167, 168, 169, 170, 172, 173, 175, 177, 178, 180, 183, 186, 187, 188, 190, 191, 193, 195, 197, 199, 200, 202, 205, 206, 207, 208, 211, 212, 215, 216, 217, 218, 220, 222, 223, 224, *[Head]* 240, 250, 252, 257, 264, 265, 269, 270, 300, 377, 379, 385, 386, *[Eye]* 389, 390, 391, 394, 401, 402, 404, 408, 415, 431, 433, 436, 438, 439, *[Visi]* 443, 456, *[Ear]* 461,

Index of words

cities *[Drea]* **1679**

clairaudience *[Hear]* **501**

clairaudient *[Mind]* **31**

clairvoyance *[Mind]* **31**, *[Visi]* **444**

clairvoyant *[Drea]* **1679**

clairvoyant state *[Slee]* **1641**

clammy *[Mout]* **608**, *[Pers]* **1737**, *[Skin]* **1749**

clarity *[Mind]* **31**, *[Visi]* **444**

claudicatio intermittens *[Extr]* **1356**

claustrophobia *[Mind]* **31**, 103

clavicles *[Ches]* 1177, 1179, 1180, 1188, 1191, 1192, 1199, 1200, 1202, 1220, 1258, 1261, *[Back]* 1299

clawing *[Stom]* **729**, *[Ches]* **1181**

claw-like *[Extr]* **1356**

clay *[Mout]* 619, *[Stoo]* 948, *[Urin]* 1002, 1008, *[Expe]* 1174, *[Chil]* 1708, *[Gene]* 1854

clay colored *[Stoo]* **940**

clayish *[Stoo]* **940**

clean t *[Mout]* **608**

cleaning *[Coug]* **1140**

cleaning teeth *[Gene]* **1811**

cleanness *[Mind]* **31**

clear *[Visi]* **444**, *[Gene]* **1811**

clearer *[Visi]* **444**

clearing *[Thro]* **685**

clearness *[Mind]* **31**

cleft *[Mout]* **608**

clenched *[Face]* **546**

clenching *[Teet]* **662**, *[Extr]* **1356**, *[Gene]* **1811**

clever *[Mind]* **31**

climacteric period *[Mind]* **31**

climbing *[Mind]* **31**, *[Drea]* **1679**

clinging *[Mind]* **31**

clitoris *[Fema]* 1044, 1047, 1048, 1051, 1059, 1075, 1089, 1090, **1092**

clock *[Coug]* **1140**

clogged *[Uret]* **985**

closed *[Vert]* **228**, *[Eye]* **391**, *[Ear]* **461**, *[Mout]* **608**, *[Lary]* **1093**, *[Extr]* **1356**

closed c *[Mind]* **32**

closer *[Visi]* **444**

closet *[Drea]* **1679**

closing *[Face]* **546**, *[Resp]* **1119**, *[Coug]* **1140**, *[Gene]* **1811**

closing eyes *[Mind]* **32**

closing the eyes *[Vert]* **228**, *[Head]* **240**, *[Eye]* **391**, *[Visi]* **444**, *[Pers]* **1738**

cloth around; tying *[Extr]* **1356**

clothes *[Mind]* 11, 16, 25, **32**, 32, 54, 55, 85, 118, 122, 133, 151, 167, 207, *[Head]* 295, 383, *[Exte]* 715, 716, *[Stom]* 729, 745, 763, 768, 775, 777, 781, *[Abdo]* **804**, 807, 810, 820, 841, 852, 858, 875, 884, *[Uret]* 996, *[Male]* 1032, 1035, *[Fema]* 1054, 1057, 1060, 1066, 1082, *[Resp]* 1123, 1125, 1127, 1129, *[Ches]* 1184, 1214, 1232, 1258, *[Back]* **1269**, 1303, 1332, *[Extr]* 1437, 1539, *[Drea]* **1679**, 1691, *[Chil]* 1705, *[Skin]* 1770, 1782, 1784, *[Gene]* **1811**, 1842, 1895, 1916, 1934, 1951

clothes agg *[Coug]* **1140**

clothing *[Mind]* 32, 69, *[Head]* 283, 308, 342, *[Thro]* 684, *[Exte]* **715**, *[Stom]* **729**, 729, 745, 785, *[Abdo]* **804**, 812, 831, *[Rect]* 930, 935, *[Kidn]* 978, *[Male]* 1040, *[Fema]* 1064, 1080, *[Resp]* **1119**, *[Ches]* **1181**, 1203, 1255, *[Extr]* 1515, 1569, *[Skin]* **1749**, *[Gene]* **1811**, 1811, 1962

cloudiness *[Mind]* **32**

cloudy *[Mind]* 7, **32**, 140, 162, 186, 218, 223, *[Head]* 309, *[Visi]* **444**, 449, *[Re⬛ ⬛ ⬛*, *[Urin]* **1001**, 1008, 1010, *[Resp⬛ ⬛]* 117⬛ 1973, 1975

clown *[Mind]* **32**

clubbing *[Extr]* **1356**

clubfoot *[Extr]* **1356**

clucking *[Head]* **240**, *[Face]* **546**, *[Thro]* **685**, *[Stom]* **729**, *[Abdo]* **805**, *[Ches]* **1181**, *[Extr]* **1356**, *[Gene]* **1811**

clumsiness *[Extr]* **1356**

clumsy *[Mind]* **32**, *[Mout]* **608**

cluster *[Head]* **240**

clutching *[Fema]* **1045**, *[Ches]* **1181**, *[Gene]* **1812**

coal *[Coug]* **1140**, *[Skin]* **1749**

coal gas *[Gene]* **1812**

coal tar *[Gene]* **1812**

coated *[Mout]* **608**, *[Teet]* **662**, *[Thro]* **685**, *[Lary]* **1093**, *[Ches]* **1181**

cobweb *[Face]* **546**, *[Abdo]* **805**, *[Extr]* **1356**, *[Skin]* **1749**, *[Gene]* **1812**

cobwebs *[Visi]* **444**, *[Nose]* **507**, *[Coug]* **1140**

coccygodynia *[Back]* **1270**

coccyx *[Back]* **1348**

cochlea *[Ear]* **498**

cod-liver oil *[Gene]* **1812**

coffee *[Mind]* 1, 9, 16, 38, 96, 138, 161, 188, *[Vert]* **228**, *[Head]* **240**, 240, 245, 257, 261, 283, 295, 317, 346, 384, *[Ear]* 468, *[Nose]* 529, 538, *[Face]*

Index of words

Index of words

complicated *[Drea]* **1679**

comply *[Mind]* **35**

comprehension *[Mind]* **35**

compression *[Back]* **1272**, *[Extr]* **1365**

compulsions *[Mind]* **35**

compulsive disorders *[Mind]* **35**

compulsive neurosis *[Mind]* **35**

computers *[Mind]* **35**

conceit *[Mind]* **35**

concentration *[Mind]* **35**

conception *[Fema]* **1046**

conceptual thinking *[Mind]* **36**

concerned *[Mind]* **36**

conclusions *[Mind]* **36**

concretions *[Thro]* **685**, *[Extr]* **1365**

concussion *[Vert]* **228**, *[Head]* **244**, *[Back]* **1272**

concussive *[Coug]* **1141**

condescending *[Mind]* **36**

condiments *[Coug]* **1141**

condition *[Gene]* **1817**

condylomata *[Eye]* **393**, *[Nose]* **507**, *[Mout]* **609**,
 [Thro] **685**, *[Rect]* **898**, *[Male]* **1014**, *[Fema]* **1046**,
 [Lary] **1093**, *[Skin]* **1750**, 1773, *[Gene]* **1817**, 1945

conference *[Drea]* **1679**

confidence *[Mind]* **36**

confident *[Mind]* **37**

confiding *[Mind]* **37**

confinement *[Fema]* **1046**

conflagration *[Drea]* **1679**

conflict *[Mind]* **37**

conformism *[Mind]* **37**

confounding *[Mind]* **37**

confused *[Visi]* **447**, *[Slee]* **1641**, *[Drea]* **1679**

confusion *[Mind]* **37**, *[Head]* **244**

congested *[Extr]* **1365**

congestion *[Mind]* 17, 18, 46, 177, 201, *[Vert]* 227,
 228, *[Head]* 241, **244**, 244, 261, 282, 284, 297,
 346, *[Eye]* 390, **393**, 415, *[Visi]* 453, *[Ear]* **463**,
 [Nose] 506, **507**, 508, 521, 522, *[Face]* **548**, 553,
 [Mout] **609**, *[Teet]* 668, *[Thro]* 683, **685**, 714,
 [Exte] **715**, *[Stom]* 729, **730**, 756, 766, 791, 792,
 [Abdo] **807**, 807, 855, 895, *[Rect]* **898**, 899, 916,
 917, 918, *[Blad]* 959, *[Kidn]* **973**, 973, *[Pros]* **981**,
 [Male] **1014**, *[Fema]* **1046**, 1046, 1051, 1067,
 1068, 1090, 1092, *[Resp]* 1122, *[Ches]* **1183**,
 1183, 1193, 1194, 1251, 1260, 1265, *[Back]* **1273**,
 1284, *[Extr]* 1528, 1622, *[Slee]* 1643, 1659, 1662,
 1669, *[Chil]* 1710, *[Skin]* **1750**, 1753, 1783, *[Gene]*

1802, **1817**, 1821, 1822, 1828, 1834, 1868, 1901,
 1918, 1942, 1959

congestive *[Chil]* **1706**

congestive heart failure *[Ches]* **1183**

conical *[Eye]* **393**, *[Skin]* 1757, 1773, 1790

conjunctiva *[Eye]* **439**

conjunctivitis *[Eye]* **393**

connected *[Drea]* **1679**

connection *[Mind]* **40**

connective tissue *[Gene]* **1817**

conscience *[Mind]* 17, 55, 115, 130, 177, *[Drea]*
 1680

conscientious *[Mind]* **40**

conscious *[Fema]* **1046**, *[Ches]* **1183**, *[Slee]* **1642**,
 [Drea] **1679**

consciousness *[Mind]* **41**, *[Vert]* **228**, *[Coug]* **1141**

conservative *[Mind]* **41**

consolation *[Mind]* **41**, 138, 183, 191, 220, *[Coug]*
 1141

conspiracies *[Drea]* **1679**

constant *[Stoo]* **940**, *[Coug]* **1141**, *[Expe]* **1171**

constantly high temperature *[Feve]* **1722**

constipation *[Mind]* 7, 17, 46, 183, *[Vert]* **228**,
 [Head] 245, **246**, 258, 276, 284, 320, *[Nose]* 506,
 [Face] 560, *[Mout]* 608, 611, 616, 629, *[Stom]* 730,
 752, 758, 768, 791, *[Abdo]* 807, 810, 816, 817,
 818, 819, 821, 832, 875, 884, 886, 888, 889, 893,
 894, *[Rect]* 897, **898**, 905, 915, 916, 917, 918,
 924, 931, 934, 937, *[Stoo]* 944, *[Blad]* 958, 965,
 [Pros] 983, *[Uret]* 988, *[Urin]* 1000, *[Male]* 1041,
 [Fema] 1046, 1053, 1086, *[Coug]* **1141**, *[Ches]*
 1264, *[Back]* 1284, 1319, *[Extr]* 1411, *[Feve]* 1731,
 [Skin] 1753, 1770, 1777, *[Gene]* 1801, **1817**, 1823,
 1830, 1840, 1901, 1918

constituents *[Urin]* **1003**

constitution *[Gene]* **1817**

constricted *[Drea]* **1679**

constriction *[Head]* **246**, *[Ear]* **463**, *[Nose]* **508**,
 [Face] **549**, *[Mout]* **609**, *[Thro]* **685**, *[Exte]* **715**,
 [Stom] **730**, *[Abdo]* **807**, *[Rect]* **901**, *[Blad]* **951**,
 [Uret] **985**, *[Male]* **1014**, *[Fema]* **1046**, *[Lary]*
 1093, *[Coug]* **1141**, *[Ches]* **1183**, *[Back]* **1273**,
 [Extr] **1365**, *[Gene]* **1817**

constringing *[Male]* **1014**

consumption *[Gene]* **1818**

contact *[Mind]* **41**

contempt *[Drea]* **1679**

contemptuous *[Mind]* **41**

Index of words

content *[Mind]* **41**

contentious *[Mind]* **41**

continuation *[Drea]* 1679

continued *[Coug]* 1141, *[Feve]* 1722

continuous *[Vert]* **228**, *[Coug]* 1141, *[Drea]* 1679

contorted *[Eye]* **393**

contortion *[Face]* 549

contortions *[Extr]* 1365

contraband *[Drea]* 1679

contracted *[Visi]* 447, *[Kidn]* 973

contraction *[Head]* **249**, *[Eye]* **393**, *[Ear]* **463**, *[Nose]* 508, *[Face]* 549, *[Mout]* **609**, *[Thro]* **686**, *[Stom]* **731**, *[Abdo]* **807**, *[Blad]* **951**, *[Uret]* **985**, *[Male]* 1014, *[Ches]* 1186, *[Extr]* **1366**, *[Skin]* 1750

contractions *[Fema]* 1046, *[Back]* 1273, *[Gene]* 1818

contractive *[Eye]* **393**

contradiction *[Mind]* 4, 9, **41**, **41**, 43, 96, 128, 135, 138, 162, 172, 217, 220, 223, *[Head]* 258, 284, *[Face]* 556, 581, *[Stom]* 733, 745, 768, *[Abdo]* 810, *[Extr]* 1612, *[Gene]* 1821, 1938

contradictory *[Mind]* **41**, *[Gene]* 1818

contrary *[Mind]* **41**

contrast *[Visi]* 447

controlling *[Mind]* **42**

convalescence *[Gene]* 1818

conversation *[Mind]* 9, 17, 36, 38, **42**, 42, 91, 96, 103, 107, 130, 138, 177, 183, 201, 221, *[Vert]* **229**, *[Head]* **249**, 284, 382, *[Face]* 594, *[Stom]* 758, 789, *[Abdo]* 832, *[Fema]* 1077, *[Ches]* 1203, *[Extr]* 1611, *[Slee]* 1646, 1651, 1654, 1655, 1657, 1662, 1673, *[Drea]* 1679, 1682, 1691, *[Feve]* **1723**, *[Pers]* **1738**, *[Gene]* **1819**, 1881, 1949, 1953, 1967, 1974

conversations *[Drea]* 1679

convulsion *[Extr]* **1367**

convulsions *[Head]* **249**, *[Face]* 549, *[Mout]* **609**, *[Thro]* **686**, *[Coug]* 1141, *[Ches]* 1186, *[Slee]* 1642, *[Drea]* **1680**, *[Chil]* **1706**, *[Feve]* **1723**, *[Pers]* **1738**, *[Gene]* **1819**

convulsions; before epileptic *[Vert]* **229**

convulsive *[Eye]* **393**, *[Nose]* 508, *[Resp]* 1119, *[Gene]* 1828

cooking *[Drea]* 1680

cool *[Expe]* 1171

copious *[Stoo]* **940**, *[Urin]* **1003**, *[Expe]* 1171, *[Pers]* **1739**

copper *[Gene]* 1828

coquettish *[Mind]* **42**

cord *[Abdo]* **808**, *[Rect]* **902**, *[Skin]* **1750**

cornea *[Eye]* 389, 390, 391, 393, 394, 395, 397, 399, 403, 405, 409, 425, 430, 432, 434, 436, 437, 438, **439**, *[Skin]* 1762, *[Gene]* 1870

corns *[Extr]* 1369, 1511

coronation *[Drea]* 1680

corpse reviver *[Gene]* **1828**

corpses *[Drea]* 1680

corroded sensation *[Teet]* 663

corrosive *[Expe]* 1171, *[Ches]* 1186

corrugated *[Extr]* 1369

corrugated t *[Mout]* **609**

coryza *[Vert]* **229**, *[Nose]* 508, *[Chil]* **1706**, *[Gene]* 1828

cosmetics *[Gene]* 1828

cosmopolitan *[Mind]* **42**

cotton *[Mout]* **609**, *[Thro]* **686**, *[Fema]* 1047, *[Ches]* 1186, *[Gene]* 1828

cough *[Vert]* **229**, *[Head]* **249**, *[Eye]* **393**, *[Visi]* 447, *[Ear]* **463**, *[Face]* 549, *[Thro]* **686**, *[Abdo]* **808**, *[Rect]* **902**, *[Blad]* **951**, *[Lary]* 1094, *[Resp]* 1119, *[Coug]* 1141, *[Ches]* 1186, *[Back]* 1273, *[Extr]* 1369, *[Drea]* 1680, *[Chil]* **1706**, *[Pers]* **1739**, *[Gene]* 1828

coughing *[Feve]* **1723**

counting *[Mind]* **42**

country *[Drea]* 1680

countryside *[Mind]* **42**

courageous *[Mind]* **42**

cover *[Mout]* **609**, *[Extr]* 1369

covered *[Chil]* **1706**, *[Pers]* **1739**

covered parts *[Feve]* **1733**

covering *[Eye]* **393**, *[Nose]* 513, *[Abdo]* **808**, *[Coug]* 1141, *[Feve]* **1723**, *[Gene]* 1828

covering the mouth or nose *[Resp]* 1119

covers *[Head]* **249**, *[Gene]* 1828

covetous *[Mind]* **42**

cowardice *[Mind]* **42**

cow-dung *[Stoo]* **940**

coxitis *[Extr]* 1369

crab lice *[Male]* 1014

cracked *[Head]* 251, *[Ear]* 465, *[Face]* 549, 590, *[Mout]* 605, 607, **609**, 611, 624, 635, 658, *[Rect]* 912, *[Male]* 1021, *[Lary]* 1106, 1107, *[Ches]* 1197, *[Extr]* 1355, **1369**, 1385, 1388, 1389, 1391, 1397, 1399, 1443, 1620, 1635, *[Feve]* 1731, 1732, 1733, *[Skin]* 1748, 1750, 1757, 1765, 1767, 1771, 1790, *[Gene]* 1831, 1876, 1950

Index of words

cracking *[Mind]* 53, 70, *[Head]* 270, *[Ear]* 473, *[Hear]* 501, *[Face]* 550, *[Teet]* 663, *[Thro]* 686, *[Exte]* 715, *[Abdo]* 808, *[Ches]* 1186, *[Back]* 1273, *[Extr]* 1351, **1370**, 1497, *[Skin]* 1754, *[Gene]* 1829

crackling *[Head]* 249, *[Nose]* 513, *[Mout]* 610, *[Skin]* **1750**

cracklings *[Gene]* 1829

cracks *[Head]* 251, *[Eye]* 393, *[Ear]* 463, 465, 466, *[Nose]* 513, *[Face]* 562, *[Mout]* 610, *[Abdo]* 808, *[Rect]* 902, *[Uret]* 985, *[Male]* 1014, *[Fema]* 1047, *[Ches]* 1186, 1186, 1189, *[Extr]* 1354, 1390, *[Slee]* 1648, *[Skin]* 1750, 1750, 1775

cradle cap *[Head]* 249

crafty *[Mind]* 42

cramp *[Eye]* 393, *[Face]* 550, *[Thro]* 686, *[Exte]* 715, *[Stom]* 731, *[Abdo]* 808, *[Rect]* 902, *[Blad]* 951, *[Uret]* 985, *[Ches]* 1186, *[Back]* 1273

cramped *[Gene]* 1829

cramps *[Nose]* 513, *[Mout]* 610, *[Coug]* 1141, *[Extr]* 1371, *[Gene]* 1829

crash *[Drea]* 1680

crawling *[Mind]* 42, *[Head]* 249, *[Eye]* 393, *[Ear]* 463, *[Nose]* 513, *[Face]* 550, *[Mout]* 610, *[Teet]* 663, *[Thro]* 686, *[Exte]* 715, *[Stom]* 731, *[Abdo]* 808, *[Rect]* 902, *[Blad]* 951, *[Uret]* 985, *[Male]* 1014, *[Fema]* 1047, *[Lary]* 1094, *[Coug]* 1141, *[Ches]* 1186, *[Back]* 1273, *[Extr]* 1377, *[Skin]* 1750, *[Gene]* 1829

crazy *[Mind]* **42**, *[Drea]* **1680**

creaking *[Extr]* 1377

cream colored *[Stoo]* 940

cream-like *[Expe]* 1171

creatinine *[Urin]* 1005

creative *[Mind]* 42

credulous *[Mind]* 42

creeping *[Nose]* 513, *[Face]* 550, *[Extr]* 1377, *[Chil]* 1706, *[Skin]* 1750

crepitation *[Extr]* 1377

cretinism *[Mind]* 42

crime *[Drea]* 1680

crippled *[Extr]* 1377

critical *[Mind]* 42, *[Pers]* **1739**

croaking *[Mind]* 42, *[Stom]* 731, *[Abdo]* 808, *[Resp]* 1119, *[Coug]* 1142

crocodiles *[Drea]* 1680

crohn's d *[Abdo]* 808

crooked *[Visi]* 447

cross *[Mind]* **42**

crossed *[Mind]* **42**, *[Extr]* **1377**

crossing *[Vert]* 229, *[Extr]* **1377**

crossing a bridge *[Vert]* 229, *[Gene]* **1829**

crossing legs *[Fema]* 1047

crossing of limbs *[Gene]* **1829**

croup *[Mind]* 28, *[Nose]* 510, *[Face]* 550, *[Thro]* 684, 686, 706, *[Lary]* **1094**, 1108, *[Resp]* 1121, 1131, *[Coug]* 1142, *[Ches]* **1186**, *[Feve]* 1721, *[Gene]* 1819, 1821, 1870

croupy *[Coug]* **1142**

crowd *[Mind]* 17, 60, 103, 112, 208, *[Vert]* **229**, *[Head]* 284, *[Stom]* 758

crowded room *[Gene]* 1829

crowds *[Drea]* **1680**

crowing *[Resp]* 1119, *[Coug]* **1142**

crown *[Head]* 249

cruelty *[Mind]* 42, *[Drea]* **1680**

crumb *[Lary]* **1095**, *[Coug]* **1142**

crumbling *[Teet]* 663, *[Stoo]* **940**

crumbly *[Expe]* **1171**

crumbs *[Thro]* 686

crural *[Male]* 1040, *[Fema]* 1079, *[Extr]* 1440, 1512, 1523, 1548

crushed *[Drea]* **1680**

crusts *[Nose]* 513, *[Mout]* 610, *[Teet]* 663, *[Gene]* **1829**

crusty *[Eye]* 393

crying *[Mind]* 43, *[Coug]* **1142**

cryptorchism *[Male]* **1014**

cunning *[Mind]* 43

cupped *[Teet]* 663

curdled *[Stoo]* 940

curettage *[Fema]* 1047

curious *[Mind]* 43, *[Drea]* **1680**

cursing *[Mind]* 43, *[Drea]* **1680**

curvature *[Back]* **1273**, *[Extr]* 1377, *[Gene]* **1829**

curved *[Extr]* 1377

curving *[Extr]* **1377**

cushing' *[Gene]* **1829**

cut *[Mind]* 43, *[Drea]* **1680**

cuticle *[Thro]* 686, *[Urin]* 1005

cutting *[Head]* 249, *[Coug]* **1142**, *[Drea]* **1680**, *[Skin]* **1750**

cyanosis *[Mind]* 144, *[Mout]* 612, *[Resp]* 1115, *[Coug]* 1166, *[Ches]* **1186**, *[Extr]* 1378, 1381, *[Gene]* 1821, **1829**

cyanotic *[Face]* 552, *[Mout]* 613, *[Resp]* 1119, 1122, *[Ches]* 1197, *[Extr]* 1382

Index of words

Index of words

dentin *[Teet]* 665

dentition *[Mind]* 15, 17, 25, 28, 97, 138, 159, 162, 177, 192, 193, 198, 220, *[Head]* 250, 265, 286, 312, 385, *[Eye]* 393, 433, *[Ear]* 463, 473, *[Hear]* 502, *[Nose]* 528, *[Face]* 546, 553, *[Mout]* 632, 641, 642, 643, 646, 657, *[Teet]* 661, 662, **663**, 663, *[Exte]* 716, *[Stom]* 752, 792, *[Rect]* 900, 906, 907, 937, *[Stoo]* 949, *[Blad]* 962, *[Kidn]* 980, *[Coug]* **1142**, *[Ches]* 1180, *[Extr]* 1399, *[Slee]* 1662, *[Feve]* **1723**, *[Skin]* **1750**, 1762, 1766, 1776, *[Gene]* 1806, 1810, 1820, 1822, **1830**, 1874, 1895, 1919, 1949, 1956, 1967

denuded *[Mout]* **610**, *[Thro]* **686**, *[Gene]* **1830**

depapillated *[Mout]* **610**

departure *[Drea]* **1681**

dependent *[Mind]* **83**

depersonalization *[Mind]* **83**

depigmentation *[Nose]* 513, *[Skin]* **1751**

depravity *[Mind]* **83**

depression *[Mind]* **83**

depressive mania *[Mind]* **83**

dermatitis *[Skin]* **1751**

dermatographism *[Skin]* **1751**

dermatomyositis *[Gene]* **1830**

descemetitis *[Eye]* **393**

descending *[Vert]* **229**, *[Head]* **249**, *[Coug]* **1142**, *[Extr]* **1377**, *[Chil]* **1707**, *[Feve]* **1723**, *[Pers]* **1739**, *[Gene]* **1830**

desert *[Drea]* **1681**

deserted *[Mind]* **83**, *[Drea]* **1681**

desire *[Male]* **1015**, *[Fema]* **1047**

desires *[Mind]* **83**, *[Stom]* **731**

desolate *[Mind]* **84**

despair *[Mind]* **84**

despising *[Mind]* **85**

despondency *[Mind]* **85**

despotic *[Mind]* **85**

desquamation *[Nose]* **513**, *[Face]* **550**, *[Mout]* **610**, *[Extr]* **1377**, *[Skin]* **1751**

destination *[Drea]* **1681**

destruction *[Teet]* **663**

destructiveness *[Mind]* **85**

detached *[Mind]* **85**, *[Mout]* **610**, *[Extr]* **1377**

detachment *[Eye]* **393**

detail *[Mind]* **85**

determination *[Mind]* **85**

development *[Mind]* **85**, *[Fema]* **1047**, *[Gene]* **1830**

devil *[Mind]* 56, 57, 104

devils *[Drea]* **1681**

diabetes *[Mind]* 7, 17, 33, 91, 112, 121, 138, 153, 183, *[Face]* 560, *[Mout]* 609, 614, 616, 621, *[Teet]* 661, *[Stom]* 751, *[Abdo]* 811, 894, 895, *[Rect]* 898, 904, *[Kidn]* 973, *[Urin]* **1005**, *[Male]* 1019, *[Fema]* 1067, *[Resp]* 1115, *[Ches]* 1257, 1266, *[Extr]* 1431, 1443, 1528, 1598, *[Skin]* 1756, 1764, 1775, 1777, 1784, *[Gene]* 1797, 1803, 1831, 1837, 1844, 1872, 1892, 1937, 1967

diabetes insipidus *[Gene]* **1830**

diabetes mellitus *[Gene]* **1830**

diabetic *[Mind]* 178, *[Eye]* 404, *[Extr]* 1404, *[Skin]* 1785, *[Gene]* 1805

diabolical *[Mind]* 60

diaper *[Rect]* **902**

diaphragm *[Stom]* 723, 753, *[Abdo]* 803, 847, *[Resp]* 1114, 1116, 1123, 1129, *[Coug]* 1141, *[Ches]* 1185, 1193, 1196, 1204, 1214, 1222, 1256, 1260, **1264**, *[Back]* 1273, *[Gene]* 1922

diarrhea *[Mind]* **85**, *[Vert]* **229**, *[Head]* **249**, *[Abdo]* **808**, *[Rect]* **902**, *[Coug]* **1142**, *[Drea]* **1681**, *[Chil]* **1707**, *[Feve]* **1723**, *[Pers]* **1739**, *[Gene]* **1831**

dictatorial *[Mind]* **85**

died *[Drea]* **1681**

difficult *[Hear]* **501**, *[Rect]* **911**, *[Stoo]* **941**, *[Resp]* **1120**, *[Coug]* **1142**, *[Expe]* **1171**

difficulties *[Drea]* **1681**

diffusion *[Mind]* **85**

digestion *[Mind]* **85**, *[Stom]* **731**

digging *[Head]* **249**

digitalis *[Gene]* **1831**

dignified *[Mind]* **85**

dilatation *[Ear]* **463**, *[Stom]* **732**, *[Ches]* **1186**

dilated *[Vert]* **229**, *[Head]* **249**, *[Nose]* **513**

dilation *[Eye]* **393**

dim *[Visi]* **447**

dim vision *[Vert]* **229**

diminished *[Urin]* **1005**

dinner *[Vert]* **229**, *[Teet]* **663**, *[Coug]* **1142**, *[Expe]* **1171**, *[Feve]* **1723**, *[Pers]* **1739**, *[Gene]* **1831**

diphtheria *[Mind]* 104, 202, 214, *[Eye]* 428, *[Visi]* 443, 448, 450, *[Nose]* 508, 510, **513**, 522, 528, *[Mout]* 605, 611, 612, 613, 614, 615, 616, 617, 619, 626, 629, 638, 640, 641, 643, 648, *[Thro]* **686**, 687, 688, 695, 700, 712, 713, *[Exte]* 719, 721, *[Kidn]* 974, *[Urin]* 999, 1007, *[Fema]* 1062, 1064, *[Lary]* **1095**, 1095, 1098, 1108, *[Resp]* 1121, *[Extr]* 1582, *[Slee]* 1642, 1662, *[Feve]* 1719, 1726,

Index of words

[Gene] 1819, 1840, 1871, 1883, 1918, 1919, 1958, 1967, 1970

diphtheritic [Fema] 1047
diplomatic [Mind] 85
diplopia [Vert] 229, [Visi] 449
dipsomania [Mind] 85
direct [Mind] 85
direction [Mind] 85
directionless [Mind] 85
dirt [Drea] 1681
dirty [Mind] 85, [Nose] 513, [Mout] 610, [Teet] 664, [Extr] 1377, [Drea] 1681, [Skin] 1751
dirty appearance [Gene] 1831
dirty-looking [Expe] 1171
disabled [Gene] 1831
disagreeable [Mind] 86, [Stom] 732, [Drea] 1681
disappointments [Drea] 1681
disaster [Drea] 1681
discharge [Head] 249, [Nose] 513, [Mout] 610, [Teet] 664, [Thro] 687, [Abdo] 809, [Rect] 911, [Uret] 985, [Male] 1015, [Fema] 1047, [Ches] 1186
discharges [Eye] 393, [Ear] 463, [Gene] 1831
discipline [Mind] 86
discoloration [Eye] 394, [Ear] 464, [Nose] 518, [Face] 550, [Mout] 610, [Teet] 664, [Thro] 687, [Exte] 715, [Stom] 732, [Abdo] 809, [Rect] 911, [Uret] 987, [Male] 1015, [Fema] 1047, [Lary] 1095, [Ches] 1187, [Back] 1273, [Extr] 1377, [Skin] 1751, [Gene] 1832
discomfort [Mind] 86
disconcerted [Mind] 86
disconnected [Drea] 1681
disconnected feeling [Mind] 86
disconnected thinking [Mind] 86
discontented [Mind] 86
discordant [Feve] 1723
discords [Mind] 87
discouraged [Mind] 87
discrimination [Mind] 87
discuss [Mind] 87
disease [Drea] 1681
disgust [Mind] 87
disgusted [Drea] 1681
disgusting [Drea] 1681
dishonest [Mind] 88
dislocated [Ches] 1187, [Extr] 1382
dislocation [Face] 559, [Back] 1273, [Extr] 1382
dislocation; easy [Extr] 1383

disobedience [Mind] 88
disorder [Mind] 88
disordered [Stom] 732, [Chil] 1707
disorderly [Mind] 88
disorganized [Mind] 88
disoriented [Mind] 88
displacement [Fema] 1047
displeased [Mind] 88
disposing [Mind] 88
dispute [Mind] 88, [Drea] 1682
disruption [Mind] 88
dissatisfied [Mind] 88
dissecting [Drea] 1682
dissociation [Mind] 88
distances [Mind] 88
distant [Visi] 450, [Hear] 501
distant things [Drea] 1682
distended [Blad] 952, [Fema] 1047
distension [Head] 249, [Ear] 465, [Nose] 519, [Thro] 688, [Exte] 715, [Stom] 732, [Abdo] 809, [Rect] 911, [Ches] 1187, [Extr] 1383, [Gene] 1832
distorted [Eye] 396, [Visi] 450, [Exte] 715, [Extr] 1383, [Drea] 1682
distortion [Face] 559, [Gene] 1832
distracting [Coug] 1142
distraction [Mind] 88
distressing [Coug] 1142
distrustful [Mind] 88
disturbed [Mind] 88, [Slee] 1643
disturbing [Drea] 1682
diversion [Mind] 88
diverticulosis [Abdo] 812
dizziness [Gene] 1833
docility [Mind] 88
doctors [Drea] 1682
dogmatic [Mind] 88
dogs [Drea] 1682
dog's [Stoo] 941
domestic [Mind] 17, 28, 92, 101, 130, 183, [Abdo] 896, [Rect] 907, [Slee] 1662
dominated [Mind] 88
domineering [Mind] 88
dorsal region [Back] 1348
dotage [Mind] 88
double [Visi] 450, [Nose] 519, [Resp] 1127
double checking [Mind] 88
doubling up [Gene] 1833
doubtful [Mind] 88

Index of words

down *[Coug]* **1142**
down' *[Gene]* **1833**
downward *[Vert]* **229**
downy *[Lary]* **1095**
dozing *[Slee]* **1644**
draft *[Coug]* **1142**
draft of air *[Head]* **249**
dragging *[Head]* **249**, *[Abdo]* **812**, *[Rect]* **911**, *[Extr]* **1383**, *[Gene]* **1833**
dragons *[Drea]* **1682**
drainage *[Nose]* **519**
drama *[Mind]* **88**
draw *[Rect]* **911**
drawing *[Mind]* **88**, *[Eye]* **396**, *[Ches]* **1187**, *[Back]* **1273**, *[Extr]* **1383**, *[Skin]* **1754**
drawing in *[Abdo]* **812**, *[Gene]* **1833**
drawing s *[Male]* **1015**
drawing up *[Gene]* **1833**
drawn *[Head]* **249**, *[Face]* **559**, *[Mout]* **619**, *[Thro]* **688**, *[Abdo]* **812**, *[Male]* **1015**, *[Lary]* **1095**, *[Ches]* **1187**, *[Extr]* **1383**
drawn backward *[Eye]* **396**
drawn in *[Abdo]* **812**
drawn inward *[Nose]* **519**
drawn together *[Eye]* **396**, *[Gene]* **1833**
drawn up *[Nose]* **519**
drawn upwards *[Eye]* **396**
dread *[Mind]* **89**
dream *[Mind]* **89**
dreaminess *[Mind]* **89**
dreaming *[Slee]* **1644**
dreamless *[Slee]* **1645**
dreams *[Slee]* **1645**, *[Drea]* **1682**
dress *[Mind]* **89**
dressing *[Coug]* **1142**
dribbling *[Male]* **1015**
dried albuminous substance *[Skin]* **1754**
drinking *[Mind]* **89**, *[Vert]* **229**, *[Head]* **250**, *[Ear]* **465**, *[Thro]* **688**, *[Stom]* **733**, *[Abdo]* **812**, *[Coug]* **1142**, *[Expe]* **1171**, *[Back]* **1273**, *[Drea]* **1682**, *[Chil]* **1707**, *[Feve]* **1723**, *[Pers]* **1739**, *[Gene]* **1833**
dripping *[Nose]* **519**, *[Rect]* **911**
driven *[Mind]* **89**
driving *[Mind]* **89**, *[Vert]* **229**, *[Coug]* **1143**, *[Drea]* **1682**
dromomania *[Mind]* **89**
drooping *[Eye]* **396**, *[Face]* **559**
drop *[Uret]* **987**

dropping *[Face]* **559**, *[Mout]* **619**, *[Uret]* **987**, *[Extr]* **1383**
drops *[Visi]* **450**, *[Blad]* **952**, *[Ches]* **1187**, *[Back]* **1274**, *[Extr]* **1383**, *[Gene]* **1833**
dropsical *[Male]* **1039**, *[Fema]* **1090**, *[Extr]* **1598**, 1601, 1602, 1621, *[Skin]* **1783**
dropsy *[Head]* **250**, *[Mout]* **614**, *[Stom]* **753**, 786, 787, *[Abdo]* **807**, **812**, 894, 896, *[Rect]* **905**, *[Kidn]* 980, *[Fema]* **1047**, 1067, 1072, *[Resp]* **1121**, 1122, *[Ches]* **1187**, 1264, 1265, 1266, *[Extr]* **1383**, *[Slee]* 1655, *[Skin]* 1752, 1753, 1754, 1784, *[Gene]* 1801, 1830, **1833**, 1833, 1834, 1893, 1919, 1967
drowned *[Drea]* **1682**
drowning *[Drea]* **1682**
drowsiness *[Eye]* **396**, *[Slee]* **1645**
drowsy *[Mind]* **89**
drugs *[Mind]* **89**, *[Gene]* **1835**
drumming *[Ches]* **1187**
drunk *[Gene]* **1835**
drunkards *[Mind]* 46, 105, 133, 183, *[Vert]* **229**, *[Head]* 286, *[Visi]* 448, *[Hear]* 502, *[Nose]* 519, 522, 525, *[Face]* 560, *[Stom]* 724, 729, **733**, 737, 738, 741, 742, 746, 750, 752, 753, 758, 770, 783, 793, 796, 797, 800, *[Abdo]* 813, *[Rect]* 907, 918, 933, *[Uret]* 997, *[Lary]* 1093, *[Resp]* 1117, *[Coug]* 1143, *[Ches]* 1188, 1197, *[Extr]* 1611, *[Slee]* 1663, *[Skin]* 1764, 1778, 1786, *[Gene]* 1822, 1868, 1967
drunken *[Mind]* **89**, *[Drea]* **1682**
drunkenness *[Mind]* 30, **89**, 142, 170, 172, 183, 190, 192, 209, 221, *[Slee]* 1663
dry *[Teet]* **664**, *[Stoo]* **941**, *[Coug]* **1143**, *[Feve]* **1723**, *[Skin]* **1754**, *[Gene]* **1835**
dryness *[Head]* **250**, *[Eye]* **396**, *[Ear]* **465**, *[Nose]* **519**, *[Face]* **559**, *[Mout]* **619**, *[Thro]* **688**, *[Stom]* **733**, *[Rect]* **911**, *[Uret]* **988**, *[Male]* **1015**, *[Fema]* **1047**, *[Lary]* **1095**, *[Coug]* **1145**, *[Ches]* **1187**, *[Extr]* **1383**, *[Gene]* **1835**
duality *[Mind]* **89**
duchenne-friedrich syndrome *[Gene]* **1835**
duels *[Drea]* **1682**
dull *[Teet]* **664**, *[Coug]* **1146**, *[Slee]* **1645**
dullness *[Mind]* **89**, *[Head]* **250**, *[Eye]* **397**, *[Mout]* **622**
duodenum *[Abdo]* **893**
duplicity *[Mind]* **92**
dupuytren's *[Extr]* **1384**
dust *[Eye]* **397**, *[Thro]* **689**, *[Lary]* **1095**, *[Resp]* **1127**, *[Coug]* **1146**, *[Expe]* **1171**, *[Gene]* **1835**

Index of words

duty *[Mind]* 17, 58, 70, 73, **92**, 92
dwarfed *[Teet]* **664**
dwarfishness *[Fema]* **1047**, *[Gene]* **1835**
dwells *[Mind]* **92**
dying *[Drea]* **1682**
dynamic *[Mind]* **92**
dysenteric *[Feve]* **1724**
dysentery *[Rect]* **911**
dyslexia *[Mind]* **92**
dysmenorrhea *[Fema]* **1047**
dyspareunia *[Male]* **1015**, *[Fema]* **1047**
dyspepsia *[Stom]* **733**
dyspnea *[Nose]* **520**, *[Pers]* **1739**
dystonia *[Gene]* **1835**
dystrophy *[Gene]* **1835**
dysuria *[Blad]* **952**

E

earache *[Ear]* **465**
eardrum *[Ear]* **465**
earlier *[Stoo]* **941**
early *[Mind]* **93**
earnestness *[Mind]* **93**
ears *[Drea]* **1682**
earthquake *[Drea]* **1682**
earthy *[Mind]* **93**, *[Stoo]* **941**
earwax *[Ear]* **465**
ease *[Mind]* **93**
easier *[Expe]* **1171**
easily *[Pers]* **1739**
easy *[Expe]* **1171**
eating *[Mind]* **93**, *[Vert]* **229**, *[Head]* **250**, *[Face]* **560**, *[Mout]* **622**, *[Teet]* **664**, *[Stom]* **733**, *[Abdo]* **812**, *[Resp]* **1127**, *[Coug]* **1146**, *[Expe]* **1172**, *[Back]* **1274**, *[Extr]* **1384**, *[Drea]* **1682**, *[Chil]* **1707**, *[Feve]* **1724**, *[Pers]* **1739**, *[Gene]* **1835**
ebullition *[Ches]* **1187**, *[Gene]* **1836**
ebullitions *[Head]* **250**
eccentric *[Drea]* **1682**
eccentricity *[Mind]* **93**
ecchymoses *[Mout]* **622**, *[Ches]* **1187**, 1187, *[Back]* **1274**, *[Extr]* 1378, **1384**, 1420, *[Skin]* **1754**
ecchymosis *[Mind]* 33, *[Eye]* **397**, *[Ear]* **465**
eclampsia *[Fema]* **1047**, *[Gene]* **1836**
ecstasy *[Mind]* **93**, *[Drea]* **1682**
ecstatic *[Mind]* **93**
ectopia *[Male]* **1015**

ectropion *[Eye]* **397**
eczema *[Mind]* 17, *[Head]* 251, *[Eye]* 397, 398, *[Ear]* 464, 465, 466, 467, *[Hear]* 502, *[Face]* 563, 564, 568, *[Stom]* 730, *[Abdo]* 813, 894, *[Rect]* 912, *[Blad]* 964, *[Male]* 1020, 1021, *[Fema]* 1048, *[Resp]* 1115, 1116, 1117, *[Ches]* 1188, 1189, 1190, 1266, *[Back]* 1274, *[Extr]* 1385, 1386, 1387, 1388, 1389, 1390, 1391, 1392, 1393, 1395, 1396, 1397, 1398, 1443, 1483, 1497, 1601, 1636, *[Skin]* 1758, 1760, 1783, *[Gene]* 1816, 1819, 1830, 1844, 1871, 1903, 1933, 1959
edema *[Mind]* 213, *[Vert]* 227, *[Head]* **250**, 281, *[Nose]* **520**, *[Face]* **560**, *[Thro]* 689, *[Abdo]* **812**, 812, *[Rect]* 905, *[Kidn]* **973**, 973, 974, *[Lary]* **1096**, *[Resp]* 1115, 1123, *[Ches]* 1192, 1266, *[Extr]* **1384**, 1448, 1595, *[Skin]* 1756, 1769, *[Gene]* 1833, **1836**
edema; pulmonary *[Ches]* **1187**
edematous *[Head]* 264, *[Eye]* 434, *[Ear]* 496, *[Nose]* 541, *[Face]* 570, 597, 598, *[Mout]* 647, *[Thro]* 712, 713, *[Kidn]* 973, *[Male]* 1039, *[Fema]* 1090, *[Ches]* 1194, *[Extr]* 1433, 1598, 1599, 1601, 1602, 1603, *[Gene]* 1946
edge *[Teet]* **664**
edges *[Teet]* **664**
effeminate *[Mind]* **93**
efficiency *[Gene]* **1836**
efficient *[Mind]* **93**
effusion *[Ear]* **465**, *[Ches]* **1188**, *[Gene]* **1836**
egg *[Stom]* **734**
egg white *[Face]* **560**
eggs *[Stoo]* **941**
egocentric *[Mind]* **93**
egoism *[Mind]* **93**
egotism *[Mind]* **93**
ejaculation *[Head]* **250**, *[Male]* **1015**, *[Drea]* **1682**
elasticity *[Skin]* **1754**
elated *[Mind]* **93**
elbow *[Extr]* **1632**
electric *[Skin]* **1754**
electrical *[Extr]* **1384**
electricity *[Gene]* **1836**
electroshock *[Gene]* **1836**
elegance *[Mind]* **94**
elephantiasis *[Male]* **1016**, *[Extr]* 1415, *[Gene]* **1836**
elevated *[Vert]* **229**
elevated temperature *[Feve]* **1724**
elevation *[Mind]* **94**, *[Extr]* **1384**
elevator *[Drea]* **1682**

Index of words

elongated *[Head]* **250**, *[Thro]* **689**, *[Back]* **1274**

elongated p *[Coug]* **1146**

elongated u *[Coug]* **1146**

elongation *[Mout]* **622**, *[Teet]* **664**, *[Extr]* **1384**

eloquent *[Mind]* **94**

emaciated *[Drea]* **1682**

emaciation *[Mind]* 59, 133, *[Head]* 257, 267, *[Face]* **560**, *[Mout]* **622**, *[Exte]* **715**, *[Stom]* **726**, *[Abdo]* 806, 809, 810, **812**, 813, 814, *[Rect]* **900**, *[Coug]* 1137, 1144, *[Ches]* **1188**, 1257, *[Back]* **1274**, *[Extr]* **1384**, 1407, *[Pers]* **1737**, *[Skin]* **1755**, 1791, *[Gene]* **1801**, **1807**, 1830, **1836**, 1837, 1922, 1947, 1948, 1965, 1967

embarrassed *[Mind]* **94**

embarrassment *[Mind]* **94**, *[Drea]* **1682**

embittered *[Mind]* **94**

embolism *[Eye]* **397**, *[Ches]* **1188**, *[Gene]* **1838**

embraces *[Mind]* **94**

emission *[Pros]* **981**, *[Drea]* **1682**

emissions *[Vert]* **229**, *[Pers]* **1739**

emissions seminal *[Gene]* **1838**

emotional *[Mind]* **94**, *[Vert]* **229**

emotions *[Mind]* **94**, *[Stom]* **734**, *[Coug]* **1146**

emphysema *[Resp]* **1115**, 1123, *[Coug]* 1137, *[Ches]* **1188**, 1195

emprosthotonos *[Back]* **1274**

emptiness *[Mind]* **94**, *[Thro]* **689**, *[Stom]* **734**, *[Abdo]* **812**, *[Rect]* **912**, *[Blad]* **952**, *[Ches]* **1188**, *[Gene]* **1838**

empty *[Head]* **250**, *[Rect]* **912**

empyema *[Face]* **560**, *[Ches]* **1188**, 1213

empyocele *[Male]* **1016**

enamel *[Teet]* **664**

encaged *[Gene]* **1838**

encephalitis *[Mind]* 46, *[Head]* **250**, 264, *[Gene]* 1819

encephaloma *[Gene]* 1807, 1955

enchondroma *[Extr]* 1615, *[Gene]* 1955

encircled *[Drea]* **1682**

encopresis *[Mind]* **94**, *[Rect]* **912**

end stage of a disease *[Gene]* **1838**

endangered *[Mind]* **94**

endarteritis obliterans *[Gene]* **1838**

endless *[Drea]* **1682**

endocarditis *[Ches]* **1188**

endometriosis *[Fema]* **1047**, *[Gene]* **1838**

enemies *[Drea]* **1682**

enemy *[Mind]* **94**

energized *[Mind]* **94**

energy *[Gene]* **1838**

enervation *[Gene]* **1838**

enjoyment *[Male]* **1016**, *[Fema]* **1048**

enlarged *[Head]* **250**, *[Eye]* **397**, *[Nose]* **520**, *[Face]* **560**, *[Mout]* **622**, *[Stom]* **735**, *[Abdo]* **813**, *[Male]* **1016**, *[Fema]* **1048**, *[Ches]* **1188**, *[Gene]* **1838**

enlargement *[Eye]* **397**, *[Thro]* **689**, *[Pros]* **981**, *[Ches]* **1188**, *[Extr]* **1384**

ennui *[Mind]* **94**

enough *[Slee]* **1645**

entering *[Vert]* **229**

enteritis *[Abdo]* **813**

enteroptosis *[Abdo]* **813**

entertainment *[Mind]* **94**, *[Drea]* **1682**

enthusiasm *[Mind]* **94**

entropion *[Eye]* **397**

enuresis *[Blad]* **952**

enuresis nocturna *[Blad]* **952**

environmental *[Mind]* **94**

envy *[Mind]* **94**

eosinophilia *[Gene]* **1838**

epidemic *[Drea]* **1682**

epigastrium *[Stom]* **801**, *[Coug]* **1146**

epiglottis *[Lary]* **1110**

epilepsy *[Vert]* **229**, *[Abdo]* **813**, *[Drea]* **1682**, *[Gene]* **1838**

epileptic *[Vert]* **229**, *[Stom]* **735**, *[Fema]* **1048**, *[Back]* **1274**, *[Extr]* **1385**

epistaxis *[Mind]* **94**, *[Vert]* **229**, *[Head]* **251**, *[Nose]* **520**, *[Ches]* **1188**

epithelioma *[Eye]* 390, 436, *[Nose]* 505, *[Face]* 545, *[Mout]* 607, 614, 625, *[Male]* 1013, *[Fema]* 1044, *[Ches]* 1180, *[Skin]* 1748, 1773, *[Gene]* 1807

epithelium *[Expe]* **1172**

epulis *[Mout]* **622**

erection *[Rect]* **912**

erections *[Vert]* **229**, *[Male]* **1016**, *[Drea]* **1682**

erethism *[Mind]* **94**

ergasiaphobia *[Mind]* **94**

ergot *[Gene]* **1838**

erosion *[Mout]* **622**, *[Thro]* **689**, *[Fema]* **1048**

erosive gnawing *[Extr]* **1385**

erotic *[Mind]* **94**

erratic *[Mind]* **94**

errors *[Drea]* **1682**

Index of words

eructations *[Vert]* **229**, *[Ear]* **465**, *[Thro]* **689**, *[Abdo]* **813**, *[Resp]* **1127**, *[Coug]* **1146**, *[Ches]* **1188**, *[Back]* **1274**, *[Extr]* **1385**, *[Gene]* **1838**

eructations; type of *[Stom]* **738**

eruptions *[Mind]* **94**, *[Vert]* **229**, *[Head]* **251**, *[Eye]* **397**, *[Ear]* **465**, *[Nose]* **524**, *[Face]* **560**, *[Mout]* **622**, *[Thro]* **689**, *[Exte]* **715**, *[Stom]* **744**, *[Abdo]* **813**, *[Rect]* **912**, *[Uret]* **988**, *[Male]* **1020**, *[Fema]* **1048**, *[Coug]* **1146**, *[Ches]* **1188**, *[Back]* **1274**, *[Extr]* **1385**, *[Drea]* **1682**, *[Skin]* **1754**

eruptive *[Feve]* **1724**

erysipelas *[Head]* **253**, *[Ear]* **467**, *[Nose]* **524**, *[Face]* **569**, 570, *[Mout]* 614, 616, 644, 656, *[Abdo]* **814**, *[Fema]* **1048**, *[Resp]* 1117, *[Ches]* **1190**, *[Back]* **1276**, *[Extr]* **1399**, *[Slee]* 1663, *[Skin]* 1759, 1769, **1772**, *[Gene]* 1819, 1871

erysipelatous *[Eye]* **398**

escape *[Mind]* **94**

esophagitis *[Thro]* **689**

esophoria *[Eye]* **398**

estranged *[Mind]* **95**

euphoria *[Mind]* **95**

euphoric *[Drea]* **1682**

eustachian *[Head]* 270, *[Ear]* 461, 462, 467, 468, 469, 485, 489, 492, 496, *[Hear]* 502, *[Nose]* 524, *[Thro]* 694, *[Exte]* 717

eustachian tube *[Ear]* **498**

euthanasia *[Gene]* **1838**

evacuated *[Rect]* **913**

evading *[Mind]* **95**

evening *[Vert]* **226**, *[Coug]* 1136, *[Expe]* 1169, *[Chil]* **1701**, *[Feve]* **1718**, *[Pers]* 1736, *[Gene]* 1795

events *[Drea]* **1682**

eversion *[Eye]* **398**

everted *[Face]* 570, *[Uret]* **988**

everything *[Ear]* **467**

evil *[Drea]* **1683**

exact *[Mind]* **95**

exacting *[Mind]* **95**

exaggerating *[Mind]* **95**

exaltation *[Mind]* **95**

examination fear *[Mind]* **95**

examinations *[Drea]* **1683**

exanthematous *[Feve]* **1724**

exasperated *[Mind]* **95**

exasperation *[Drea]* **1683**

excelling *[Drea]* **1683**

excessive *[Slee]* **1645**

excitability *[Male]* **1021**, *[Fema]* **1048**

excitement *[Mind]* 5, 6, 7, 10, 13, 17, 39, 45, 49, 83, 85, 90, **95**, 96, 97, 99, 106, 109, 126, 127, 130, 136, 145, 150, 169, 172, 173, 179, 182, 183, 185, 188, 199, 203, 205, 210, 213, 214, 221, 222, *[Vert]* **229**, *[Head]* 245, 260, 266, 287, 318, 338, 358, 373, *[Ear]* 467, 476, 495, *[Nose]* 511, 519, *[Face]* 556, 559, 574, 582, *[Mout]* 626, 645, 646, *[Teet]* 664, 666, 671, *[Thro]* 701, 710, *[Exte]* 716, 720, *[Stom]* 723, 732, 733, 737, 759, 771, 783, 793, *[Abdo]* 807, 836, 841, 891, *[Rect]* 907, 918, 920, 933, *[Blad]* 965, *[Urin]* 1000, *[Male]* 1016, 1018, 1019, **1021**, 1024, 1032, 1035, 1039, *[Fema]* 1043, **1048**, 1051, 1052, 1056, 1057, 1058, 1061, 1062, 1063, 1065, 1066, 1069, 1070, 1072, 1077, 1078, 1088, *[Lary]* 1100, *[Resp]* 1117, 1123, *[Coug]* **1146**, *[Ches]* 1178, 1183, 1191, 1193, 1194, 1198, 1200, 1202, 1205, 1210, 1224, 1230, 1242, 1252, 1254, 1255, 1262, 1266, *[Back]* 1277, 1339, 1345, *[Extr]* 1357, 1358, 1360, 1361, 1378, 1382, 1407, 1413, 1430, 1431, 1434, 1440, 1523, 1562, 1570, 1579, 1608, 1610, 1611, *[Slee]* 1642, 1646, 1654, 1656, 1663, 1666, 1671, *[Chil]* **1707**, 1708, *[Feve]* **1724**, *[Pers]* **1739**, *[Skin]* 1748, 1753, 1770, 1774, 1778, 1781, *[Gene]* 1808, 1810, 1820, 1824, 1825, 1826, 1827, 1837, 1841, 1883, 1895, 1900, 1918, 1919, 1924, 1926, 1927, 1953, 1954, 1968, 1971, 1974

exciting *[Drea]* **1683**

exclaiming *[Mind]* **98**

exclusive *[Mind]* **98**

excoriating *[Stoo]* **941**, *[Urin]* **1005**

excoriation *[Eye]* **398**, *[Ear]* **467**, *[Nose]* **524**, *[Face]* **570**, *[Mout]* **623**, *[Thro]* **689**, *[Exte]* **716**, *[Rect]* **913**, *[Uret]* **988**, *[Male]* **1021**, *[Fema]* **1048**, *[Ches]* **1190**, *[Back]* **1276**, *[Extr]* **1399**, *[Skin]* **1773**, *[Gene]* **1838**

excoriations *[Abdo]* **814**

excrements *[Drea]* **1683**

excrescence *[Abdo]* **814**

excrescences *[Eye]* **398**, *[Mout]* **623**, *[Uret]* **988**, *[Male]* **1021**, *[Fema]* **1049**, *[Extr]* 1388, 1390, 1397, **1399**, 1635, *[Drea]* **1683**, *[Skin]* **1773**

execution *[Mind]* **98**

exercise *[Mind]* **98**

exertion *[Mind]* **98**, *[Vert]* **229**, *[Head]* **253**, *[Eye]* **398**, *[Visi]* **450**, *[Teet]* **664**, *[Resp]* 1127, *[Coug]*

Index of words

1146, *[Ches]* **1190**, *[Back]* **1276**, *[Drea]* **1683**, *[Chil]* **1707**, *[Feve]* **1724**, *[Pers]* **1739**, *[Gene]* **1838**

exertion of the eyes *[Vert]* **230**, *[Visi]* **450**

exfoliation *[Mout]* **623**, *[Teet]* **664**, *[Extr]* **1399**

exhalations *[Nose]* **524**

exhausted *[Mind]* **98**

exhausting *[Coug]* **1146**, *[Slee]* **1645**, *[Drea]* **1683**

exhaustion *[Gene]* **1839**

exhibitionism *[Mind]* **98**

exhilaration *[Mind]* **98**

exophoria *[Eye]* **398**

exophthalmos *[Eye]* **398**

exostosis *[Head]* **253**, *[Ear]* **467**, *[Nose]* **524**, *[Face]* **570**, *[Mout]* **623**, *[Ches]* **1190**, *[Back]* **1276**, *[Extr]* **1399**, *[Gene]* **1839**, 1948

expanded *[Head]* **253**

expanding *[Ches]* **1190**

expansion *[Head]* **253**, *[Nose]* **524**, *[Ches]* **1190**, *[Extr]* **1399**, *[Gene]* **1839**

expansive *[Mind]* **98**

expectoration *[Resp]* **1127**, *[Coug]* **1146**, *[Drea]* **1683**, *[Gene]* **1839**

expiration *[Coug]* **1147**, *[Gene]* **1839**

expirations *[Nose]* **524**

explosion *[Drea]* **1683**

explosive *[Stoo]* **941**, *[Coug]* **1147**

exposing *[Drea]* **1683**

exposure *[Chil]* **1707**

expressing *[Mind]* **98**

expression *[Face]* **570**

expressionless *[Eye]* **398**

expulsion *[Skin]* **1774**

expulsive power *[Ches]* **1190**

extend the arms *[Extr]* **1399**

extended *[Extr]* **1399**

extending *[Abdo]* **814**, *[Chil]* **1708**

extension *[Extr]* **1399**

external *[Chil]* **1708**, *[Feve]* **1724**

extravagance *[Mind]* **98**

extremes *[Mind]* **98**

extroverted *[Mind]* **98**

exuberance *[Mind]* **98**

exudates *[Gene]* **1839**

exudation *[Ear]* **467**, *[Mout]* **623**, *[Thro]* **689**, *[Ches]* **1190**

exultant *[Mind]* **98**

eye gum *[Eye]* **398**

eyeballs *[Eye]* **439**

eyebrows *[Eye]* **439**

eyelashes *[Eye]* **439**

eyelids *[Eye]* **439**

eyes *[Mind]* **99**, *[Head]* **253**, *[Drea]* **1683**

F

face *[Drea]* **1683**, *[Pers]* **1739**

faces *[Mind]* **99**

facetiousness *[Mind]* **99**

fade *[Visi]* **450**

fail *[Mind]* 60, 215, *[Ear]* 475, *[Resp]* 1116, 1123, *[Extr]* 1612, *[Gene]* 1825, 1827, 1932

failure *[Mind]* 4, 5, 19, 27, 33, 37, 60, **99**, 102, 106, 133, 150, 169, *[Stom]* 732, 751, 756, *[Ches]* 1188, **1190**, 1266, *[Gene]* 1801, 1833, **1839**, 1840, 1872, 1929, 1936, 1937, 1958, 1966, 1979

failures *[Drea]* **1683**

faint *[Abdo]* **814**, *[Ches]* **1190**

fainting *[Drea]* **1683**

faint-like *[Vert]* **230**

faintness *[Stom]* **744**, *[Gene]* **1839**

fair *[Gene]* **1844**

faithless *[Mind]* **99**

fall *[Vert]* **230**, *[Extr]* **1399**, *[Gene]* **1844**

falling *[Head]* **253**, *[Eye]* **399**, *[Face]* **572**, *[Teet]* **664**, *[Stom]* **744**, *[Abdo]* **814**, *[Stoo]* **941**, *[Ches]* **1190**, *[Drea]* **1683**, *[Gene]* **1844**

falling asleep *[Slee]* **1645**

falling out *[Extr]* **1400**

falling; as if *[Vert]* **230**

falls *[Blad]* **952**, *[Gene]* **1844**

false step *[Stom]* **744**

faltering *[Mind]* **99**

familiarity *[Mind]* **99**

family *[Mind]* 1, 2, 18, 23, 29, 34, 37, 42, 52, 56, 57, 61, 69, 75, 77, 95, 105, 106, 107, 121, 131, 138, 149, 154, 170, 204, 206, 215, 217, *[Exte]* 716, *[Rect]* 910, *[Resp]* 1118, *[Extr]* 1499, *[Drea]* 1681, **1684**

family history *[Gene]* **1844**

famine *[Drea]* **1684**

fanaticism *[Mind]* **99**

fancies *[Mind]* **99**

fan-like *[Nose]* **524**

fanned *[Extr]* **1400**, *[Gene]* **1844**

fanning *[Resp]* **1127**

Index of words

fantastic *[Drea]* **1684**

fantasy *[Mind]* **100**

far *[Mind]* **100**

farming *[Drea]* **1684**

far-sighted *[Visi]* **450**

fascinating *[Mind]* **100**

fastidious *[Mind]* **100**

fasting *[Head]* **254**, *[Stom]* **744**, *[Abdo]* **814**, *[Coug]* 1147, *[Ches]* **1190**, *[Gene]* **1844**

fat *[Eye]* **399**, *[Abdo]* **814**, *[Ches]* **1190**

fat food *[Abdo]* **814**, *[Coug]* 1147

fat people *[Gene]* **1844**

fatalistic *[Mind]* **100**

father *[Drea]* **1684**

fatigue *[Gene]* **1844**

fatiguing *[Coug]* 1147, *[Drea]* **1684**

fatty *[Head]* **254**, *[Stoo]* **941**, *[Kidn]* **973**, *[Urin]* **1005**, *[Ches]* **1190**, *[Back]* **1276**, *[Extr]* **1400**

fatty degeneration *[Abdo]* **814**, *[Skin]* **1774**, *[Gene]* **1844**

faultfinding *[Mind]* **100**

fear *[Mind]* **100**, *[Stom]* **744**, *[Coug]* 1147, *[Extr]* **1400**, *[Drea]* **1684**

fearless *[Mind]* **114**

feasting *[Mind]* **114**, *[Drea]* **1684**, *[Gene]* **1844**

feather *[Thro]* **689**, *[Coug]* 1147

feather bed *[Gene]* **1844**

feathers *[Gene]* **1844**

feathery *[Visi]* **450**

fecal *[Stoo]* **941**

feces *[Mind]* **114**, *[Rect]* **913**, *[Skin]* **1774**

feeble *[Resp]* **1128**

feeble power *[Expe]* **1172**

feel *[Gene]* **1844**

feeling *[Face]* **572**

feelings *[Mind]* **114**

feet *[Mind]* **114**, *[Vert]* **230**, *[Extr]* **1633**, *[Pers]* **1739**

feigned *[Slee]* **1647**

feigning *[Mind]* **114**

felon *[Extr]* **1400**, 1400, 1636, *[Gene]* 1949

fermentation *[Stom]* **744**, *[Abdo]* **814**

fermented *[Stoo]* **941**

fervent *[Mind]* **114**

festering *[Pros]* **981**, *[Skin]* **1774**

fetid breath *[Mout]* **623**

fetus *[Fema]* **1049**

fever *[Vert]* **230**, *[Stom]* **744**, *[Abdo]* **814**, *[Coug]* 1147, *[Extr]* **1400**, *[Drea]* **1684**, *[Chil]* **1708**, *[Feve]* **1717**, *[Pers]* **1739**, *[Gene]* **1845**

feverish *[Drea]* **1684**

fibroid *[Exte]* 721, *[Fema]* 1091, *[Ches]* 1262, *[Extr]* 1615, *[Gene]* 1955

fibrosis *[Abdo]* **814**, *[Ches]* **1190**

fibrositis *[Back]* **1276**, *[Extr]* **1400**, *[Gene]* **1845**

fickle *[Mind]* **114**

fidgety *[Mind]* **114**

field *[Visi]* **450**

fiery *[Mind]* **114**, *[Visi]* **450**

fight *[Mind]* **114**

fighting *[Drea]* **1684**

fights *[Drea]* **1684**

filaments *[Stoo]* **941**

filling *[Coug]* 1147

fills *[Mind]* **114**

filmy *[Eye]* **399**

filthy *[Extr]* **1400**, *[Skin]* **1774**

filthy t *[Mout]* **623**

final stage of a disease *[Gene]* **1845**

finances *[Mind]* **114**

finery *[Mind]* **114**

fingers *[Mind]* **114**, *[Mout]* **623**, *[Extr]* **1633**, *[Drea]* **1684**

fire *[Mind]* **114**, *[Eye]* **399**, *[Visi]* **451**, *[Coug]* 1147, *[Drea]* **1684**

firmness *[Mind]* **114**, *[Male]* **1021**

fish *[Coug]* 1147, *[Drea]* **1684**

fishbone *[Thro]* **689**

fishing *[Mind]* **114**, *[Drea]* **1684**

fissure *[Eye]* **399**, *[Rect]* **913**

fissured *[Mout]* **623**, *[Thro]* **689**

fissures *[Head]* **254**, *[Lary]* **1096**, *[Skin]* **1774**

fist *[Mout]* **623**

fists *[Mind]* **114**

fistula *[Eye]* **399**, *[Face]* **572**, 576, *[Mout]* **623**, *[Teet]* **664**, *[Rect]* **913**, *[Fema]* **1049**, *[Ches]* 1182, 1202, 1251, 1253, 1257

fistulae *[Exte]* 716, *[Abdo]* **814**, *[Coug]* 1154, *[Back]* **1276**, *[Gene]* **1845**, 1877

fistulous *[Male]* **1021**, *[Ches]* **1190**, *[Extr]* **1400**

fit *[Drea]* **1684**

fitful *[Mind]* **114**

fixed *[Mind]* **114**, *[Eye]* **399**, *[Drea]* **1684**

flabbiness *[Stom]* **744**, *[Skin]* **1774**

Index of words

flabby *[Mout]* **623**, *[Abdo]* **814**, *[Ches]* **1190**, *[Gene]* **1845**

flaccidity *[Male]* **1021**

flakes *[Expe]* **1172**

flaky *[Stoo]* **941**, *[Urin]* **1005**

flames *[Visi]* **451**

flapping *[Ear]* **467**, *[Nose]* **524**, *[Face]* **572**, *[Lary]* **1096**

flashback *[Mind]* **114**

flashes *[Visi]* **451**

flat *[Mind]* **114**, *[Mout]* **623**, *[Stoo]* **941**

flat foot *[Extr]* **1401**

flattened *[Head]* **254**, *[Abdo]* **814**

flattered *[Mind]* **114**

flattering *[Mind]* **114**

flatulence *[Mind]* **19**, **138**, **184**, *[Vert]* **230**, *[Head]* **243**, **277**, **279**, **288**, *[Face]* **601**, *[Mout]* **616**, *[Stom]* **736**, **744**, **751**, **772**, **774**, *[Abdo]* **810**, **814**, **822**, **832**, **833**, **834**, **835**, **836**, **840**, **849**, **852**, **856**, **870**, **874**, **878**, **879**, *[Rect]* **900**, **918**, **920**, *[Resp]* **1117**, **1124**, **1129**, *[Ches]* **1184**, **1203**, **1210**, **1213**, **1232**, **1243**, **1244**, **1246**, **1253**, *[Back]* **1304**, **1317**, **1319**, *[Extr]* **1613**, *[Slee]* **1643**, **1663**, **1669**, *[Skin]* **1753**, *[Gene]* **1800**, **1822**, **1824**, **1841**, **1845**

flatulent *[Stoo]* **941**

flatus *[Head]* **254**, *[Rect]* **913**, *[Stoo]* **941**, *[Uret]* **988**, *[Fema]* **1049**, *[Pers]* **1739**

flatus; passing *[Abdo]* **817**, *[Coug]* **1147**, *[Back]* **1276**, *[Gene]* **1845**

flayed *[Drea]* **1684**

fleeing *[Drea]* **1684**

fleeing away *[Mind]* **114**

flesh *[Lary]* **1096**

flexed *[Extr]* **1401**

flexibility *[Mind]* **114**

flexible *[Extr]* **1401**

flickering *[Visi]* **451**

flies *[Expe]* **1172**, *[Pers]* **1739**

flirtation *[Drea]* **1684**

flirting *[Mind]* **114**

floating *[Mind]* **114**, *[Vert]* **230**, *[Visi]* **452**, *[Stom]* **744**, *[Stoo]* **941**, *[Kidn]* **973**, *[Ches]* **1190**, *[Extr]* **1401**, *[Drea]* **1684**, *[Gene]* **1845**

flocculi *[Stoo]* **941**

flood *[Drea]* **1684**

flora *[Abdo]* **817**

florid *[Gene]* **1845**

flowers *[Mind]* **114**, *[Drea]* **1684**, *[Chil]* **1708**

flowing *[Gene]* **1845**

flu *[Gene]* **1845**

fluctuation *[Head]* **254**, *[Ches]* **1190**

fluid *[Head]* **254**

fluid retention *[Gene]* **1845**

fluids *[Nose]* **524**, *[Coug]* **1147**, *[Gene]* **1845**

flushed *[Face]* **572**

flushes *[Mind]* **9**, **16**, **18**, **184**, *[Head]* **258**, **260**, **276**, **279**, **370**, *[Eye]* **400**, *[Ear]* **468**, *[Nose]* **522**, *[Face]* **549**, **553**, **556**, **574**, *[Exte]* **716**, *[Abdo]* **820**, *[Fema]* **1049**, **1068**, *[Ches]* **1193**, **1251**, **1264**, *[Back]* **1277**, *[Extr]* **1405**, **1406**, **1407**, **1408**, **1409**, **1612**, *[Slee]* **1663**, *[Chil]* **1701**, **1703**, **1705**, *[Feve]* **1719**, **1725**, **1725**, *[Skin]* **1778**, *[Gene]* **1823**, **1830**, **1841**, **1845**, **1865**, **1866**, **1968**

flushes of heat *[Fema]* **1049**

fluttering *[Stom]* **744**, *[Abdo]* **817**, *[Kidn]* **973**, *[Ches]* **1190**, *[Back]* **1276**, *[Extr]* **1401**, *[Gene]* **1845**

flying *[Drea]* **1684**, *[Gene]* **1845**

foam *[Mout]* **623**

foamy *[Urin]* **1005**

focal *[Visi]* **452**

focus *[Mind]* **115**, *[Eye]* **399**

foetus *[Fema]* **1049**

fogged *[Mind]* **115**

foggy *[Visi]* **452**

folded *[Mout]* **623**

folds *[Abdo]* **817**

followed *[Vert]* **230**

followed by *[Coug]* **1147**, *[Drea]* **1684**, *[Chil]* **1708**, *[Pers]* **1739**

fontanelles *[Head]* **254**

food *[Nose]* **524**, *[Mout]* **623**, *[Thro]* **689**, *[Stom]* **744**, *[Lary]* **1096**, *[Coug]* **1147**, *[Drea]* **1684**, *[Pers]* **1740**, *[Gene]* **1845**

food poisoning *[Stom]* **744**, *[Rect]* **915**, *[Gene]* **1863**

foolish *[Mind]* **115**, *[Drea]* **1684**

foot *[Drea]* **1684**

foppish *[Mind]* **115**

forced *[Mind]* **115**, *[Gene]* **1863**

forcible *[Stoo]* **941**, *[Resp]* **1128**, *[Coug]* **1147**

forcing himself *[Mind]* **115**

forearm *[Extr]* **1633**

forebodings *[Mind]* **115**

forehead *[Vert]* **230**, *[Head]* **385**, *[Face]* **602**

foreign *[Head]* **254**, *[Nose]* **524**, *[Thro]* **690**, *[Stom]* **744**, *[Rect]* **915**, *[Lary]* **1096**, *[Coug]* **1147**

foreign bodies *[Skin]* **1774**, *[Gene]* **1863**

Index of words

foreign body *[Eye]* **399**, *[Ear]* **467**, *[Ches]* **1191**

foreign country *[Drea]* **1684**

forenoon *[Vert]* **225**, *[Coug]* **1135**, *[Expe]* **1169**, *[Chil]* **1699**, *[Feve]* **1717**, *[Pers]* **1735**, *[Gene]* **1794**

forest *[Drea]* **1684**

forests *[Gene]* **1863**

forger *[Mind]* **115**

forgetful *[Mind]* **115**

forgetting *[Mind]* **116**

forgiving *[Mind]* **116**

forgotten *[Mind]* **116**, *[Drea]* **1684**

formal *[Mind]* **116**

formication *[Head]* **254**, *[Ear]* **467**, *[Nose]* **524**, *[Face]* **572**, *[Mout]* **623**, *[Teet]* **664**, *[Thro]* **690**, *[Exte]* **716**, *[Stom]* **744**, *[Abdo]* **817**, *[Rect]* **915**, *[Kidn]* **973**, *[Male]* **1021**, *[Fema]* **1049**, *[Ches]* **1191**, *[Back]* **1276**, *[Extr]* **1401**, *[Skin]* **1774**, *[Gene]* **1863**

forms *[Drea]* **1684**

forsaken *[Mind]* **116**, *[Drea]* **1684**

forsaking *[Mind]* **116**

foundering *[Drea]* **1684**

fractures *[Head]* **255**, *[Extr]* **1403**, *[Gene]* **1863**

fragile *[Mind]* **116**, *[Gene]* **1863**

frail *[Mind]* **116**, *[Gene]* **1863**

frantic *[Mind]* **116**

fraternized *[Mind]* **116**

freckles *[Nose]* **524**, *[Face]* **572**, *[Ches]* 1187, *[Extr]* 1378, *[Skin]* **1774**

freedom *[Mind]* **116**

free-spirited *[Mind]* **116**

freethinker *[Mind]* **116**

freezing *[Ear]* **467**, *[Extr]* **1403**, *[Drea]* **1684**, *[Chil]* **1708**

frenzy *[Mind]* **116**

frequent *[Stoo]* **941**, *[Urin]* **1005**, *[Expe]* **1172**, *[Chil]* **1708**

fresh air *[Gene]* **1863**

fretful *[Mind]* **116**

fretting *[Male]* **1022**, *[Coug]* **1147**

friendly *[Mind]* **116**, *[Drea]* **1684**

friends *[Drea]* **1684**

friendship *[Mind]* **116**

fright *[Mind]* **4**, **5**, **9**, **13**, **18**, **51**, **62**, 106, 107, 111, 115, **117**, 117, 126, 133, 181, 199, 203, 211, *[Vert]* **230**, *[Head]* 245, **255**, 258, 288, 350, *[Visi]* 455, *[Hear]* 503, *[Face]* 557, *[Mout]* 626, 629, 646, *[Thro]* 691, *[Exte]* 721, *[Stom]* 772, 793, *[Abdo]* 837, *[Rect]* 900, 908, 920, 935, *[Blad]* 958, 959, 964, 965, *[Male]* 1019, *[Fema]* 1043, 1058, 1065, 1066, 1067, 1069, 1070, 1087, *[Lary]* 1108, 1109, *[Resp]* 1117, 1124, *[Coug]* **1147**, *[Ches]* 1253, *[Extr]* 1356, 1407, 1411, 1425, 1441, 1579, 1580, 1582, 1594, 1611, 1612, 1617, 1628, *[Slee]* 1656, 1663, 1670, *[Chil]* **1708**, 1712, *[Feve]* 1720, **1725**, *[Pers]* **1740**, *[Skin]* 1753, 1760, 1764, *[Gene]* 1799, 1808, 1810, 1812, 1824, 1825, 1831, 1837, 1841, 1892, 1919, 1953, 1956, 1968

frightened *[Mind]* **117**

frightening *[Coug]* **1147**

frightful *[Mind]* **17**, **47**, **50**, **61**, **62**, **65**, **66**, **99**, 118, 140, 141, 208, 214, *[Head]* 279, 371, *[Eye]* **399**, *[Face]* 559, *[Resp]* 1123, *[Slee]* 1643, 1644, 1651, *[Drea]* **1685**, 1690, 1695

frigidity *[Fema]* **1049**

fringe *[Eye]* **399**

fritters *[Mind]* **117**

frivolous *[Mind]* **117**

frog *[Stoo]* **942**, *[Drea]* **1685**

frostbite *[Extr]* 1353, *[Gene]* **1863**

frostbitten *[Nose]* **524**

frosty *[Gene]* **1863**

froth *[Mout]* **623**

frothy *[Stoo]* **942**, *[Urin]* **1005**, *[Expe]* **1172**

frown *[Mind]* **117**

frowning *[Head]* 288, *[Face]* 571, **572**, *[Ches]* 1197

frozen *[Head]* **255**, *[Ear]* **467**, *[Extr]* **1403**

fruit *[Teet]* **664**, *[Abdo]* **817**, *[Coug]* **1147**

fruits *[Drea]* **1685**

frustrated *[Mind]* **117**

fullness *[Vert]* **230**, *[Head]* **255**, *[Eye]* **399**, *[Ear]* **467**, *[Nose]* **524**, *[Face]* **572**, *[Thro]* **690**, *[Exte]* **716**, *[Stom]* **744**, *[Abdo]* **817**, *[Rect]* **915**, *[Blad]* **952**, *[Pros]* **981**, *[Male]* **1022**, *[Fema]* **1049**, *[Lary]* **1096**, *[Coug]* **1147**, *[Ches]* **1191**, *[Extr]* **1403**, *[Gene]* **1863**

fumes *[Nose]* **524**, *[Gene]* **1864**

funerals *[Drea]* **1685**

fungoid *[Blad]* **952**, *[Uret]* **988**, *[Gene]* **1864**

fungoid growth *[Gene]* **1864**

fungous *[Ear]* **467**

fungus *[Head]* **256**, *[Eye]* **399**, *[Face]* **572**

fungus haematodes *[Extr]* **1404**, *[Skin]* **1774**

fur *[Mind]* **117**, *[Gene]* **1864**

fur- *[Face]* **572**

furor *[Mind]* **117**

Index of words

furrows *[Face]* **572**
furry *[Mout]* **624**, *[Lary]* **1096**
fury *[Mind]* **117**
fussy *[Mind]* **117**
future *[Mind]* 1, 18, 23, 45, 84, 87, 89, 106, 121, 143, 158, 168, 184, 196, 206, 208, 209, 221, *[Slee]* 1643, *[Drea]* 1682
fuzziness *[Mind]* **117**, *[Head]* **256**, *[Extr]* **1404**
fuzzy *[Teet]* **664**

G

gagging *[Mout]* **624**, *[Stom]* **745**, *[Coug]* **1147**
gait reeling *[Gene]* **1864**
galactorrhea *[Ches]* **1192**
gallstone colic *[Abdo]* **818**
gallstones *[Abdo]* **818**, *[Gene]* **1864**
gambling *[Mind]* **117**
ganglia *[Skin]* **1774**
ganglion *[Ches]* 1195, *[Extr]* **1404**, *[Gene]* 1955
gangrene *[Mind]* 47, *[Eye]* **399**, *[Nose]* **524**, *[Face]* **572**, *[Thro]* **690**, *[Stom]* **745**, *[Abdo]* **818**, *[Blad]* **952**, *[Male]* **1022**, 1033, *[Fema]* **1049**, *[Ches]* 1180, **1192**, *[Extr]* **1404**, *[Feve]* **1725**, *[Skin]* 1759, **1775**, *[Gene]* 1830, 1873, 1978, 1979
gangrenous *[Mout]* **624**
gardening *[Mind]* **117**
gardens *[Drea]* **1685**
gargling *[Vert]* **230**, *[Gene]* **1864**
garment *[Drea]* **1685**
gas *[Abdo]* **818**, *[Blad]* **952**
gasping *[Resp]* **1128**
gasses *[Gene]* **1864**
gassy *[Urin]* **1005**
gastric *[Stom]* **745**, *[Coug]* **1147**
gastric fever *[Feve]* **1725**
gastritis *[Stom]* **745**
gastrointestinal *[Stom]* **745**, *[Abdo]* **818**
gathered together *[Gene]* **1864**
gauze *[Visi]* **452**
gay *[Mind]* **117**
gelatinous *[Stoo]* **942**, *[Urin]* **1005**, *[Expe]* **1172**
generous *[Mind]* **117**
gentleness *[Mind]* **117**
genu valgum *[Extr]* **1404**
genu varum *[Extr]* **1404**
genupectoral *[Slee]* 1649
gestation *[Fema]* **1049**

gestures *[Mind]* **117**
get oneself together *[Mind]* **120**
ghosts *[Drea]* **1685**
giants *[Drea]* **1685**
giddiness *[Vert]* **230**
gifted *[Mind]* **120**
giggling *[Mind]* **120**
gingival fistula *[Mout]* **624**, *[Teet]* **664**
gingivitis *[Mout]* **624**
girl *[Drea]* **1685**
girls *[Mind]* 23, 90, 126, 128, 140, 151, 170, 184, 188, 190, 195, *[Head]* 300, *[Nose]* 522, *[Face]* 561, *[Mout]* 629, *[Stom]* 797, *[Abdo]* 884, *[Rect]* 906, 910, *[Male]* 1035, *[Fema]* 1053, 1054, 1059, 1061, 1062, 1063, 1065, 1067, 1069, 1088, 1089, *[Ches]* 1202, *[Extr]* 1458, *[Slee]* 1663, *[Drea]* 1685, 1689, *[Skin]* 1790, *[Gene]* 1801, 1826, 1924
give way *[Extr]* **1404**
glairy *[Expe]* **1172**, *[Gene]* **1864**
glanders *[Gene]* **1864**
glands *[Ear]* **498**, *[Gene]* **1980**
glandular *[Feve]* **1725**
glandular swelling *[Mout]* **624**
glans *[Male]* **1041**
glass *[Gene]* **1864**
glassy *[Eye]* **399**
glaucoma *[Eye]* **399**, 400, 414, 416
glazed *[Eye]* **399**, *[Mout]* **624**, *[Thro]* **690**
gleet *[Uret]* **988**, *[Male]* **1022**
gliding *[Back]* **1276**
glimmering *[Visi]* **452**
glistening *[Eye]* **399**, *[Mout]* **624**, *[Thro]* **690**, *[Coug]* **1147**, *[Extr]* **1404**
glittering *[Visi]* **452**
globular *[Expe]* **1172**
globus *[Thro]* **690**
gloomy *[Mind]* **120**, *[Drea]* **1685**
glorification of oneself *[Drea]* **1685**
glossitis *[Mout]* **624**
glossy t *[Mout]* **624**
glow *[Extr]* **1404**
glowing *[Face]* **572**
glue *[Ear]* **467**
glued *[Mout]* **624**
gluey *[Thro]* **690**
glutinous *[Mout]* **624**, *[Expe]* **1172**
gluttony *[Mind]* **120**
glycogen storage diseases *[Gene]* **1864**

Index of words

gnawing *[Uret]* **988**, *[Skin]* **1775**

god *[Drea]* **1685**

godless *[Mind]* 120

going out *[Mind]* 120

goitre *[Exte]* 716

gonadotrophic hormone *[Urin]* 1005

goneness *[Stom]* 745, *[Abdo]* 818

gonorrhea *[Head]* 385, *[Eye]* 391, *[Face]* 582, *[Mout]* 642, *[Abdo]* 804, *[Rect]* 908, *[Blad]* 951, 960, *[Kidn]* 976, 980, *[Pros]* 982, *[Uret]* 985, **988**, 988, 989, 991, 997, *[Urin]* 1000, *[Male]* 1018, 1019, 1023, 1032, 1036, 1039, 1040, *[Fema]* 1050, 1077, 1088, *[Coug]* 1145, **1147**, *[Extr]* 1414, 1443, 1448, 1498, 1513, 1602, *[Gene]* 1819, 1844, **1864**, 1871, 1945

gonorrheal *[Eye]* 402, 403, *[Blad]* 953, *[Uret]* 986, 997, *[Male]* 1022, *[Fema]* 1055, *[Gene]* 1874, 1875, 1903

good for nothing *[Mind]* 120

good health *[Gene]* **1864**

good-humored *[Mind]* 120

goose *[Drea]* **1685**

goose flesh *[Head]* **256**, *[Abdo]* **818**, *[Back]* **1276**, *[Extr]* **1404**, *[Chil]* **1708**, *[Skin]* **1775**

gossiping *[Mind]* 120

gourmand *[Mind]* 120

gout *[Mind]* 113, *[Eye]* 390, *[Ear]* 474, *[Hear]* 502, 504, *[Teet]* 672, *[Thro]* 695, *[Stom]* 730, 751, 766, 791, *[Rect]* 905, *[Urin]* 999, *[Resp]* 1115, 1116, *[Coug]* **1147**, *[Ches]* 1266, *[Extr]* **1404**, 1453, 1603, 1625, *[Slee]* 1663, *[Feve]* 1726, *[Skin]* 1758, *[Gene]* 1830, 1844, 1945, 1968

gouty *[Mind]* 16, *[Head]* 280, 288, 316, *[Eye]* 401, *[Ear]* 470, 492, *[Face]* 582, 588, *[Mout]* 625, *[Thro]* **690**, *[Stom]* **745**, 753, *[Abdo]* **818**, 825, *[Rect]* 900, 908, *[Ches]* **1192**, 1211, *[Extr]* 1414, 1434, 1435, 1448, 1457, 1462, 1473, 1484, 1486, 1491, 1497, 1503, 1509, 1513, 1523, 1553, 1555, 1558, 1559, 1560, 1574, 1576, 1594, 1595, 1600, 1602, *[Gene]* 1900, 1901

gracious *[Mind]* 120

grand mal *[Gene]* **1864**

granular *[Eye]* **399**, *[Nose]* **524**, *[Stoo]* **942**, *[Expe]* **1172**

granulated *[Thro]* **690**

granulation *[Fema]* 1049

granuloma *[Ches]* **1192**

grasped *[Lary]* **1096**

grasping *[Mout]* **624**, *[Exte]* **716**, *[Coug]* **1147**, *[Ches]* **1192**, *[Extr]* **1404**

grasping objects *[Gene]* **1864**

grasps *[Vert]* **230**

graves *[Drea]* **1685**

graves' disease *[Gene]* **1864**

gravity *[Mind]* 120, *[Urin]* 1005

gray *[Stoo]* **942**

grayish *[Expe]* **1172**

grease *[Coug]* **1147**

greasy *[Face]* **572**, *[Mout]* **624**, *[Stoo]* **942**, *[Skin]* **1775**, *[Gene]* **1864**

great leaps *[Drea]* **1685**

greatness *[Drea]* **1685**

greed *[Mind]* 120

green *[Stoo]* **942**

greenish *[Eye]* **399**, *[Expe]* **1172**

grief *[Mind]* 4, 5, 7, 18, 26, 30, 63, 98, 107, **120**, 126, 133, 138, 144, 149, 153, 169, 170, 171, 184, 203, 217, *[Head]* 245, 250, 260, 288, 338, 366, 386, *[Visi]* 454, 458, *[Nose]* 525, *[Face]* 593, 603, *[Stom]* 733, 737, 752, 772, 790, *[Abdo]* 810, 822, *[Rect]* 908, 920, *[Kidn]* 980, *[Fema]* 1043, 1045, 1047, 1058, 1059, 1061, 1063, 1065, 1067, *[Resp]* 1117, *[Coug]* **1147**, *[Ches]* 1185, 1224, 1253, *[Back]* 1287, 1341, *[Extr]* 1581, *[Slee]* 1656, 1663, *[Drea]* **1685**, *[Chil]* **1708**, *[Skin]* 1764, *[Gene]* 1801, 1808, 1810, 1825, 1831, 1837, 1841, 1956, 1968

grimaces *[Mind]* 121, *[Drea]* **1685**

grinding *[Teet]* **664**, *[Gene]* **1864**

griping *[Abdo]* **818**

grippe *[Gene]* **1864**

gritty *[Eye]* **399**

groaning *[Mind]* 121, *[Resp]* 1128

groping *[Mind]* 121

grotesque *[Drea]* **1685**

grounded *[Mind]* 121

growing *[Drea]* **1685**

growing pains *[Extr]* **1404**

growling *[Mind]* 121, *[Ches]* **1192**, *[Gene]* **1864**

growth *[Extr]* **1404**, *[Gene]* **1864**

growths *[Mout]* **624**

grudge *[Mind]* 121

grumbling *[Mind]* 121, *[Rect]* **915**, *[Back]* **1276**

grumous *[Stoo]* **942**

grunting *[Mind]* 121

guillain-barré syndrome *[Gene]* **1864**

Index of words

guilt *[Mind]* 121, *[Drea]* 1685
gullible *[Mind]* 121
gulping up *[Thro]* 690
gumboil *[Mout]* 624
gums *[Mout]* 659
gunning *[Drea]* 1685
gurgling *[Head]* 256, *[Thro]* 690, *[Stom]* 745, *[Abdo]* 818, *[Rect]* 915, *[Pros]* 981, *[Male]* 1022, *[Ches]* 1192, *[Extr]* 1404
gushing *[Abdo]* 819, *[Stoo]* 942
gymnastic *[Drea]* 1685

H

hacking *[Stom]* 746, *[Coug]* 1147
haggard *[Eye]* 399, *[Face]* 572
hair *[Mind]* 121, *[Vert]* 230, *[Head]* 385, *[Eye]* 439, *[Visi]* 452, *[Nose]* 525, *[Mout]* 624, *[Thro]* 690, *[Stoo]* 942, *[Male]* 1022, *[Fema]* 1049, *[Lary]* 1096, *[Coug]* 1148, *[Ches]* 1192, *[Back]* 1276, *[Extr]* 1404, *[Drea]* 1685, *[Skin]* 1775, *[Gene]* 1864
hairy *[Mout]* 624
half asleep *[Slee]* 1647
hallucinations *[Mind]* 121
halo *[Visi]* 452
hammering *[Ear]* 467, *[Abdo]* 819, *[Gene]* 1864
hand *[Gene]* 1864
handicapped *[Drea]* 1685, *[Gene]* 1864
handled *[Mind]* 121
handling *[Fema]* 1049
handling genitals *[Male]* 1022
hands *[Head]* 256, *[Abdo]* 819, *[Coug]* 1148, *[Extr]* 1633, *[Drea]* 1685
hands and knees; on *[Coug]* 1148
handyman *[Mind]* 121
hang down *[Resp]* 1128, *[Ches]* 1192, *[Extr]* 1404, *[Gene]* 1864
hanging *[Eye]* 399, *[Face]* 572, *[Thro]* 690, *[Stom]* 746, *[Abdo]* 819, *[Male]* 1022, *[Ches]* 1192
hangnails *[Extr]* 1405
hangover *[Gene]* 1865
haphephobia *[Mind]* 121
happen *[Drea]* 1686
happy *[Mind]* 121, *[Coug]* 1148, *[Drea]* 1686
harassing *[Coug]* 1148, *[Drea]* 1686
hard *[Mind]* 121, *[Head]* 256, *[Mout]* 624, *[Thro]* 691, *[Stom]* 746, *[Abdo]* 819, *[Stoo]* 942, *[Uret]* 988, *[Coug]* 1148, *[Expe]* 1172, *[Ches]* 1192, *[Skin]* 1775
hard bed *[Gene]* 1865
hardhearted *[Mind]* 121
hardness *[Eye]* 399, *[Ear]* 467, *[Nose]* 524, *[Face]* 572, *[Stom]* 746, *[Pros]* 981, *[Uret]* 988, *[Male]* 1022, *[Fema]* 1049, *[Ches]* 1192, *[Extr]* 1405, *[Gene]* 1865
harmony *[Mind]* 121
harsh *[Mind]* 121
hastiness *[Mind]* 121
hat *[Head]* 256, *[Feve]* 1725, *[Gene]* 1865
hatred *[Mind]* 122
haughty *[Mind]* 122
hawk *[Thro]* 691
hawked *[Expe]* 1172
hawking *[Coug]* 1149, *[Ches]* 1192
hawks *[Thro]* 691
hay fever *[Nose]* 524
hazelnuts *[Stoo]* 943
hazy *[Mind]* 122
head *[Drea]* 1686, *[Feve]* 1725, *[Pers]* 1740
headache *[Vert]* 230, *[Head]* 256, *[Coug]* 1149, *[Drea]* 1686, *[Chil]* 1708, *[Pers]* 1740
head-banging *[Mind]* 122
headless *[Head]* 256
headstrong *[Mind]* 122
health *[Mind]* 18, 19, 43, 64, 84, 86, 92, 107, 149, 184, 221, *[Gene]* 1862
hearing *[Drea]* 1686
heart *[Coug]* 1149, *[Ches]* 1192
heartbeat *[Ches]* 1192
heartburn *[Stom]* 746, *[Coug]* 1149
heat *[Vert]* 231, *[Head]* 256, *[Eye]* 399, *[Ear]* 467, *[Nose]* 525, *[Face]* 572, *[Mout]* 624, *[Teet]* 664, *[Thro]* 691, *[Exte]* 716, *[Stom]* 747, *[Abdo]* 819, *[Rect]* 915, *[Blad]* 952, *[Kidn]* 973, *[Pros]* 981, *[Uret]* 988, *[Male]* 1022, *[Fema]* 1049, *[Lary]* 1096, *[Coug]* 1149, *[Ches]* 1192, *[Back]* 1277, *[Extr]* 1405, *[Slee]* 1647, *[Chil]* 1708, *[Feve]* 1725, *[Skin]* 1775, *[Gene]* 1865
heat stroke *[Gene]* 1868
heat; flushes of *[Fema]* 1050
heated *[Head]* 260, *[Extr]* 1409, *[Gene]* 1868
heaviness *[Mind]* 122, *[Head]* 260, *[Eye]* 400, *[Ear]* 468, *[Nose]* 525, *[Mout]* 625, *[Teet]* 665, *[Stom]* 747, *[Abdo]* 820, *[Rect]* 915, *[Blad]* 952, *[Kidn]* 973, *[Pros]* 981, *[Uret]* 988, *[Male]* 1022, *[Fema]*

Index of words

1050, *[Lary]* **1096**, *[Ches]* **1193**, *[Back]* **1278**, *[Extr]* **1409**, *[Gene]* **1868**

heaving *[Head]* **264**

heavy *[Face]* **575**, *[Abdo]* **821**, *[Stoo]* **943**, *[Urin]* **1005**, *[Expe]* **1172**, *[Slee]* **1647**, *[Drea]* **1686**

hectic *[Coug]* **1149**

hectic fever *[Feve]* **1725**

heedless *[Mind]* **122**

held *[Mind]* **122**, *[Drea]* **1686**, *[Chil]* **1708**

helping *[Drea]* **1686**

helping others *[Mind]* **122**

helpless *[Drea]* **1686**

helplessness *[Mind]* **122**

hematemesis *[Stom]* **748**

hematocele *[Male]* **1022**, *[Fema]* **1050**

hematoma *[Ear]* **468**, *[Gene]* **1868**

hematophobia *[Mind]* **123**

hematuria *[Blad]* **952**, *[Urin]* **1005**

hemeralopia *[Visi]* **453**

hemiballism *[Extr]* **1413**

hemicrania *[Mind]* 159, *[Head]* 346, *[Visi]* 453

hemiopia *[Vert]* 226, *[Eye]* 390, *[Visi]* 452, **453**

hemiplegia *[Extr]* 1579, *[Gene]* 1844, **1868**

hemming *[Lary]* **1096**

hemophilia *[Gene]* **1868**

hemophobia *[Mind]* **123**

hemoptysis *[Mind]* 212, *[Nose]* 522, *[Resp]* 1124, *[Expe]* **1172**, *[Ches]* 1183, **1193**, 1197, *[Extr]* 1443, *[Drea]* **1686**, *[Feve]* **1725**, *[Gene]* 1825, 1841

hemorrhage *[Head]* **264**, *[Eye]* **401**, *[Mout]* **625**, *[Stom]* **748**, *[Abdo]* **821**, *[Rect]* **915**, *[Blad]* **952**, *[Uret]* **988**, *[Fema]* **1050**, *[Ches]* **1193**, *[Back]* **1278**, *[Drea]* **1686**, *[Feve]* **1725**, *[Gene]* **1868**

hemorrhoids *[Mind]* **123**, *[Vert]* **231**, *[Rect]* **916**, *[Blad]* **952**, *[Coug]* **1149**, *[Back]* **1278**, *[Gene]* **1870**

hepatic *[Chil]* **1708**

hepatitis *[Abdo]* **821**, *[Gene]* **1870**

hepatization *[Ches]* **1194**

hepatomegaly *[Abdo]* **821**

hernia *[Abdo]* 811, 862, 863, 864, 865, 872, 879, 885, *[Rect]* 899, *[Male]* **1022**

hernia; abdominal *[Abdo]* **821**

herpes *[Mind]* 189, *[Head]* 252, 276, *[Eye]* 397, 398, *[Ear]* 465, 466, 467, *[Face]* 563, 564, *[Mout]* 622, **625**, *[Exte]* 715, *[Stom]* 730, *[Abdo]* 813, *[Rect]* 912, 913, *[Coug]* 1160, 1166, *[Ches]* 1182, 1188, 1189, 1190, 1211, 1228, *[Back]* 1274, 1287, *[Extr]* 1385, 1386, 1387, 1388, 1389, 1390, 1391, 1392, 1393, 1394, 1395, 1396, 1397, 1398, *[Skin]* 1758, 1760, 1781, *[Gene]* 1900, 1947

herpes zoster ophthalmicus *[Eye]* **401**

herpetic *[Eye]* 403, *[Ear]* 466, *[Mout]* 657, *[Thro]* 693, *[Rect]* 912, *[Male]* 1020, 1021, 1022, *[Fema]* 1048, *[Extr]* 1621, *[Skin]* 1760, 1761, 1786, *[Gene]* 1900

hesitating *[Mind]* **123**

hiccough *[Stom]* **748**, *[Ches]* **1194**, *[Drea]* **1686**, *[Gene]* **1870**

hiccup *[Stom]* **750**

hidebound *[Skin]* **1776**

hiding *[Mind]* **123**

hidradenitis *[Gene]* **1870**

high *[Vert]* **231**, *[Visi]* **453**, *[Drea]* **1686**, *[Gene]* **1870**

high fever *[Feve]* **1725**

high places *[Mind]* **123**

highly seasoned food *[Coug]* **1149**

high-spirited *[Mind]* **123**

hilarity *[Mind]* **123**

hill *[Gene]* **1870**

hindered *[Mind]* **123**

hip *[Abdo]* **893**, *[Extr]* **1634**

hip dysplasia *[Extr]* **1413**

hip joint *[Extr]* **1413**

hippocratic *[Face]* **575**

hippus *[Eye]* **401**

hirsutism *[Gene]* **1870**

hissing *[Resp]* **1128**, *[Coug]* **1149**

historic *[Drea]* **1686**

history *[Gene]* **1870**

hoarfrost *[Gene]* **1871**

hoarse *[Coug]* **1149**

hoarseness *[Lary]* **1096**

hodgkin's *[Gene]* **1871**

hold *[Mind]* **123**, *[Head]* **264**, *[Coug]* **1149**, *[Ches]* **1194**

holding *[Mind]* **123**, *[Abdo]* **821**, *[Lary]* **1096**, *[Resp]* **1128**, *[Extr]* **1413**, *[Chil]* **1708**, *[Gene]* **1871**

holds *[Ches]* **1194**

holes *[Drea]* **1686**

hollow *[Head]* **264**, *[Teet]* **665**, *[Thro]* **691**, *[Stom]* **750**, *[Abdo]* **821**, *[Coug]* **1149**, *[Ches]* **1194**, *[Gene]* **1872**

hollowness *[Ear]* **468**

Index of words

home *[Mind]* 18, 19, 25, 43, 47, 54, 61, 65, 102, 108, **123**, 123, 139, *[Rect]* 900, *[Drea]* **1686**, 1688, 1692

homeless *[Drea]* **1686**

homeopathy *[Mind]* **123**

homesickness *[Mind]* **123**, *[Drea]* **1686**

homophobia *[Mind]* **123**

homosexuality *[Mind]* **123**

honest *[Mind]* **123**

honor *[Mind]* **123**

hoop *[Extr]* **1413**

hopeful *[Mind]* **123**

hopeless *[Mind]* **124**

hordeolum *[Eye]* **401**

horny *[Extr]* **1413**

horrible *[Mind]* **124**, *[Stom]* **750**, *[Drea]* **1686**

horripilation *[Head]* **264**, *[Abdo]* **821**, *[Extr]* **1413**

horror *[Mind]* **124**

horror movies *[Mind]* **124**

horse *[Mind]* 65, 73, **134**, *[Vert]* 234, *[Head]* 299, *[Nose]* 529, *[Mout]* 629, *[Abdo]* 841, 864, *[Rect]* 913, *[Stoo]* 945, *[Blad]* 954, 970, *[Urin]* 1006, *[Fema]* 1056, *[Resp]* 1117, 1125, *[Ches]* 1214, 1243, *[Back]* 1289, *[Extr]* 1532, 1549, 1591, *[Slee]* 1657, *[Drea]* 1677, 1683, 1686, 1693, *[Gene]* 1881, 1933

horseback *[Gene]* **1872**

horses *[Mind]* 12, 47, 65, 107, *[Drea]* **1686**, 1691, *[Pers]* 1741

hot *[Head]* **264**, *[Stoo]* **943**, *[Urin]* **1005**, *[Resp]* **1128**, *[Expe]* **1172**, *[Pers]* **1740**, *[Skin]* **1776**

house *[Mind]* **124**, *[Vert]* **231**, *[Coug]* **1149**, *[Expe]* **1172**, *[Drea]* **1686**, *[Gene]* **1872**

household *[Mind]* 19, 87, 131, 164, *[Drea]* **1686**

housekeeping *[Mind]* **124**

housemaid's *[Extr]* **1413**

howling *[Mind]* **124**

hugging *[Mind]* **124**

humankind *[Mind]* **124**

humble *[Mind]* **124**

humid *[Coug]* **1149**

humiliated *[Mind]* **124**

humiliation *[Drea]* **1686**

humility *[Mind]* **124**

humming *[Ear]* **468**, *[Face]* **575**, *[Extr]* **1413**

humor *[Mind]* **124**

humorous *[Mind]* **124**

hung *[Drea]* **1686**

hunger *[Thro]* **691**, *[Stom]* **750**, *[Coug]* **1149**, *[Drea]* **1686**, *[Gene]* **1872**

hungry *[Vert]* **231**

hunting *[Mind]* **124**, *[Drea]* **1686**

hurried *[Mind]* **124**

hurry *[Mind]* **124**, *[Drea]* **1686**

hurt *[Mind]* **125**

hurting *[Mind]* **125**

husband *[Mind]* **125**

hydrocele *[Male]* **1022**

hydrocephalus *[Mind]* 97, 107, 192, 203, 214, *[Head]* **264**, *[Face]* **547**, *[Rect]* **908**, *[Urin]* **1005**, *[Gene]* **1825**

hydrometra *[Fema]* **1050**

hydronephrosis *[Kidn]* **974**

hydropericardium *[Ches]* **1194**

hydrophobia *[Mind]* **125**, *[Drea]* **1686**

hydrops *[Ear]* **468**

hydrosalpingitis *[Fema]* **1050**

hydrosalpinx *[Fema]* **1050**

hydrothorax *[Mind]* 65, *[Resp]* 1124, *[Ches]* 1184, **1194**, 1213, *[Extr]* **1599**

hygroma patellae *[Extr]* **1413**

hyperactive children *[Mind]* **125**

hyperchlorhydria *[Stom]* **751**, *[Resp]* 1116

hyperemia *[Eye]* 397, **401**, 404

hyperesthesia *[Head]* **264**, *[Eye]* **401**, *[Back]* **1278**, *[Extr]* **1413**, *[Skin]* **1776**

hyperlipidemia *[Gene]* **1872**

hypermetropia *[Visi]* **453**

hyperphoria *[Eye]* **401**

hypertension *[Mind]* 184, *[Head]* 272, *[Face]* 555, *[Kidn]* 973, **974**, 975, *[Urin]* 999, *[Ches]* 1186, 1195, *[Gene]* 1802, 1831, **1872**

hyperthyroidism *[Exte]* **716**, *[Gene]* **1872**

hypertrophy *[Eye]* **401**, *[Mout]* **625**, *[Ches]* **1194**, *[Extr]* **1413**, *[Gene]* **1872**

hyperventilation *[Resp]* **1128**, *[Ches]* **1195**

hypnotics *[Gene]* **1872**

hypochondria *[Abdo]* **893**

hypochondriasis *[Mind]* **125**

hypocrisy *[Mind]* **125**

hypogammaglobulinemia *[Gene]* **1872**

hypoglycemia *[Gene]* **1872**

hypopyon *[Eye]* **401**

hypotension *[Kidn]* 973, *[Ches]* 1192, *[Gene]* **1872**, 1928

hypothermia *[Gene]* **1872**

Index of words

hypothyreosis *[Gene]* **1872**
hypothyroidism *[Exte]* **716**, *[Gene]* **1872**
hypotony *[Gene]* **1872**
hysteria *[Mind]* **125**
hysterical *[Vert]* **231**, *[Resp]* **1128**, *[Coug]* **1149**

I

ice *[Skin]* **1776**
ice cream *[Coug]* **1149**
ice-water *[Feve]* **1725**
ichthyosis *[Skin]* **1776**
icy *[Coug]* **1149**
icy coldness *[Chil]* **1708**
ideal *[Mind]* **126**
idealistic *[Mind]* **126**
ideas *[Mind]* **126**
identity *[Mind]* 39, 40, 65, *[Drea]* 1679
idiocy *[Mind]* **127**
idiopathic *[Feve]* **1725**
idleness *[Mind]* **127**, *[Gene]* **1872**
ileocecal *[Abdo]* 811, 859, 888
ileus *[Stom]* 791, *[Abdo]* **821**, 821
iliac region *[Abdo]* **894**
ill *[Mind]* **127**
ill feeling *[Gene]* **1872**
ill humor *[Mind]* **127**
illnesses *[Gene]* **1872**
ill-treatment *[Drea]* **1686**
illuminations *[Drea]* **1686**
illusions *[Visi]* **453**, *[Hear]* **501**
images *[Visi]* **453**
imaginary *[Mind]* **127**
imaginations *[Mind]* **127**
imbecility *[Mind]* **127**
imitation *[Mind]* **127**
immaturity *[Gene]* **1872**
immobile *[Abdo]* **821**, *[Back]* **1278**
immobility *[Eye]* **401**
immovable *[Ches]* **1195**
impacted *[Rect]* **919**
impaction *[Abdo]* **821**
impaired *[Visi]* **453**, *[Hear]* **501**
impatience *[Mind]* **127**
impeded *[Resp]* **1128**
imperceptible *[Resp]* **1129**
imperious *[Mind]* **128**
impertinence *[Mind]* **128**

impetigo *[Head]* 252, *[Face]* 563, 564, *[Back]* 1274, *[Extr]* 1385, 1387, *[Skin]* **1761**
impetuous *[Mind]* **128**
impolite *[Mind]* **128**
important *[Mind]* **128**
importunate *[Mind]* **128**
impossible *[Expe]* **1172**
impotence *[Male]* **1022**
impressionable *[Mind]* **128**
impressions *[Skin]* **1776**, *[Gene]* **1872**
impressive *[Drea]* **1686**
imprinted *[Mout]* **625**
imprisonment *[Drea]* **1686**
improvident *[Mind]* **128**
imprudence *[Mind]* **128**
impudent *[Mind]* **128**
impulse *[Mind]* **128**, *[Ches]* **1195**
impulsive *[Mind]* **129**
inability *[Coug]* **1149**
inactivity *[Mind]* **129**, *[Stom]* **751**, *[Abdo]* **821**, *[Rect]* **919**, *[Blad]* **952**, *[Skin]* **1776**
inadvertence *[Mind]* **129**
inattentive *[Mind]* **129**
incense *[Mind]* **129**
incessant *[Coug]* **1149**
incest *[Mind]* **129**
incisors *[Teet]* **681**
inciting *[Mind]* **129**
inclination *[Male]* **1022**
inconsolable *[Mind]* **129**
inconstancy *[Mind]* **129**
incontinence *[Blad]* **952**
incoordination *[Extr]* **1413**
increasing and decreasing suddenly *[Pers]* **1740**
incrustations *[Teet]* **665**
indecent behavior *[Drea]* **1686**
indecision *[Mind]* **129**
indented *[Mout]* 618, 622, **625**, 625, 647, *[Extr]* **1413**, *[Skin]* 1761, **1776**, 1790, *[Gene]* 1807
independent *[Mind]* **129**
indians *[Drea]* **1686**
indican *[Urin]* **1005**
indifference *[Mind]* **129**
indigestion *[Stom]* **751**
indignation *[Mind]* **132**
indiscretion *[Mind]* **132**
indolence *[Mind]* **132**, *[Gene]* **1872**

Index of words

induration *[Eye]* **401**, *[Ear]* **468**, *[Mout]* **625**, *[Thro]* **691**, *[Exte]* **716**, *[Stom]* **752**, *[Abdo]* **821**, *[Rect]* **919**, *[Blad]* **952**, *[Pros]* **981**, *[Uret]* **988**, *[Male]* **1022**, *[Fema]* **1050**, *[Ches]* **1195**, *[Extr]* **1413**

indurations *[Face]* **575**, *[Skin]* **1776**, *[Gene]* **1873**

industrious *[Mind]* **132**, *[Drea]* **1686**

ineffectual *[Rect]* **919**

inelasticity *[Skin]* **1776**

inertia *[Fema]* **1050**

inexorable *[Mind]* **132**

infantile *[Mind]* **132**, *[Abdo]* **821**

infantilism *[Fema]* **1050**

infants *[Mind]* 129, 138, *[Head]* 257, 370, *[Eye]* **401**, 401, *[Ear]* 484, *[Nose]* 509, 522, 528, 541, *[Face]* 563, *[Mout]* 605, 631, *[Thro]* 700, *[Stom]* 794, *[Abdo]* 803, 813, 822, 823, 892, *[Rect]* 899, 900, 906, 912, 913, 916, 933, *[Stoo]* 939, *[Blad]* 958, 959, 969, *[Kidn]* 980, *[Urin]* 1000, 1006, *[Resp]* 1116, *[Coug]* 1166, *[Ches]* 1196, 1197, 1198, 1230, *[Extr]* 1384, 1394, 1603, *[Slee]* 1649, 1662, *[Drea]* 1680, *[Skin]* 1759, 1766, 1776, *[Gene]* 1821, 1824, 1829, 1837, 1844, 1852, 1876, 1882, 1919, 1920, 1936, 1949

infarction *[Ches]* **1195**

infectious *[Gene]* **1873**

inferiority *[Mind]* **132**

infertility *[Male]* **1023**, *[Fema]* **1050**

infiltration *[Eye]* **401**, *[Extr]* **1413**, *[Gene]* **1873**

infirmity *[Gene]* **1873**

inflammation *[Head]* **264**, *[Eye]* **401**, *[Ear]* **468**, *[Nose]* **525**, *[Face]* **576**, *[Teet]* **665**, *[Thro]* **692**, *[Exte]* **716**, *[Stom]* **753**, *[Abdo]* **821**, *[Rect]* **919**, *[Blad]* **952**, *[Kidn]* **974**, *[Pros]* **981**, *[Uret]* **988**, *[Male]* **1023**, *[Fema]* **1050**, *[Lary]* **1096**, *[Resp]* **1129**, *[Ches]* **1195**, *[Back]* **1278**, *[Extr]* **1413**, *[Skin]* **1776**, *[Gene]* **1873**

inflammatory *[Feve]* **1725**

inflexible *[Mind]* **132**

influenza *[Mind]* 39, 122, 131, 169, 218, *[Head]* 244, 265, 289, 338, *[Eye]* 403, 417, *[Ear]* 461, *[Hear]* 504, *[Nose]* 512, *[Face]* 556, 570, *[Mout]* 605, 609, 612, 616, *[Thro]* 692, *[Stom]* 753, 782, 794, 796, *[Abdo]* 818, 894, *[Rect]* 908, *[Kidn]* 974, *[Fema]* 1043, *[Lary]* 1096, *[Coug]* **1149**, *[Ches]* 1196, 1197, 1198, 1199, 1235, 1251, 1253, 1264, 1266, *[Back]* 1272, *[Extr]* 1411, 1441, 1529, *[Slee]* 1656, 1663, *[Chil]* 1702, 1705, *[Pers]* 1742, *[Gene]*

1819, 1871, **1876**, 1887, 1900, 1907, 1916, 1917, 1932, 1968, 1970

infrequent *[Expe]* **1172**

ingrowing eyelashes *[Eye]* **404**

ingrowing nails *[Extr]* **1415**

inguinal *[Abdo]* **894**

inhaling *[Coug]* **1150**

inheritance *[Gene]* **1876**

inhibition *[Mind]* **132**

inhumanity *[Mind]* **132**

initiative *[Mind]* **132**

injected *[Eye]* **404**

injuries *[Mind]* 5, 47, 91, **132**, 133, 153, 156, 169, 180, 184, 193, 214, *[Vert]* **231**, *[Head]* 264, **265**, 265, 289, 312, 346, *[Eye]* 390, 395, 399, 401, 402, 403, **405**, 428, 430, 433, *[Visi]* 450, 455, 457, *[Hear]* 503, *[Nose]* 522, 538, *[Face]* **576**, 577, 594, *[Mout]* **626**, *[Thro]* 693, *[Stom]* **753**, *[Rect]* 900, 908, 916, *[Blad]* 953, 959, 965, *[Kidn]* **975**, *[Male]* **1023**, 1040, *[Fema]* 1043, 1047, 1050, **1051**, 1067, 1069, *[Lary]* **1097**, *[Coug]* **1150**, *[Ches]* 1180, 1194, **1199**, 1199, 1258, *[Back]* **1279**, 1279, 1287, 1301, 1320, *[Extr]* 1357, 1400, **1415**, 1430, 1441, 1529, 1581, 1584, 1585, 1636, *[Slee]* 1656, 1663, 1673, *[Drea]* **1686**, *[Pers]* 1739, *[Skin]* 1751, 1773, 1775, **1776**, *[Gene]* 1815, 1819, 1822, 1824, 1825, 1829, 1834, 1839, 1870, 1873, 1874, 1875, **1876**, 1893, 1900, 1908, 1917, 1919, 1937, 1968

injuring *[Mind]* **132**

injury *[Mind]* 12, 35, 39, 59, 66, 85, 108, 126, 148, 202, 203, 208, 215, *[Eye]* 393, *[Ear]* **469**, *[Hear]* 503, 504, *[Teet]* **665**, 673, *[Abdo]* 822, **823**, 823, *[Blad]* **953**, *[Resp]* 1117, **1129**, *[Ches]* 1257, 1262, *[Back]* 1279, *[Extr]* 1358, 1361, 1437, *[Skin]* 1787, *[Gene]* 1830, 1841, 1871

injustice *[Mind]* **132**

innocent *[Mind]* **132**

innovative *[Mind]* **132**

inquisitive *[Mind]* **132**

insane *[Drea]* **1686**

insanity *[Mind]* **132**, *[Coug]* **1150**

insects *[Drea]* **1686**

insecure *[Extr]* **1416**

insecurity *[Mind]* **135**, *[Rect]* **919**

insensibility *[Mind]* **135**, *[Eye]* **405**, *[Stom]* **753**, *[Abdo]* **823**, *[Rect]* **919**, *[Blad]* **953**, *[Fema]* **1051**, *[Lary]* **1097**, *[Ches]* **1199**, *[Back]* **1279**, *[Extr]* **1416**, *[Gene]* **1877**

Index of words

insensible *[Mout]* **626**
insidious *[Feve]* **1725**
insignificant *[Mind]* **135**
insolence *[Mind]* **135**
inspiration *[Vert]* **231**, *[Coug]* **1150**, *[Gene]* **1877**
instability *[Mind]* **135**
instability of body *[Gene]* **1878**
insufficiency; renal *[Kidn]* **975**
insufficient *[Stoo]* **943**, *[Slee]* **1647**
insulin secretion *[Gene]* **1878**
insulting *[Mind]* **135**
insults *[Drea]* **1687**
insurrections *[Drea]* **1687**
intellect *[Mind]* **135**
intellectual *[Mind]* **135**, *[Drea]* **1687**
intelligent *[Mind]* **135**
intemperance *[Mind]* **135**
intense *[Mind]* **135**, *[Feve]* **1726**
intercostal *[Ches]* **1199**
interference *[Mind]* **135**
intermittent *[Resp]* **1129**, *[Feve]* **1726**, *[Pers]* **1740**
intermitting *[Coug]* **1150**
internal *[Chil]* **1708**, *[Feve]* **1726**
internal parts *[Gene]* **1980**
interrupted *[Resp]* **1130**, *[Coug]* **1150**, *[Slee]* **1647**
interruption *[Mind]* **10**, **39**, **127**, **135**, 135, **162**, **207**
intertrigo *[Abdo]* **823**, *[Extr]* **1416**, *[Skin]* **1776**
intestines *[Stoo]* **943**
intimidating *[Drea]* **1687**
intolerance *[Mind]* **135**
intoxicated *[Eye]* **405**
intoxicated; as if *[Vert]* **231**
intoxication *[Mind]* **135**, *[Head]* **265**, *[Gene]* **1878**
intriguer *[Mind]* **135**
intrigues *[Drea]* **1687**
introspection *[Mind]* **135**
introverted *[Mind]* **135**
intruders *[Drea]* **1687**
intuitive *[Mind]* **135**
intussusception *[Mout]* **616**, *[Stom]* **750**, **798**, *[Abdo]* **823**
invaders *[Drea]* **1687**
invention *[Drea]* **1687**
inversion *[Eye]* **405**, *[Ches]* **1199**, *[Extr]* **1416**
inverted *[Visi]* **453**, *[Face]* **576**, *[Slee]* **1647**
involuntarily *[Face]* **576**
involuntary *[Rect]* **919**, *[Blad]* **953**, *[Urin]* **1005**, *[Fema]* **1051**

involvement *[Mind]* **135**
iodine *[Urin]* **1005**, *[Gene]* **1878**
irascibility *[Mind]* **135**
iris *[Eye]* **440**
iritis *[Eye]* **405**
irksome *[Mind]* **135**
iron *[Gene]* **1878**
ironing *[Head]* **265**
irony *[Mind]* **135**
irrational *[Mind]* **135**
irregular *[Teet]* **665**, *[Resp]* **1130**, *[Chil]* **1709**, *[Feve]* **1727**
irreligious *[Mind]* **136**
irrepressible *[Coug]* **1150**
irresistible *[Coug]* **1150**
irresolution *[Mind]* **136**
irritability *[Mind]* **136**, *[Gene]* **1878**
irritable *[Coug]* **1150**
irritable bladder *[Blad]* **953**
irritable bowel syndrome *[Abdo]* **823**
irritable heart *[Ches]* **1199**, *[Gene]* **1878**
irritating *[Urin]* **1005**, *[Coug]* **1150**
irritation *[Head]* **265**, *[Eye]* **405**, *[Nose]* **525**, *[Face]* **576**, *[Thro]* **693**, *[Stom]* **753**, *[Abdo]* **823**, *[Rect]* **920**, *[Kidn]* **975**, *[Pros]* **982**, *[Uret]* **988**, *[Male]* **1024**, *[Fema]* **1051**, *[Lary]* **1097**, *[Coug]* **1150**, *[Ches]* **1199**, *[Back]* **1279**, *[Extr]* **1416**, *[Skin]* **1776**
irritative *[Feve]* **1727**
ischias *[Extr]* **1416**
isolation *[Mind]* **140**
itch *[Coug]* **1151**
itching *[Head]* **265**, *[Eye]* **405**, *[Ear]* **469**, *[Nose]* **525**, *[Face]* **576**, *[Mout]* **626**, *[Teet]* **665**, *[Thro]* **694**, *[Exte]* **717**, *[Stom]* **753**, *[Abdo]* **823**, *[Rect]* **920**, *[Blad]* **953**, *[Uret]* **988**, *[Male]* **1024**, *[Fema]* **1051**, *[Lary]* **1097**, *[Coug]* **1151**, *[Ches]* **1199**, *[Back]* **1279**, *[Extr]* **1416**, *[Skin]* **1776**, *[Gene]* **1878**

J

jar *[Head]* **266**, *[Blad]* **953**, *[Back]* **1280**, *[Gene]* **1878**
jarring *[Abdo]* **824**
jars *[Head]* **266**
jaundice *[Mind]* **10**, **214**, *[Head]* **290**, *[Face]* **577**, *[Mout]* **616**, **628**, *[Stom]* **760**, **791**, *[Abdo]* **804**, **824**, *[Rect]* **908**, *[Ches]* **1266**, *[Extr]* **1419**, *[Skin]* **1753**, **1778**, **1780**, *[Gene]* **1834**, **1968**
jaws *[Drea]* **1687**

Index of words

jealousy *[Mind]* **140**

jellylike *[Stoo]* **943**, *[Expe]* **1172**

jerk *[Eye]* **406**, *[Lary]* **1098**

jerking *[Head]* 266, *[Eye]* **406**, *[Nose]* **526**, *[Face]* **577**, *[Thro]* **694**, *[Stom]* **753**, *[Abdo]* **824**, *[Pros]* **982**, *[Uret]* **989**, *[Male]* **1025**, *[Fema]* **1052**, *[Resp]* **1130**, *[Coug]* **1151**, *[Back]* **1280**, *[Extr]* **1423**, *[Gene]* **1879**

jerks *[Teet]* **665**, *[Exte]* **717**, *[Ches]* **1199**

jesting *[Mind]* **141**

jet airplane *[Drea]* **1687**

jet lag *[Gene]* **1879**

job *[Drea]* **1687**

joints *[Gene]* **1980**

joke *[Drea]* **1687**

joking *[Mind]* **141**

journeys *[Mind]* **141**, *[Drea]* **1687**

jovial *[Mind]* **141**

joy *[Mind]* 5, 16, 44, 67, 93, 97, 131, 137, **141**, 141, 145, 221, *[Head]* 290, *[Face]* **582**, *[Teet]* **672**, *[Rect]* 908, *[Fema]* 1051, *[Ches]* 1253, *[Slee]* 1664, *[Gene]* 1808, 1953, 1956

joyless *[Mind]* **141**

joyous *[Mind]* **141**, *[Drea]* **1687**

jump *[Visi]* **453**

jumping *[Mind]* **141**, *[Stom]* **753**, *[Coug]* **1151**, *[Ches]* **1200**, *[Extr]* **1425**, *[Drea]* **1687**, *[Gene]* **1879**

jumping up *[Mind]* **142**

jumpy *[Mind]* **142**

justice *[Mind]* **142**

K

keep *[Eye]* **406**

keloid *[Skin]* 1748, 1778, **1780**, *[Gene]* 1955

keratitis *[Eye]* **406**

keratoconus *[Eye]* **406**

keratoses *[Skin]* **1780**

kicking *[Mind]* **142**

kill *[Mind]* **142**

killed *[Mind]* **142**, *[Drea]* **1687**

killing *[Drea]* **1687**

kimmelstiel-wilson *[Gene]* **1879**

kindness *[Mind]* **142**

kissing *[Mind]* **142**

kleptomania *[Mind]* **142**

kneading *[Vert]* **231**, *[Abdo]* **824**

knee *[Drea]* **1687**

kneeling *[Mind]* 134, **142**, 168, 214, *[Vert]* 231, 235, *[Head]* **267**, *[Face]* 582, *[Stom]* 760, *[Rect]* 918, 925, 933, *[Resp]* 1124, **1130**, *[Coug]* **1151**, *[Ches]* 1253, *[Back]* 1287, 1320, 1329, *[Extr]* 1426, 1435, 1503, 1504, 1509, 1523, 1529, 1596, 1605, 1606, 1610, 1614, 1628, 1629, 1630, *[Slee]* 1649, *[Gene]* 1841, **1879**

knees *[Extr]* **1634**, *[Gene]* **1879**

knell *[Drea]* **1687**

knife *[Mind]* **142**

knitting *[Extr]* **1425**

knives *[Drea]* **1687**

knobby *[Nose]* **526**, *[Extr]* **1425**

knock knee *[Extr]* **1425**

knocked *[Extr]* **1425**

knocking *[Head]* **267**

knots *[Expe]* **1172**

knotted *[Abdo]* **824**, *[Fema]* **1052**, *[Gene]* **1879**

knotty *[Stoo]* **943**, *[Uret]* **989**

korsakoff *[Mind]* **142**

kraurosis vulvae *[Fema]* **1052**

L

labor *[Fema]* **1052**, *[Coug]* **1151**

labor pains *[Fema]* **1052**

laboratory *[Gene]* **1879**

labored *[Resp]* **1130**

laborious *[Drea]* **1687**

labyrinth *[Ear]* **498**

lacerated t *[Mout]* **626**

laceration *[Nose]* **526**

lachrymal glands *[Eye]* **440**

lachrymation *[Eye]* **406**

lack *[Gene]* **1880**

laconic *[Mind]* **142**

lactatio falsa *[Gene]* **1880**

lactation *[Fema]* **1052**, *[Coug]* **1151**, *[Ches]* **1200**, *[Gene]* **1880**

laid *[Mind]* **142**

lame *[Mout]* **626**, *[Gene]* **1880**

lameness *[Kidn]* **975**, *[Back]* **1280**, *[Extr]* **1425**

lamenting *[Mind]* **143**, *[Coug]* **1151**

languages *[Mind]* **143**

languor *[Extr]* **1427**

laparotomy *[Blad]* 951, 958

174

Index of words

large *[Eye]* **408**, *[Visi]* **453**, *[Face]* **577**, *[Mout]* **626**, *[Teet]* **665**, *[Stoo]* **943**, *[Ches]* **1200**, *[Extr]* **1427**
large field *[Visi]* **453**
large size *[Head]* **267**
larger *[Face]* **577**
laryngismus *[Lary]* **1098**
laryngitis *[Lary]* **1098**
larynx *[Lary]* **1110**, *[Drea]* **1687**
lascivious *[Mind]* **143**, *[Drea]* **1687**
lassitude *[Extr]* **1427**, *[Gene]* **1880**
late *[Mind]* **143**
later *[Stoo]* **943**
latin; speaking *[Drea]* **1687**
laughed at *[Drea]* **1687**
laughing *[Mind]* **3**, **5**, **8**, **23**, **30**, 39, 44, 47, 88, 133, 135, 137, **143**, 143, 144, 145, 148, 150, 151, 159, 161, 162, 171, 172, 182, 184, 190, 191, 192, 194, 205, 216, 219, 220, 221, 222, *[Head]* 247, 248, 258, **267**, 290, 319, 334, 338, 344, 373, *[Eye]* 407, *[Ear]* **470**, 470, 485, *[Face]* 550, 559, **577**, 582, 588, *[Thro]* 694, *[Stom]* 750, 772, 783, *[Abdo]* **824**, 837, 851, 863, 867, 872, 879, *[Rect]* 920, **921**, *[Blad]* 965, *[Kidn]* 976, *[Fema]* 1068, *[Lary]* 1099, 1108, *[Resp]* 1117, 1124, **1130**, *[Coug]* **1151**, 1164, *[Ches]* **1200**, 1203, 1212, 1236, 1242, 1247, 1253, *[Back]* **1280**, 1287, 1320, 1331, *[Extr]* **1427**, 1491, 1529, 1570, 1589, 1627, 1631, *[Slee]* 1646, 1656, 1662, 1665, *[Drea]* **1687**, *[Skin]* 1788, *[Gene]* 1821, 1825, **1881**, 1881
lawsuits *[Drea]* **1687**
laxatives *[Gene]* **1881**
laziness *[Mind]* **145**
lead *[Abdo]* **824**, *[Gene]* **1881**
leaf *[Thro]* **694**, *[Lary]* **1098**, *[Gene]* **1881**
lean *[Head]* **267**, *[Gene]* **1881**
leaning *[Vert]* **231**, *[Head]* **267**, *[Back]* **1280**, *[Gene]* **1882**
learning *[Mind]* **147**
leather *[Mout]* **626**
lecherous *[Mind]* **147**
lecture *[Drea]* **1687**
leeches *[Skin]* **1780**, *[Gene]* **1882**
left *[Chil]* **1699**, *[Pers]* **1735**
leg *[Drea]* **1687**
legs *[Extr]* **1634**
leishmaniasis *[Gene]* **1882**
lemon-colored *[Expe]* **1173**
lens *[Eye]* **408**

leper *[Drea]* **1687**
lepra *[Gene]* **1882**
lethargy *[Mind]* **147**, *[Drea]* **1687**
letters *[Visi]* **453**
letting go *[Mind]* **147**
leukemia *[Gene]* **1882**
leukocytosis *[Gene]* **1882**
leukoplakia *[Mout]* **626**
leukorrhea *[Abdo]* **824**, *[Fema]* **1052**, *[Back]* **1280**, *[Gene]* **1882**
levitation *[Mind]* **147**
lewdness *[Mind]* **147**
liar *[Mind]* **147**
libertinism *[Mind]* **147**
lice *[Head]* 266, **267**, *[Drea]* **1687**, *[Skin]* **1774**
licking *[Mind]* **147**, *[Face]* **577**, *[Gene]* **1882**
licks *[Mout]* **626**
lids *[Eye]* **440**
lie *[Mind]* **147**
lie down *[Coug]* **1151**, *[Gene]* **1882**
lienteric *[Stoo]* **943**
life *[Mind]* **147**
lifeless *[Mind]* **147**
lifting *[Vert]* **231**, *[Head]* **267**, *[Thro]* **694**, *[Stom]* **753**, *[Abdo]* **824**, *[Kidn]* **975**, *[Coug]* **1151**, *[Ches]* **1200**, *[Back]* **1280**, *[Extr]* **1427**, *[Gene]* **1882**
light *[Mind]* **147**, *[Vert]* **231**, *[Eye]* **408**, *[Visi]* **453**, *[Coug]* **1151**, *[Slee]* **1647**, *[Gene]* **1882**
light colored *[Stoo]* **943**
light on *[Slee]* **1648**
light-headed *[Vert]* **231**
lightness *[Head]* **267**, *[Extr]* **1427**, *[Gene]* **1883**
lightning *[Vert]* **231**, *[Visi]* **453**, *[Drea]* **1687**, *[Gene]* **1883**
lightning-like *[Ear]* **470**
limbs *[Drea]* **1687**
limpid *[Urin]* **1005**
limping *[Extr]* **1427**
line *[Eye]* **408**, *[Visi]* **454**
linea *[Face]* **577**
lions *[Drea]* **1687**
lipoma *[Nose]* **526**, *[Extr]* **1427**, *[Gene]* **1955**
liquid *[Head]* **267**, *[Stoo]* **944**
liquids *[Nose]* **526**, *[Thro]* **694**, *[Lary]* **1098**, *[Coug]* **1151**, *[Expe]* **1173**
listened to *[Mind]* **147**
listless *[Mind]* **147**
literary work *[Mind]* **147**

Index of words

litigious *[Mind]* **147**
lively *[Mind]* **147**
liver *[Vert]* **231**, *[Abdo]* **894**
liver-colored *[Expe]* **1173**
livid *[Mout]* **626**, *[Gene]* **1883**
living *[Stom]* **753**, *[Ches]* **1200**
loathing *[Mind]* **147**, *[Stom]* **753**
lobes *[Ear]* **498**
locality *[Mind]* **148**
location *[Mind]* **148**, *[Teet]* **665**
lochia *[Fema]* **1058**
lockjaw *[Face]* **577**, *[Gene]* **1824**
locomotor ataxia *[Extr]* **1427**, *[Gene]* **1883**
logical thinking *[Mind]* **148**
lolling *[Mout]* **626**
loneliness *[Mind]* **148**
long *[Eye]* **408**, *[Nose]* **526**, *[Face]* **577**, *[Mout]* **626**, *[Teet]* **665**, *[Stoo]* **944**, *[Resp]* **1130**, *[Slee]* **1648**, *[Drea]* **1687**, *[Feve]* **1727**
long lasting *[Chil]* **1709**
longer *[Extr]* **1427**, *[Gene]* **1883**
longing *[Mind]* **148**
long-lasting *[Pers]* **1740**
looked at *[Mind]* **148**
looking *[Mind]* **148**, *[Vert]* **231**, *[Head]* **267**, *[Eye]* **408**, *[Visi]* **454**, *[Back]* **1280**, *[Drea]* **1687**, *[Gene]* **1883**
loose *[Eye]* **408**, *[Abdo]* **824**, *[Stoo]* **944**, *[Coug]* **1151**, *[Ches]* **1200**, *[Back]* **1280**, *[Extr]* **1427**, *[Skin]* **1780**
looseness *[Head]* **267**, *[Teet]* **665**, *[Extr]* **1427**
looting *[Drea]* **1687**
loquacity *[Mind]* **148**
losing *[Mind]* **149**
losing one's temper *[Mind]* **149**
loss *[Vert]* **231**, *[Extr]* **1427**, *[Drea]* **1687**, *[Gene]* **1884**
loss of vision *[Visi]* **454**
loss of voice *[Lary]* **1098**
lost *[Hear]* **504**, *[Drea]* **1687**
lottery *[Drea]* **1688**
loud *[Resp]* **1130**
lousiness *[Skin]* **1780**
love *[Mind]* **5, 10, 12, 28, 35, 47, 84, 85, 117, 121, 124, 126, 133, 140, 149, 149, 168, 184, 196, 203,** *[Fema]* **1067, 1088,** *[Ches]* **1224,** *[Gene]* **1808, 1825, 1969**
low fever *[Feve]* **1727**

lower limbs *[Extr]* **1635**, *[Pers]* **1740**
low-fever states *[Gene]* **1884**
low-minded *[Mind]* **149**
low-spirited *[Mind]* **149**
loyal *[Mind]* **149**
lucid *[Drea]* **1688**
lucidity *[Mind]* **149**
ludicrous *[Mind]* **149**, *[Drea]* **1688**
lumbago *[Back]* **1280**
lumbar region *[Back]* **1349**
luminous *[Visi]* **456**, *[Pers]* **1740**
lump *[Head]* **267**, *[Eye]* **408**, *[Nose]* **526**, *[Thro]* **694**, *[Stom]* **754**, *[Abdo]* **824**, *[Rect]* **921**, *[Pros]* **982**, *[Lary]* **1098**, *[Coug]* **1152**
lumps *[Ear]* **470**, *[Face]* **577**, *[Mout]* **626**, *[Exte]* **717**, *[Abdo]* **824**, *[Stoo]* **944**, *[Ches]* **1200**, *[Back]* **1280**, *[Extr]* **1427**
lumpy *[Stoo]* **944**, *[Expe]* **1173**
lungs *[Ches]* **1200**
lupus *[Head]* **267**, *[Eye]* **408**, *[Ear]* **467, 470**, *[Nose]* **526**, *[Face]* **545, 577**, *[Extr]* **1427**, *[Skin]* **1780**, *[Gene]* **1807, 1955**
lusterless *[Eye]* **408**, *[Skin]* **1780**
lustful *[Mind]* **149**
luxury *[Mind]* **149**
lying *[Vert]* **231**, *[Head]* **267**, *[Ear]* **470**, *[Nose]* **526**, *[Teet]* **665**, *[Thro]* **695**, *[Stom]* **754**, *[Abdo]* **824**, *[Blad]* **953**, *[Kidn]* **975**, *[Fema]* **1058**, *[Resp]* **1130**, *[Coug]* **1152**, *[Expe]* **1173**, *[Ches]* **1200**, *[Back]* **1281**, *[Extr]* **1427**, *[Drea]* **1688**, *[Chil]* **1709**, *[Pers]* **1740**, *[Gene]* **1884**
lying down *[Vert]* **232**, *[Kidn]* **975**, *[Coug]* **1153**, *[Ches]* **1200**, *[Chil]* **1709**
lying-in *[Fema]* **1059**
lyme disease *[Gene]* **1886**
lymphangitis *[Gene]* **1886**
lymphatic *[Gene]* **1886**
lymphatic glands *[Gene]* **1886**
lymphoma *[Gene]* **1886**
lypothymia *[Mind]* **150**

M

macular degeneration *[Eye]* **408**
madness *[Mind]* **150**
magic *[Drea]* **1688**
magnesia *[Gene]* **1886**
magnetic *[Mind]* **150**

Index of words

magnetism *[Gene]* **1886**
magnetized *[Mind]* **150**
maidens *[Teet]* **665**
making fun *[Mind]* **150**
malaise *[Gene]* **1886**
malaria *[Feve]* **1727**, *[Gene]* **1886**
malformation *[Face]* **577**, *[Abdo]* **824**, *[Gene]* **1886**
malicious *[Mind]* **150**
malignant *[Gene]* **1886**
malingering *[Mind]* **150**
malnutrition *[Gene]* **1886**
mammae *[Ches]* **1267**
man *[Drea]* **1688**
mania *[Mind]* **150**
mania a potu *[Mind]* **151**
manic-depressive *[Mind]* **151**
manipulative *[Mind]* **151**
mankind *[Mind]* **151**
mannerly *[Mind]* **151**
mannish *[Mind]* **151**
manual *[Gene]* **1886**
manual labor *[Coug]* **1153**, *[Back]* **1281**
manual work *[Mind]* **151**
many *[Drea]* **1688**
many symptoms *[Gene]* **1886**
mapped *[Mout]* **626**, *[Gene]* **1886**
marasmus *[Gene]* **1886**
marble *[Head]* **268**
marbled *[Face]* **577**, *[Skin]* **1780**
margin of hair *[Face]* **603**
marriage *[Mind]* 3, 23, 68, 108, **151**, 151, 184, 208
marriages *[Drea]* **1688**
masks *[Drea]* **1688**
masochism *[Mind]* **152**
masses *[Expe]* **1173**
mastitis *[Ches]* **1200**
mastoid *[Ear]* **498**
masturbation *[Pros]* **982**, *[Male]* **1025**, *[Fema]* **1059**, *[Gene]* **1886**
materialistic *[Mind]* **152**
maternal instinct; exaggerated *[Mind]* **152**
mathematics *[Mind]* **152**
mature *[Mind]* **152**
maturity *[Fema]* **1059**
meadow *[Drea]* **1688**
mealy *[Stoo]* **944**, *[Ches]* **1200**
measles *[Mind]* 105, 188, *[Head]* 244, 264, 292, 385, *[Eye]* 397, 402, 407, 430, 431, 433, 438,

[Visi] 449, 450, *[Ear]* 464, **470**, *[Hear]* 503, 504, *[Nose]* 506, 508, 522, *[Mout]* 612, 624, 642, 643, *[Thro]* 686, *[Stom]* 794, *[Rect]* 908, *[Fema]* 1049, *[Lary]* 1093, 1108, *[Resp]* 1117, 1124, *[Coug]* 1145, **1153**, *[Ches]* 1183, 1198, 1266, 1267, *[Back]* 1279, *[Extr]* 1385, 1390, 1397, 1437, *[Slee]* 1664, 1666, *[Feve]* 1724, *[Skin]* 1760, 1762, 1763, *[Gene]* 1808, 1819, 1825, 1871, 1874, **1887**, 1903
measly *[Back]* **1274**
meat *[Coug]* **1153**, *[Drea]* **1688**
meatus *[Ear]* **498**
meddlesome *[Mind]* **152**
medicine *[Mind]* **152**, *[Gene]* **1887**
meditating *[Mind]* **152**
meditation *[Mind]* **152**
meeting of souls *[Mind]* **152**
megacolon *[Abdo]* **825**
megalomania *[Mind]* 134, **152**
melancholy *[Mind]* **152**
melanoma *[Gene]* **1807**
melanosis *[Eye]* **408**, *[Skin]* **1780**
melt *[Eye]* **408**
membrane *[Eye]* **408**, *[Nose]* **526**, *[Face]* **577**, *[Mout]* **626**, *[Thro]* **695**, *[Lary]* **1098**
membranes *[Gene]* **1887**
membranous *[Stoo]* **944**, *[Expe]* **1173**
memory *[Mind]* **152**, *[Drea]* **1688**
men *[Mind]* **154**, *[Drea]* **1688**
menarche *[Mind]* **185**, *[Fema]* **1059**
mendacity *[Mind]* **154**
ménière's *[Ear]* **470**
ménière's disease *[Vert]* **232**
meningitis *[Head]* **268**
menopause *[Mind]* 19, 95, 97, 103, 108, 110, 111, 116, 126, 134, 139, 145, 149, 151, **154**, 162, 164, 178, 184, 188, 193, 204, 221, *[Vert]* **232**, *[Head]* 258, 260, 292, 367, 386, *[Eye]* 438, *[Ear]* 475, 486, *[Nose]* 523, 538, *[Face]* 556, 570, 574, *[Mout]* 643, *[Thro]* 694, *[Stom]* 727, 735, 760, 784, 794, 799, *[Abdo]* 838, 895, *[Rect]* 908, 912, 916, 918, *[Blad]* 969, *[Uret]* 991, *[Urin]* 1006, *[Fema]* 1045, 1055, **1059**, 1061, 1062, 1064, 1065, 1069, 1081, 1088, *[Coug]* **1153**, *[Ches]* 1183, 1194, 1195, 1212, 1213, 1230, 1234, 1254, 1261, *[Extr]* 1406, 1407, 1457, 1465, 1469, 1484, 1487, 1498, 1571, 1621, *[Slee]* 1664, *[Pers]* 1736, 1738, **1740**, 1742, *[Skin]* 1770, 1778, 1789, *[Gene]* 1810, 1817, 1819, 1826, 1830, 1834, 1841, 1866, 1867, 1870, 1872,

Index of words

1887, 1893, 1894, 1901, 1936, 1953, 1954, 1969, 1974

menorrhagia *[Fema]* **1059**

menses *[Mind]* **154**, *[Vert]* **232**, *[Head]* **268**, *[Eye]* **408**, *[Visi]* **456**, *[Teet]* **665**, *[Thro]* **695**, *[Stom]* **754**, *[Abdo]* **825**, *[Blad]* **953**, *[Fema]* **1059**, *[Coug]* **1153**, *[Ches]* **1200**, *[Back]* **1281**, *[Extr]* **1428**, *[Drea]* **1688**, *[Chil]* **1709**, *[Feve]* **1727**, *[Pers]* **1740**, *[Skin]* **1780**, *[Gene]* **1887**

mentagra *[Gene]* **1888**

mental *[Mind]* **224**

mental deterioration *[Mind]* **155**

mental exertion *[Mind]* **155**, *[Vert]* **232**, *[Head]* **268**, *[Coug]* **1153**, *[Back]* **1281**, *[Drea]* **1688**, *[Chil]* **1709**, *[Feve]* **1727**, *[Pers]* **1740**, *[Gene]* **1888**

mental overstimulation *[Mind]* **156**

mental power *[Mind]* **156**

mental shock *[Pers]* **1740**

mental symptoms *[Mind]* **156**

mental work *[Mind]* **156**

mentally *[Mind]* **156**

menthol *[Gene]* **1888**

mercurial *[Mout]* **626**

mercury *[Mout]* **626**, *[Gene]* **1888**

merging of self *[Mind]* **156**

merry *[Mind]* **156**, *[Drea]* **1688**

mesmerized *[Mind]* **156**

metallic *[Coug]* **1153**

metastasis *[Thro]* **695**, *[Abdo]* **825**, *[Male]* **1025**, *[Extr]* **1428**, *[Gene]* **1888**

metastatic *[Coug]* **1153**

meteorism *[Abdo]* **825**

meticulous *[Mind]* **156**

metrorrhagia *[Fema]* **1068**

mice *[Drea]* **1688**

microcephaly *[Head]* **268**

micturition *[Gene]* **1888**

migraine *[Head]* **268**

mildness *[Mind]* **156**

milk *[Head]* **268**, *[Stom]* **754**, *[Abdo]* **825**, *[Stoo]* **944**, *[Coug]* **1153**, *[Ches]* **1200**, *[Gene]* **1888**

milk fever *[Ches]* **1201**

milk leg *[Extr]* **1428**

milky *[Urin]* **1005**, *[Expe]* **1173**

minerals *[Gene]* **1888**

mining *[Gene]* **1888**

minute *[Coug]* **1153**

mirage *[Visi]* **456**

mirror *[Vert]* **232**

mirth *[Mind]* **59**, **90**, **132**, **137**, **141**, **150**, **156**, **182**, **191**, **205**, **220**, *[Ches]* **1251**

misanthropy *[Mind]* **157**

miscarriage *[Fema]* **1071**, *[Drea]* **1688**

mischievous *[Mind]* **157**

miserable *[Mind]* **157**

miserly *[Mind]* **157**

misery *[Mind]* **157**

misfortune *[Mind]* **157**, *[Drea]* **1688**

missing *[Extr]* **1428**, *[Drea]* **1688**

mist *[Visi]* **456**

mistakes *[Mind]* **157**, *[Visi]* **456**, *[Drea]* **1688**

moaning *[Mind]* **159**, *[Resp]* **1130**

mobility *[Gene]* **1888**

mocking *[Mind]* **160**

modesty *[Mind]* **160**

moist *[Nose]* **526**, *[Mout]* **626**, *[Coug]* **1153**

moisture *[Ear]* **470**, *[Abdo]* **825**, *[Rect]* **922**, *[Uret]* **989**, *[Male]* **1025**, *[Fema]* **1071**, *[Ches]* **1201**, *[Skin]* **1780**

molars *[Teet]* **681**

moles *[Fema]* **1071**, **1071**, *[Back]* **1281**, *[Skin]* **1780**

money *[Mind]* **6**, **19**, **28**, **69**, **77**, **117**, **118**, **121**, **142**, **185**, **198**, *[Drea]* **1682**, **1688**, **1688**, **1691**

monkey *[Drea]* **1688**

monomania *[Mind]* **160**

mononucleosis *[Abdo]* **825**, *[Gene]* **1888**

mons pubis *[Abdo]* **895**

mons veneris *[Abdo]* **895**

monsters *[Drea]* **1688**

monstrous *[Drea]* **1688**

monthly *[Chil]* **1709**

mood *[Mind]* **160**

moon *[Coug]* **1153**, *[Gene]* **1888**

moon agg *[Skin]* **1780**

moonlight *[Mind]* **160**, *[Eye]* **408**, *[Gene]* **1888**

moping *[Mind]* **160**

moral feeling *[Mind]* **160**

morning *[Vert]* **225**, *[Coug]* **1135**, *[Expe]* **1169**, *[Chil]* **1699**, *[Feve]* **1717**, *[Pers]* **1735**, *[Gene]* **1794**

morose *[Mind]* **161**

morphine *[Gene]* **1888**

morphinism *[Mind]* **162**

mortification *[Vert]* **232**, *[Coug]* **1153**, *[Drea]* **1688**

moss *[Stoo]* **944**

mother *[Drea]* **1689**

mother complex *[Mind]* **162**

Index of words

nates *[Extr]* **1637**

native country *[Drea]* **1689**

nature *[Mind]* **163**

nausea *[Vert]* **233**, *[Thro]* **697**, *[Stom]* **754**, *[Abdo]* **825**, *[Ches]* **1201**, *[Drea]* **1689**, *[Chil]* **1709**, *[Pers]* **1740**

near *[Eye]* **409**

nearer *[Visi]* **456**

neat *[Mind]* **163**

neck *[Back]* **1281**

necrophobia *[Mind]* **163**

necrosis *[Head]* **270**, *[Eye]* **404**, *[Ear]* **470**, *[Nose]* **526**, *[Face]* **578**, *[Mout]* **628**, *[Thro]* **697**, *[Lary]* **1099**, *[Ches]* **1201**, *[Back]* **1281**, *[Extr]* **1383**, **1430**, *[Skin]* **1787**, *[Gene]* **1892**

need of sleep *[Slee]* **1648**

negative *[Mind]* **163**

neglected *[Drea]* **1689**

neglecting *[Mind]* **163**

nephritis *[Kidn]* **975**, *[Gene]* **1892**

nephrocalcinosis *[Kidn]* **975**

nephrosis *[Kidn]* **975**

nephrotic syndrome *[Kidn]* **975**

nerves *[Teet]* **682**, *[Gene]* **1980**

nervous *[Mind]* **164**, *[Vert]* **233**, *[Coug]* **1153**, *[Extr]* **1430**, *[Chil]* **1709**, *[Feve]* **1727**, *[Pers]* **1740**

nervous bladder *[Blad]* **953**

net *[Visi]* **456**

netted capillaries *[Gene]* **1892**

network *[Skin]* **1780**

neuralgia *[Eye]* **409**, *[Abdo]* **825**, *[Slee]* **1648**, *[Gene]* **1892**

neurocirculatory asthenia *[Ches]* **1201**, *[Gene]* **1892**

neurodermatitis *[Skin]* **1780**

neurological *[Gene]* **1892**

neuropathy *[Gene]* **1893**

neurosis *[Mind]* **164**

neutral *[Urin]* **1006**

never *[Pers]* **1740**

never well since *[Gene]* **1893**

nevi *[Face]* **578**, 602, *[Skin]* **1780**, *[Gene]* **1955**

new *[Mind]* **164**

newborns *[Mind]* 19, 220, *[Head]* 240, 252, *[Eye]* 394, 401, 404, 433, 438, *[Nose]* 509, 541, *[Face]* 571, 575, 577, 602, *[Thro]* 711, *[Stom]* 727, 797, *[Abdo]* 809, 814, 821, 823, 831, 892, *[Rect]* 899, 901, 906, 912, 913, 920, *[Stoo]* 939, *[Blad]* 958, 959, *[Urin]* 999, *[Male]* 1020, *[Fema]* 1048, *[Resp]*

1114, 1123, *[Ches]* 1202, *[Extr]* 1356, 1381, 1395, *[Slee]* 1643, 1662, *[Drea]* 1679, *[Chil]* 1705, *[Skin]* 1757, 1763, 1772, 1773, *[Gene]* 1809, 1821, 1822, 1825, 1834, 1837, 1966

news *[Mind]* **164**, *[Pers]* **1740**

nibble *[Mind]* **164**

nibbling *[Stom]* **763**

nicotinism *[Gene]* **1893**

night *[Vert]* **226**, *[Coug]* **1136**, *[Expe]* **1169**, *[Chil]* **1702**, *[Feve]* **1718**, *[Pers]* **1736**, *[Gene]* **1796**

night blindness *[Visi]* **456**

night watching *[Mind]* 19, 70, *[Head]* 295, 301, *[Ches]* 1200, *[Slee]* 1664

nightmares *[Drea]* **1689**

night-terror *[Mind]* **164**

nihilistic attitude *[Mind]* **164**

nitrate of silver *[Gene]* **1893**

nitrogen *[Urin]* **1006**

no *[Mind]* **164**

no desire for stool *[Rect]* **922**

no dreams *[Drea]* **1689**

no perspiration *[Pers]* **1740**

nodding *[Head]* **270**

node *[Uret]* **989**

nodes *[Ear]* **470**, *[Lary]* **1099**, *[Extr]* **1430**

nodosities *[Nose]* **527**, *[Face]* **578**, *[Mout]* **628**, *[Extr]* **1430**, *[Skin]* **1780**, *[Gene]* **1893**

nodules *[Head]* **270**, *[Eye]* **409**, *[Face]* **578**, *[Male]* **1025**, *[Fema]* **1071**, *[Ches]* **1201**, *[Back]* **1281**, *[Extr]* **1430**

noise *[Mind]* **164**, *[Vert]* **233**, *[Ear]* **471**, *[Face]* **578**, *[Teet]* **665**, *[Coug]* **1154**, *[Extr]* **1430**, *[Drea]* **1689**, *[Chil]* **1709**, *[Feve]* **1727**

noises *[Head]* **270**, *[Ear]* **471**, *[Abdo]* **825**, *[Ches]* **1202**, *[Gene]* **1893**

noisy *[Mind]* **164**, *[Stoo]* **945**, *[Resp]* **1130**

noma *[Mout]* **628**

none *[Drea]* **1689**

noon *[Vert]* **225**, *[Coug]* **1136**, *[Expe]* **1169**, *[Chil]* **1700**, *[Feve]* **1717**, *[Pers]* **1735**, *[Gene]* **1794**

nose *[Drea]* **1689**

nosophobia *[Mind]* **164**

nostalgia *[Mind]* **164**

nostalgic *[Drea]* **1689**

nostrils *[Nose]* **527**

not refreshed *[Slee]* **1648**

notched *[Teet]* **665**

nothingness *[Mind]* **164**

Index of words

numbness *[Head]* **270**, *[Eye]* **409**, *[Ear]* **480**, *[Nose]* **527**, *[Face]* **578**, *[Mout]* **629**, *[Teet]* **665**, *[Thro]* **697**, *[Exte]* **717**, *[Abdo]* **825**, *[Rect]* **922**, *[Blad]* **953**, *[Kidn]* **975**, *[Uret]* **989**, *[Male]* **1025**, *[Fema]* **1071**, *[Lary]* **1099**, *[Ches]* **1202**, *[Back]* **1281**, *[Extr]* **1430**, *[Skin]* **1780**, *[Gene]* **1893**

nursed *[Mind]* **164**

nursing *[Teet]* **666**, *[Fema]* **1071**, *[Coug]* **1154**, *[Ches]* **1202**, *[Back]* **1281**, *[Gene]* **1894**

nursing others *[Mind]* **164**

nurslings *[Gene]* **1894**

nyctalopia *[Visi]* **456**

nyctophobia *[Mind]* **164**

nymphomania *[Mind]* **164**, *[Fema]* **1071**

nystagmus *[Eye]* **409**

O

obedience *[Mind]* **164**

obesity *[Exte]* **716**, **721**, *[Stom]* **751**, **752**, *[Abdo]* **825**, *[Fema]* **1064**, *[Resp]* **1115**, 1121, 1134, *[Ches]* 1264, *[Gene]* **1894**, 1965

objective *[Mind]* **164**

objects *[Vert]* **233**, *[Visi]* **456**, *[Drea]* **1689**

obligations *[Mind]* **164**

obliged *[Mind]* **164**

obliquity *[Visi]* **456**

obscene *[Mind]* **164**, *[Drea]* **1689**

obscuration *[Visi]* **456**

obsequious *[Mind]* **164**

observant *[Mind]* **164**

observer *[Mind]* **164**

obsession *[Mind]* **164**

obstinate *[Mind]* **164**, *[Gene]* **1894**

obstructed *[Resp]* **1130**

obstruction *[Eye]* **409**, *[Ear]* **480**, *[Nose]* **527**, *[Face]* **578**, *[Thro]* **697**, *[Stom]* **763**, *[Abdo]* **825**, *[Blad]* **953**, *[Ches]* **1202**, *[Gene]* **1894**

obtunded *[Mind]* **165**

occipital *[Vert]* **233**

occiput *[Head]* **387**

occultism *[Mind]* **165**

occupation *[Mind]* **165**, *[Pers]* **1740**

occupied *[Mind]* **165**

occurrences *[Drea]* **1689**

ocean *[Mind]* **165**

ochre *[Stoo]* **945**

odor *[Mout]* **629**, *[Teet]* **666**, *[Stoo]* **945**, *[Urin]* **1006**, *[Male]* **1025**, *[Expe]* **1173**, *[Extr]* **1437**, *[Pers]* **1740**, *[Skin]* **1781**

odor of the body *[Gene]* **1894**

odorless *[Stoo]* **946**, *[Urin]* **1006**

odors *[Vert]* **233**, *[Head]* **271**, *[Ear]* **480**, *[Nose]* **529**, *[Drea]* **1689**, *[Gene]* **1895**

odors agg *[Resp]* **1130**, *[Coug]* **1154**

oedema *[Head]* **271**, *[Nose]* **530**, *[Face]* **578**, *[Abdo]* **826**, *[Lary]* **1099**, *[Ches]* **1202**, *[Gene]* **1895**

oedipus complex *[Mind]* **165**

offended *[Mind]* **165**

offensiveness *[Gene]* **1895**

oil *[Vert]* **233**, *[Teet]* **666**

oily *[Head]* **271**, *[Nose]* **530**, *[Face]* **578**, *[Urin]* **1006**, *[Pers]* **1741**, *[Skin]* **1781**

old *[Mind]* **165**, *[Face]* **578**, *[Coug]* **1154**

old age *[Gene]* **1895**

old people *[Mind]* **31**, **90**, **91**, **108**, **116**, **123**, **134**, **148**, **158**, **193**, **195**, *[Vert]* **233**, *[Head]* **262**, **283**, **295**, **385**, *[Eye]* **389**, **391**, **393**, **402**, *[Visi]* **449**, *[Hear]* **503**, *[Nose]* **506**, **512**, **523**, *[Face]* **562**, **563**, **567**, *[Mout]* **638**, *[Thro]* **710**, *[Stom]* **752**, *[Abdo]* **816**, **821**, *[Rect]* **897**, **899**, **901**, **904**, **905**, **909**, **912**, **916**, *[Stoo]* **945**, *[Blad]* **951**, **958**, **959**, **963**, **965**, **970**, **971**, *[Pros]* **982**, **983**, *[Urin]* **1007**, *[Male]* **1017**, **1018**, **1019**, **1023**, **1035**, **1038**, *[Fema]* **1049**, **1056**, **1061**, **1091**, *[Lary]* **1093**, *[Resp]* **1118**, **1123**, **1125**, **1131**, **1133**, *[Coug]* **1157**, **1158**, **1160**, *[Expe]* **1171**, **1173**, **1174**, *[Ches]* **1179**, **1180**, **1188**, **1196**, **1198**, **1199**, **1254**, **1256**, **1258**, **1266**, **1267**, *[Extr]* **1361**, **1380**, **1404**, **1579**, *[Slee]* **1642**, **1656**, **1664**, *[Feve]* **1726**, *[Skin]* **1751**, **1752**, **1754**, **1763**, **1773**, **1775**, **1778**, **1787**, **1791**, *[Gene]* **1803**, **1805**, **1811**, **1824**, **1826**, **1829**, **1834**, **1837**, **1867**, **1873**, **1893**, **1894**, **1895**, **1919**, **1920**, **1927**, **1928**, **1953**, **1959**, **1970**, **1972**, **1974**, **1975**

older *[Mind]* **165**

oleaginous *[Expe]* **1174**

onanism *[Male]* **1025**, *[Fema]* **1071**, *[Gene]* **1895**

one idea *[Mind]* **165**

one side *[Chil]* **1699**, *[Pers]* **1735**

onions *[Coug]* **1154**

onychia *[Extr]* **1437**

onychophagy *[Extr]* **1437**

onyx *[Eye]* **409**

oophoritis *[Fema]* **1071**

Index of words

oozing *[Extr]* **1437**

opacity *[Eye]* **409**

opaque *[Expe]* **1174**

open *[Mind]* **165**, *[Head]* **271**, *[Eye]* **409**, *[Ear]* **480**, *[Nose]* **530**, *[Face]* **578**, *[Mout]* **630**, *[Stom]* **763**, *[Rect]* **922**, *[Uret]* **989**, *[Fema]* **1071**, *[Ches]* **1202**

opening *[Vert]* **233**, *[Head]* **271**, *[Eye]* **410**, *[Ear]* **480**

opening the eyes *[Gene]* **1895**

opening the mouth *[Ear]* **480**, *[Face]* **578**, *[Gene]* **1895**

openness *[Eye]* **410**

operation *[Mind]* 110, *[Eye]* 391, **410**, 419, 430, 433, *[Visi]* 453, 456, *[Ear]* **480**, *[Nose]* 523, **530**, 535, *[Teet]* **666**, 673, 680, *[Thro]* 702, *[Stom]* 750, 761, **763**, 794, *[Abdo]* 811, 816, 821, 825, **826**, 840, 884, *[Rect]* 901, 918, *[Blad]* 951, 953, 959, *[Kidn]* 975, *[Urin]* 1009, *[Coug]* **1154**, *[Ches]* 1180, 1187, **1202**, *[Back]* **1281**, *[Slee]* 1664, *[Feve]* **1727**, *[Skin]* 1748, *[Gene]* 1842, 1845, 1867, 1873, 1877, **1895**, 1901, 1937, 1970

ophidiophobia *[Mind]* **165**

ophthalmia *[Eye]* **410**

opinionated *[Mind]* **165**

opinions *[Mind]* **165**

opisthotonos *[Mind]* 33, *[Vert]* 226, *[Face]* 592, *[Abdo]* 833, *[Rect]* 897, *[Coug]* **1154**, *[Back]* **1281**, *[Gene]* 1826, 1827

oppression *[Stom]* **763**, *[Abdo]* **826**, *[Resp]* **1131**, *[Coug]* **1154**, *[Ches]* **1202**, *[Back]* **1282**

oppressive *[Coug]* **1154**, *[Slee]* **1648**

optic *[Eye]* **440**

optimistic *[Mind]* **165**

orange *[Expe]* **1174**

orbital cellulitis *[Eye]* **410**

orbits *[Eye]* **440**

orchitis *[Male]* **1025**

order *[Mind]* **165**

orderly manner *[Mind]* **165**

organic mental syndrome *[Mind]* **165**

organized *[Mind]* **165**

orgasm *[Male]* **1025**, *[Fema]* **1071**, *[Ches]* **1205**, *[Back]* **1282**, *[Extr]* **1437**, *[Drea]* **1689**, *[Gene]* **1895**

orientation *[Mind]* **165**

orphans *[Mind]* **165**

orthopnea *[Resp]* **1124**, *[Ches]* **1196**

os uteri *[Fema]* **1071**

oscillating *[Mout]* **630**

ossification *[Gene]* **1896**

osteochondrosis *[Gene]* **1896**

osteogenesis imperfecta tarda *[Gene]* **1896**

osteoma *[Gene]* 1955

osteomalacia *[Gene]* **1896**

osteomyelitis *[Gene]* **1896**

osteoporosis *[Extr]* **1437**, *[Gene]* **1896**

othematoma *[Ear]* **480**

otitis *[Ear]* **480**

otorrhea *[Ear]* **480**

otosclerosis *[Ear]* **480**

outgoing *[Mind]* **166**

ovaries *[Fema]* **1092**

ovaritis *[Gene]* **1896**

overactive *[Mind]* **166**

overactivity *[Abdo]* **826**

overbearing *[Mind]* **166**

overburdened *[Mind]* **166**

overheated *[Chil]* **1709**

overheating *[Coug]* **1154**

overlifting *[Head]* **271**, *[Back]* **1282**

overloaded *[Stom]* **764**, *[Abdo]* **826**

overpowering *[Coug]* **1154**, *[Slee]* **1648**

oversensitive *[Mind]* **166**

overshot jaw *[Face]* **578**

overuse *[Gene]* **1896**

overweening *[Mind]* **166**

overwhelmed *[Mind]* **166**

overworked *[Mind]* **166**

ovulation *[Fema]* **1071**

own *[Extr]* **1437**

oxen *[Drea]* **1689**

oysters *[Coug]* **1154**

ozena *[Nose]* **530**

P

pain *[Mind]* **166**, *[Vert]* **233**, *[Head]* **271**, *[Eye]* **410**, *[Ear]* **480**, *[Nose]* **530**, *[Face]* **578**, *[Mout]* **630**, *[Teet]* **666**, *[Thro]* **697**, *[Exte]* **717**, *[Stom]* **764**, *[Abdo]* **826**, *[Rect]* **922**, *[Blad]* **953**, *[Kidn]* **975**, *[Pros]* **982**, *[Uret]* **989**, *[Male]* **1025**, *[Fema]* **1071**, *[Lary]* **1099**, *[Coug]* **1154**, *[Ches]* **1205**, *[Back]* **1282**, *[Extr]* **1437**, *[Slee]* **1648**, *[Drea]* **1689**, *[Chil]* **1709**, *[Feve]* **1727**, *[Skin]* **1781**, *[Gene]* **1896**

painful *[Vert]* **233**, *[Stoo]* **946**, *[Resp]* **1131**, *[Coug]* **1154**, *[Expe]* **1174**, *[Pers]* **1741**

Index of words

painless *[Stoo]* **946**, *[Coug]* **1154**
painlessness *[Gene]* **1918**
pains *[Resp]* **1131**, *[Pers]* **1741**
painter's *[Abdo]* **884**
painting *[Mind]* **166**
pale *[Eye]* **428**, *[Visi]* **456**, *[Expe]* **1174**
paleness *[Thro]* **708**
palpitation *[Vert]* **233**, *[Coug]* **1154**, *[Ches]* **1250**, *[Drea]* **1690**, *[Pers]* **1741**
panaris *[Extr]* **1579**
panaritium *[Back]* **1344**, *[Extr]* **1400**, **1579**, **1636**
pancreas *[Abdo]* **895**
panic *[Mind]* **166**
pannus *[Eye]* **428**
panting *[Resp]* **1131**, *[Coug]* **1154**
papillae *[Mout]* **637**
paradoxical *[Mind]* **166**, *[Gene]* **1918**
paralysis *[Vert]* **233**, *[Head]* **370**, *[Eye]* **428**, *[Ear]* **494**, *[Face]* **593**, *[Mout]* **638**, *[Thro]* **708**, *[Exte]* **719**, *[Stom]* **781**, *[Abdo]* **884**, *[Rect]* **932**, *[Blad]* **958**, *[Lary]* **1103**, *[Resp]* **1131**, *[Ches]* **1256**, *[Back]* **1338**, *[Extr]* **1579**, *[Gene]* **1918**
paralysis agitans *[Gene]* **1920**
paralysis of senses *[Gene]* **1920**
paralytic *[Blad]* **958**
paralyzed *[Teet]* **680**
paranoia *[Mind]* **166**
paraphimosis *[Male]* **1033**
paraplegia *[Blad]* **958**, *[Urin]* **1000**, *[Gene]* **1844**, **1903**, **1919**
parasites *[Rect]* **932**
parched *[Mout]* **638**, *[Thro]* **708**
parchment *[Nose]* **537**, *[Face]* **594**, *[Skin]* **1782**
paresis *[Gene]* **1920**
parkinson's disease *[Gene]* **1920**
paronychia *[Extr]* **1583**
parotid gland *[Face]* **603**
paroxysmal *[Vert]* **234**, *[Resp]* **1131**, *[Coug]* **1154**, *[Feve]* **1727**, *[Gene]* **1920**
paroxysms *[Feve]* **1727**
partial *[Mind]* **166**, *[Chil]* **1709**, *[Pers]* **1741**
parties *[Drea]* **1690**
parturition *[Head]* **386**, *[Rect]* **918**, *[Fema]* **1044**, **1061**, **1086**, *[Slee]* **1673**, *[Gene]* **1826**, **1920**, **1970**
passion *[Drea]* **1690**
passionate *[Mind]* **166**
passivity *[Mind]* **166**

past *[Mind]* **10**, **35**, **37**, **39**, **60**, **66**, **68**, **69**, **71**, **76**, **81**, **92**, **103**, **121**, **152**, **153**, **158**, **165**, **174**, **185**, **208**, **210**, **222**, *[Resp]* **1129**, *[Drea]* **1683**, **1690**, *[Gene]* **1926**
pasty *[Mout]* **638**, *[Stoo]* **946**, *[Expe]* **1174**
patches *[Mout]* **638**
pathetic *[Mind]* **166**
patience *[Mind]* **166**
patted *[Mind]* **166**
pattern *[Slee]* **1648**
peaceful *[Drea]* **1690**
peacemaker *[Mind]* **166**
peaked *[Face]* **594**
pecking *[Mind]* **166**, *[Extr]* **1583**, *[Gene]* **1920**
pedophilia *[Mind]* **166**
peeling *[Nose]* **537**, *[Face]* **594**
peevish *[Mind]* **166**, *[Drea]* **1690**
pellagra *[Gene]* **1920**
pelvic *[Fema]* **1086**
pendulous *[Abdo]* **884**
penis *[Male]* **1041**, *[Drea]* **1690**
people *[Drea]* **1690**
pepper *[Coug]* **1155**
pepsin *[Stom]* **781**
perceptions *[Mind]* **166**
perfectionist *[Mind]* **166**
perfidious *[Mind]* **166**
perforated *[Nose]* **537**
perforation *[Ear]* **494**, *[Abdo]* **884**
perfume *[Mind]* **166**
perianal glands *[Rect]* **937**
periarteritis nodosa *[Gene]* **1920**
pericarditis *[Ches]* **1256**
perineum *[Abdo]* **859**, **866**, **883**, *[Rect]* **897**, **898**, **902**, **911**, **912**, **913**, **915**, **921**, **922**, **931**, **932**, **934**, **935**, **936**, **937**, **937**, *[Blad]* **968**, *[Pros]* **983**, *[Uret]* **994**, *[Male]* **1020**, **1025**, *[Fema]* **1048**, **1049**, **1079**, *[Back]* **1328**
periodical *[Vert]* **234**, *[Coug]* **1155**, *[Chil]* **1709**, *[Feve]* **1727**, *[Pers]* **1741**
periodicity *[Mind]* **166**, *[Head]* **370**, *[Chil]* **1710**, *[Gene]* **1920**
periodontosis *[Mout]* **638**, *[Teet]* **680**
periostitis *[Head]* **370**, *[Teet]* **680**
peristalsis *[Abdo]* **884**
peritonitis *[Abdo]* **884**
pernicious *[Chil]* **1710**
perseverance *[Mind]* **166**

Index of words

persevering *[Mind]* **166**

persistent *[Coug]* **1155**, *[Drea]* **1690**

persisting *[Mind]* **166**

personal *[Mind]* **22**

personal appearance *[Mind]* **166**

personal history *[Gene]* **1921**

persons *[Coug]* **1156**, *[Drea]* **1690**

perspective *[Visi]* **456**

perspiration *[Vert]* **234**, *[Head]* **370**, *[Eye]* **429**, *[Ear]* **494**, *[Nose]* **537**, *[Face]* **594**, *[Thro]* **708**, *[Exte]* **719**, *[Stom]* **781**, *[Abdo]* **884**, *[Rect]* **932**, *[Male]* **1033**, *[Fema]* **1086**, *[Coug]* **1156**, *[Ches]* **1256**, *[Back]* **1338**, *[Extr]* **1583**, *[Slee]* **1648**, *[Chil]* **1710**, *[Feve]* **1728**, *[Pers]* **1735**, *[Skin]* **1782**, *[Gene]* **1921**

pert *[Mind]* **166**

pertinacity *[Mind]* **166**

pertussis *[Coug]* **1156**

perverse *[Mind]* **166**

pessary *[Fema]* **1086**

pessimist *[Mind]* **166**

pest *[Gene]* **1922**

petechiae *[Ches]* **1257**, *[Extr]* 1380, 1382, 1385, 1390, 1393, 1394, 1395, 1397, *[Skin]* 1763, **1782**

petit mal *[Gene]* **1922**

pettiness *[Mind]* **166**

petulant *[Mind]* **167**

phantom *[Gene]* **1922**

pharyngitis *[Thro]* **708**

pharynx *[Thro]* **714**

pheochromocytoma *[Gene]* **1922**

philosophy *[Mind]* **167**

phimosis *[Male]* **1033**

phlegmasia alba dolens *[Extr]* **1586**

phlegmatic *[Mind]* **167**

phobia *[Mind]* **167**

phosphorescent *[Expe]* **1174**

phosphorous *[Urin]* **1006**

phosphorus *[Gene]* **1922**

photodermatosis *[Skin]* **1782**

photomania *[Mind]* **167**, *[Eye]* **429**

photophobia *[Eye]* **429**

phthisis *[Male]* **1033**, *[Lary]* **1103**, *[Ches]* **1257**

physical *[Mind]* **167**

physical symptoms *[Gene]* **1922**

physician *[Drea]* **1690**

physometra *[Fema]* **1086**

piano *[Coug]* **1156**

picking *[Mind]* **167**, *[Nose]* **537**, *[Face]* **595**, *[Mout]* **638**, *[Teet]* **680**, *[Extr]* **1586**

picky *[Mind]* **167**

picnics *[Drea]* **1690**

picture taken *[Mind]* **167**

pieces *[Expe]* **1174**

piety *[Mind]* **167**

pigmentary *[Abdo]* **884**

pimples *[Mout]* **638**, *[Thro]* **708**

pinched *[Nose]* **537**, *[Drea]* **1690**

pinching *[Mind]* **167**, *[Extr]* **1586**, *[Gene]* **1922**

pining people *[Gene]* **1922**

pins *[Drea]* **1690**

pitch-like *[Stoo]* **946**

pithy *[Head]* **372**, *[Extr]* **1586**

pities *[Mind]* **167**

pitting *[Extr]* **1586**

pityriasis *[Skin]* **1782**

placenta *[Fema]* **1086**

places *[Drea]* **1690**

placidity *[Mind]* **167**

plaintive *[Mind]* **167**

plans *[Mind]* **167**

playful *[Mind]* **167**

playing *[Mind]* **167**, *[Extr]* **1586**, *[Drea]* **1690**

playing piano *[Gene]* **1922**

pleasant *[Male]* **1033**, *[Drea]* **1690**

pleasantry *[Mind]* **167**

pleased *[Mind]* **167**

pleasing *[Mind]* **167**

pleasure *[Mind]* **167**

plethora *[Abdo]* **884**, *[Gene]* **1922**

plethoric *[Face]* **595**

pleuralgia *[Ches]* **1258**

pleurisy *[Ches]* **1258**

pleuritis *[Coug]* **1156**

pleurodynia *[Ches]* **1258**

pleuropneumonia *[Ches]* **1258**

plica polonica *[Head]* **372**

plug *[Thro]* **708**, *[Stom]* **781**, *[Abdo]* **884**, *[Rect]* **933**, *[Blad]* **958**, *[Fema]* **1086**, *[Lary]* **1103**, *[Coug]* **1156**, *[Ches]* **1258**, *[Gene]* **1922**

plummer-vinson *[Mout]* **638**

pneumonia *[Coug]* **1156**, *[Ches]* **1258**

pneumothorax *[Ches]* **1258**

poetic *[Drea]* **1690**

poetry *[Mind]* **168**

pointed *[Nose]* **537**, *[Face]* **595**

Index of words

pointed t *[Mout]* **638**

poison *[Drea]* **1690**

poison ivy *[Gene]* **1922**

poisoned *[Drea]* **1690**

poisonings *[Gene]* **1922**

police *[Mind]* 72, 73, 110, *[Drea]* **1690**, 1691

poliomyelitis *[Gene]* **1922**

polite *[Mind]* **168**

political *[Drea]* **1690**

pollution *[Ches]* **1258**, *[Back]* **1338**

pollutions *[Male]* **1033**

polyarthritis *[Gene]* **1922**

polycystic *[Kidn]* **979**

polycythemia *[Gene]* **1922**

polyopia *[Visi]* **456**

polypi *[Abdo]* **884**, *[Rect]* **933**, *[Blad]* **958**, 959, *[Lary]* **1103**, *[Resp]* 1116

polypous *[Urin]* **1006**

polypus *[Eye]* **430**, 436, *[Ear]* 463, **494**, 494, *[Nose]* **537**, *[Fema]* 1070, **1086**, *[Back]* **1338**, *[Gene]* **1922**

pompe's disease *[Gene]* **1923**

pompous *[Mind]* **168**

ponophobia *[Mind]* **168**

porphyrins *[Urin]* **1006**

portal *[Abdo]* **884**

position *[Fema]* **1086**, *[Coug]* **1156**, *[Extr]* **1586**, *[Slee]* **1648**, *[Gene]* **1923**

positiveness *[Mind]* **168**

possessiveness *[Mind]* **168**

postmenopausal bleeding *[Fema]* **1086**

postpartum hemorrhage *[Fema]* **1086**

postponing *[Mind]* **168**, *[Chil]* **1710**

potassium *[Urin]* **1006**

potatoes *[Coug]* **1156**

potbelly *[Abdo]* **884**

pott's disease *[Back]* **1338**

pounding *[Gene]* **1923**

pouting *[Uret]* **996**

powder *[Thro]* **708**

power *[Mind]* **168**

powerful *[Extr]* **1586**

powerless *[Mind]* **168**

practical *[Mind]* **168**

praised *[Mind]* **168**

praying *[Mind]* **168**, *[Drea]* **1690**

preaching *[Mind]* **168**, *[Drea]* **1690**

prearranging *[Mind]* **168**

precipice *[Drea]* **1690**

precocity *[Mind]* **168**, *[Fema]* **1086**

predicting *[Mind]* **168**

predominating *[Chil]* **1710**

pregnancy *[Mind]* **168**, *[Vert]* **234**, *[Ear]* **494**, *[Teet]* **680**, *[Stom]* **781**, *[Abdo]* **884**, *[Blad]* **958**, *[Fema]* **1086**, *[Coug]* **1156**, *[Gene]* **1923**

pregnant *[Abdo]* **884**, *[Drea]* **1690**

prejudiced *[Mind]* **168**

premenstrual *[Mind]* **168**, *[Fema]* **1086**

premonition *[Mind]* **168**

preoccupied *[Mind]* **168**

presentiment *[Mind]* **168**

presses *[Exte]* **720**

pressing *[Mout]* **638**, *[Teet]* **680**, *[Stom]* **781**

pressure *[Vert]* **234**, *[Head]* **372**, *[Eye]* **430**, *[Ear]* **494**, *[Nose]* **537**, *[Teet]* **680**, *[Stom]* **781**, *[Abdo]* **884**, *[Rect]* **933**, *[Blad]* **958**, *[Kidn]* **979**, *[Male]* **1035**, *[Fema]* **1086**, *[Lary]* **1103**, *[Resp]* **1131**, *[Coug]* **1156**, *[Ches]* **1258**, *[Back]* **1338**, *[Extr]* **1586**, *[Chil]* **1710**, *[Skin]* **1782**, *[Gene]* **1923**

pressure in the eyeball *[Eye]* **430**

presumptuous *[Mind]* **168**

pretty *[Mind]* **168**

priapism *[Male]* **1035**

prickling *[Head]* **372**, *[Eye]* **430**, *[Ear]* **494**, *[Nose]* **537**, *[Face]* **595**, *[Mout]* **638**, *[Teet]* **680**, *[Stom]* **781**, *[Abdo]* **885**, *[Rect]* **933**, *[Male]* **1035**, *[Lary]* **1103**, *[Coug]* **1156**, *[Ches]* **1258**, *[Back]* **1339**, *[Extr]* **1586**, *[Skin]* **1782**, *[Gene]* **1923**

prickly *[Thro]* **708**

pride *[Mind]* **168**

prim *[Mind]* **168**

prince *[Mind]* 73

prisoner *[Drea]* **1690**

procrastinating *[Mind]* **168**

proctitis *[Rect]* **933**

prodrome *[Coug]* **1156**

profanity *[Mind]* **168**

profound *[Slee]* **1650**, *[Drea]* **1690**

profuse *[Expe]* **1174**, *[Pers]* **1741**

prognathism *[Face]* **595**

programming *[Mind]* **168**

progressive muscular atrophy *[Gene]* **1923**

projecting *[Eye]* **430**

projects *[Drea]* **1690**

prolapsus *[Mind]* 139, *[Head]* 260, 280, *[Stom]* 724, 751, *[Abdo]* **885**, *[Rect]* 899, 926, **933**, 935, *[Blad]*

Index of words

958, 969, 970, *[Fema]* **1086**, *[Back]* **1339**, *[Extr]* 1585, *[Gene]* **1923**

prolonged *[Slee]* **1650**

prominent cheekbones *[Face]* **595**

promiscuous *[Mind]* **168**

pronation *[Extr]* **1586**

proper *[Mind]* **168**

prophesying *[Mind]* **169**

prophetic *[Drea]* **1691**

proportion *[Mind]* **169**, *[Visi]* **456**

prostatitis *[Pros]* **982**, *[Male]* **1035**

prostatorrhea *[Pros]* **982**

prostration *[Mind]* **169**, *[Coug]* **1156**, *[Gene]* **1923**

protected *[Mind]* **170**, *[Drea]* **1691**

protesting *[Mind]* **170**

protozoa *[Rect]* **933**

protruding *[Eye]* **430**, *[Face]* **595**, *[Mout]* **638**, *[Thro]* **708**, *[Coug]* **1156**

protrusion *[Eye]* **430**, *[Face]* **595**, *[Abdo]* **885**, *[Ches]* **1258**, *[Gene]* **1923**

protuberances *[Nose]* **537**

proud *[Mind]* **170**, *[Mout]* **639**, *[Teet]* **680**, *[Abdo]* **885**

proving *[Drea]* **1691**

proving oneself *[Mind]* **170**

provoked *[Drea]* **1691**

provoking *[Mind]* **170**

prude *[Drea]* **1691**

prune *[Expe]* **1174**

pruritus *[Skin]* **1782**

prying *[Mind]* **170**

psora *[Gene]* **1923**

psoriasis *[Head]* 252, 277, *[Face]* 566, 569, *[Mout]* 622, *[Male]* 1021, *[Back]* 1275, *[Extr]* 1386, 1387, 1388, 1389, 1390, 1391, 1392, 1393, 1397, *[Skin]* 1764, **1782**, *[Gene]* 1831, 1907

psychosis *[Mind]* **170**

psychotropic *[Gene]* **1924**

pterygium *[Eye]* **430**

ptomaine poisoning *[Gene]* **1924**

ptosis *[Eye]* **430**

ptyalism *[Mout]* **639**

puberty *[Mind]* **170**, *[Vert]* **234**, *[Male]* **1035**, *[Fema]* **1087**, *[Gene]* **1924**

pubic region *[Abdo]* **895**

public *[Mind]* 21, 102, 103, 110, 160, 206, 211, 212, *[Male]* 1022, 1025, *[Fema]* 1059, *[Lary]* 1103, *[Ches]* 1255, *[Drea]* 1678, 1690

puckered *[Eye]* **430**, *[Mout]* **639**

puerperal *[Fema]* **1087**

puerperal fever *[Feve]* **1728**

puffed *[Face]* **595**

puffiness *[Nose]* **537**

puffing *[Ear]* **494**, *[Resp]* **1131**

pulled *[Head]* **372**, *[Nose]* **537**

pulling *[Mind]* **170**, *[Eye]* **430**, *[Back]* **1339**, *[Extr]* **1586**

pulsating *[Head]* **372**, *[Thro]* **708**, *[Fema]* **1087**, *[Lary]* **1103**, *[Back]* **1339**

pulsation *[Eye]* **430**, *[Ear]* **494**, *[Nose]* **537**, *[Face]* **595**, *[Mout]* **639**, *[Exte]* **720**, *[Stom]* **781**, *[Abdo]* **885**, *[Rect]* **933**, *[Blad]* **958**, *[Kidn]* **979**, *[Uret]* **996**, *[Male]* **1035**, *[Ches]* **1258**, *[Extr]* **1587**, *[Gene]* **1924**

pulsations *[Teet]* **680**

pulse *[Vert]* **234**, *[Feve]* **1728**, *[Gene]* **1925**

punctilious *[Mind]* **170**

pungent *[Coug]* **1156**

punishment *[Mind]* **170**, *[Drea]* **1691**

pupils *[Eye]* **440**

purchase *[Drea]* **1691**

purgatives *[Gene]* **1930**

purging *[Gene]* **1930**

purpura *[Mout]* **639**, *[Ches]* **1259**, *[Skin]* **1782**

purpura idiopathic thrombocytopenic *[Gene]* **1930**

purring *[Lary]* **1103**, *[Coug]* **1156**, *[Ches]* **1259**, *[Extr]* **1588**

pursued *[Drea]* **1691**

purulent *[Stoo]* **946**, *[Urin]* **1007**, *[Expe]* **1174**, *[Pers]* **1743**

pus *[Gene]* **1930**

pushed *[Vert]* **234**, *[Head]* **376**, *[Extr]* **1588**

pushes *[Fema]* **1087**

pushing *[Head]* **376**, *[Abdo]* **885**

pustules *[Eye]* **431**, *[Mout]* **639**, *[Thro]* **708**

put *[Mout]* **639**

putrefaction *[Abdo]* **885**

putrid *[Mout]* **639**, *[Feve]* **1728**

putrid phenomena *[Gene]* **1930**

puts *[Thro]* **708**

putting *[Coug]* **1156**

pyemia *[Gene]* **1930**

pyometra *[Fema]* **1087**

pyorrhea alveolaris *[Mout]* **639**

pyromania *[Mind]* **170**

pyrophobia *[Mind]* **170**

Index of words

pyrosis *[Stom]* **782**
python *[Drea]* **1691**

Q

quaking *[Mind]* **170**
qualmish *[Mind]* **170**, *[Stom]* **782**
quarrelling *[Mind]* **170**
quarrels *[Drea]* **1691**
quarrelsome *[Mind]* **170**
quartan *[Chil]* **1710**
quartan fever *[Feve]* **1728**
queer *[Mind]* **171**
questions *[Mind]* **171**
quick *[Mind]* **171**, *[Resp]* **1131**
quiet *[Mind]* **171**
quieted *[Mind]* **171**
quinine *[Gene]* **1930**
quivering *[Head]* **376**, *[Eye]* **431**, *[Visi]* **456**, *[Ear]* **495**, *[Nose]* **537**, *[Face]* **595**, *[Stom]* **782**, *[Abdo]* **885**, *[Pros]* **982**, *[Ches]* **1259**, *[Back]* **1339**, *[Extr]* **1588**, *[Gene]* **1930**
quotidian *[Chil]* **1710**

R

rabies *[Drea]* **1691**, *[Gene]* **1930**
rachitis *[Extr]* **1588**, *[Gene]* **1930**
racing *[Mind]* **171**
racking *[Coug]* **1156**
radiant heat *[Gene]* **1930**
radiation therapy *[Gene]* **1930**
radium treatments *[Gene]* **1930**
rage *[Mind]* **171**, *[Pers]* **1743**
ragged *[Mout]* **639**
rain *[Mind]* **172**, *[Head]* **376**, *[Visi]* **456**, *[Gene]* **1930**
rainbow *[Visi]* **456**
rainbows *[Drea]* **1691**
raised *[Coug]* **1156**, *[Extr]* **1588**
raising *[Vert]* **234**, *[Head]* **376**, *[Fema]* **1087**, *[Back]* **1339**, *[Extr]* **1588**, *[Gene]* **1930**
raising arms *[Coug]* **1156**, *[Ches]* **1259**
rancidity *[Stom]* **782**
range *[Visi]* **456**
ranula *[Mout]* **639**
rape *[Drea]* **1691**
rapid *[Coug]* **1156**
rapidly growing *[Gene]* **1930**
rash *[Mind]* **172**, *[Drea]* **1691**

rasping *[Resp]* **1131**, *[Coug]* **1156**
rat *[Extr]* **1588**
rats *[Drea]* **1691**
rattling *[Nose]* **537**, *[Mout]* **639**, *[Abdo]* **885**, *[Lary]* **1103**, *[Resp]* **1131**, *[Coug]* **1156**, *[Ches]* **1259**
raw *[Uret]* **996**
rawness *[Ear]* **495**, *[Mout]* **639**, *[Coug]* **1157**, *[Ches]* **1259**, *[Back]* **1339**, *[Skin]* **1782**
raynaud's disease *[Extr]* **1588**
rays *[Visi]* **456**
reabsorbent *[Gene]* **1930**
reaching *[Vert]* **234**
reaching up *[Fema]* **1087**
reaction *[Gene]* **1930**
read *[Drea]* **1691**
reading *[Mind]* **172**, *[Vert]* **234**, *[Head]* **377**, *[Eye]* **431**, *[Resp]* **1132**, *[Extr]* **1588**, *[Drea]* **1691**, *[Gene]* **1931**
reading aloud *[Coug]* **1157**
ready *[Drea]* **1691**
reality *[Mind]* **173**
reason *[Mind]* **173**
reasonable *[Mind]* **173**
reassured *[Mind]* **173**
rebellious *[Mind]* **173**
rebels *[Mind]* **173**, *[Gene]* **1931**
recalling *[Drea]* **1691**
recedes *[Rect]* **934**
receding *[Visi]* **457**, *[Mout]* **639**, *[Stoo]* **946**, *[Urin]* **1007**
reckless *[Mind]* **173**
recognition *[Mind]* **173**
recognizing *[Mind]* **173**
reconciliation *[Drea]* **1691**
recovering *[Gene]* **1931**
recriminating *[Mind]* **173**
rectum *[Rect]* **937**
recurrent *[Feve]* **1728**
red *[Nose]* **537**, *[Gene]* **1931**
reddish *[Stoo]* **946**, *[Expe]* **1174**
redness *[Eye]* **431**, *[Ear]* **495**, *[Face]* **595**, *[Rect]* **934**, *[Uret]* **996**, *[Male]* **1036**, *[Fema]* **1087**, *[Ches]* **1259**, *[Back]* **1339**, *[Gene]* **1931**
re-echo *[Coug]* **1157**
reeling *[Vert]* **234**
refined *[Mind]* **173**
reflecting *[Mind]* **173**, *[Vert]* **234**, *[Head]* **377**, *[Visi]* **457**, *[Teet]* **680**, *[Coug]* **1157**, *[Drea]* **1691**

Index of words

reflex *[Coug]* **1157**
reflexes *[Extr]* **1588**, *[Gene]* **1931**
refreshing *[Slee]* **1650**
refusing *[Mind]* **173**
regions *[Drea]* **1691**
regression *[Mind]* **173**
regurgitation *[Stom]* **782**
reiter's syndrome *[Gene]* **1931**
relapsing *[Feve]* **1728**
relatives *[Mind]* 19, 28, 45, 50, 73, 95, 104, 115, 160, 172, 173, *[Drea]* 1681, **1691**, 1691
relaxation *[Vert]* **234**, *[Head]* **377**, *[Ear]* **495**, *[Thro]* **708**, *[Stom]* **782**, *[Blad]* **958**, *[Fema]* **1087**, *[Lary]* **1103**, *[Extr]* **1589**, *[Gene]* **1931**
relaxed *[Mind]* **173**, *[Face]* **595**, *[Stom]* **782**, *[Abdo]* **885**, *[Rect]* **934**, *[Male]* **1036**, *[Skin]* **1782**
relieved *[Resp]* **1132**
religion *[Mind]* 131, 173
religious *[Mind]* 4, 5, 20, 23, 24, 37, 48, 73, 85, 93, 97, 98, 99, 106, 109, 122, 134, 143, 149, 151, 168, 172, 173, 174, 185, 189, *[Male]* 1037, *[Fema]* 1088, *[Drea]* 1681, **1691**, *[Gene]* 1808, 1825, 1826
religious affections *[Mind]* **173**
remedies *[Gene]* **1932**
remembered *[Drea]* **1691**
remembering *[Mind]* **174**
remittent *[Coug]* **1157**, *[Feve]* **1728**
remorse *[Mind]* **174**, *[Drea]* **1691**
removed *[Head]* **377**, *[Lary]* **1103**
removing *[Drea]* **1691**
renal failure *[Kidn]* **979**
renunciation *[Mind]* **174**
repeating *[Mind]* **174**, *[Drea]* **1691**
repentance *[Drea]* **1691**
repenting *[Mind]* **174**
repose *[Mind]* **174**, *[Coug]* **1157**
reproached *[Mind]* **174**
reproaches *[Drea]* **1691**
reproaching *[Mind]* **174**
repugnance *[Stom]* **782**
repulsive mood *[Mind]* **174**
reputation *[Mind]* **174**
rescuing *[Drea]* **1691**
resentment *[Mind]* **174**
reserved *[Mind]* **174**
resignation *[Mind]* **175**
resolute *[Mind]* **175**
resonant *[Coug]* **1157**

respected *[Mind]* **175**
respecting *[Mind]* **175**
respiration *[Nose]* **537**
respiratory *[Ches]* **1267**, *[Drea]* **1691**
responsibility *[Mind]* **175**, *[Drea]* **1691**
responsive *[Mind]* **175**
rest *[Mind]* **175**, *[Vert]* **234**, *[Coug]* **1157**, *[Gene]* **1932**
resting *[Vert]* **234**, *[Coug]* **1157**
restless *[Eye]* **431**, *[Slee]* **1650**, *[Drea]* **1691**
restlessness *[Mind]* **175**, *[Head]* **377**, *[Stom]* **782**, *[Abdo]* **885**, *[Ches]* **1259**, *[Back]* **1339**, *[Extr]* **1589**, *[Gene]* **1932**
resurrection *[Drea]* **1692**
retardation *[Mind]* **180**
retching *[Head]* **377**, *[Stom]* **782**, *[Coug]* **1157**, *[Gene]* **1932**
retentio secundinarum *[Fema]* **1087**
retention *[Blad]* **958**
retention of stool *[Rect]* **934**
reticent *[Mind]* **180**
retinitis *[Eye]* **431**
retirement *[Mind]* **180**
retiring *[Mind]* **180**
retracted *[Ear]* **495**, *[Mout]* **639**
retraction *[Ear]* **495**, *[Face]* **595**, *[Stom]* **783**, *[Abdo]* **886**, *[Rect]* **934**, *[Male]* **1036**, *[Ches]* **1259**, *[Gene]* **1932**
revealing *[Mind]* **180**, *[Drea]* **1692**
reveling *[Mind]* **180**, *[Gene]* **1932**
revenge *[Drea]* **1692**
revengeful *[Mind]* **180**
reverberations *[Ear]* **495**
reverence *[Mind]* **180**
reveries *[Mind]* **180**
reversed *[Thro]* **708**, *[Slee]* **1651**
reversed action *[Stom]* **783**, *[Rect]* **934**
revolution *[Drea]* **1692**
revolutionist *[Mind]* **180**
revolving *[Ches]* **1259**
rhagades *[Extr]* **1590**, *[Skin]* **1782**
rheumatic *[Blad]* **959**, *[Ches]* **1259**, *[Feve]* **1728**
rheumatic arthritis *[Extr]* **1590**
rheumatic complaints *[Extr]* **1590**
rheumatism *[Mind]* **180**
rhinitis *[Nose]* **537**
rhinopharyngitis *[Thro]* **708**
rhymes *[Mind]* **180**

Index of words

ribs *[Ches]* **1267**

rickets *[Gene]* **1932**

ridiculed *[Mind]* **180**

ridiculous *[Mind]* **180**, *[Drea]* **1692**

riding *[Mind]* **180**, *[Vert]* **234**, *[Head]* **377**, *[Ear]* **495**, *[Uret]* **996**, *[Male]* **1036**, *[Coug]* **1157**, *[Drea]* **1692**, *[Chil]* **1710**, *[Feve]* **1728**, *[Gene]* **1932**

riding in a carriage *[Back]* **1339**

right *[Mind]* **180**, *[Ches]* **1259**, *[Chil]* **1699**, *[Pers]* **1735**

righteous *[Mind]* **180**

rigid *[Mind]* **180**, *[Head]* **377**

rigidity *[Thro]* **708**, *[Abdo]* **886**, *[Fema]* **1087**, *[Extr]* **1590**

rigor *[Chil]* **1710**

ringing *[Coug]* **1157**

rings *[Visi]* **457**

ringworm *[Mout]* **639**, *[Skin]* **1782**

rinsing *[Coug]* **1157**

rinsing mouth *[Gene]* **1933**

riots *[Drea]* **1692**

rise *[Slee]* **1651**

risen and dressed *[Drea]* **1692**

rising *[Vert]* **234**, *[Coug]* **1157**, *[Ches]* **1259**, *[Back]* **1339**, *[Extr]* **1590**, *[Chil]* **1710**, *[Feve]* **1729**, *[Gene]* **1933**

rising body *[Visi]* **457**

rising sensation *[Head]* **377**

rising up *[Stom]* **783**

risus *[Face]* **595**

ritualistic behavior *[Mind]* **180**

rivet *[Ches]* **1259**, *[Gene]* **1933**

roaming *[Drea]* **1692**

robbers *[Mind]* 73, 78, 111, *[Slee]* 1643, *[Drea]* 1684, 1691, **1692**, 1692

robust *[Gene]* **1933**

rocking *[Mind]* **180**, *[Vert]* **235**, *[Gene]* **1933**

rolling *[Mind]* **180**, *[Head]* **377**, *[Eye]* **431**, *[Ear]* **495**, *[Abdo]* **886**, *[Extr]* **1590**, *[Gene]* **1934**

romantic *[Mind]* **180**, *[Drea]* **1692**

romberg's *[Gene]* **1934**

room *[Vert]* **235**, *[Head]* **377**, *[Coug]* **1157**, *[Chil]* **1710**, *[Feve]* **1729**, *[Pers]* **1743**, *[Gene]* **1934**

rooms *[Drea]* **1692**

rope *[Extr]* **1590**

ropy *[Expe]* **1174**

rosy *[Expe]* **1174**

rotary *[Vert]* **235**

rough *[Mind]* **180**, *[Eye]* **431**, *[Ear]* **495**, *[Face]* **595**, *[Resp]* **1132**, *[Coug]* **1157**, *[Skin]* **1782**, *[Gene]* **1934**

roughness *[Nose]* **537**, *[Mout]* **639**, *[Teet]* **680**, *[Thro]* **708**, *[Stom]* **783**, *[Lary]* **1103**, *[Coug]* **1157**, *[Extr]* **1590**

round *[Visi]* **457**

rousing *[Drea]* **1692**

roving *[Mind]* **180**

rowdy *[Drea]* **1692**

rowing *[Drea]* **1692**

rubbed *[Head]* **377**

rubbing *[Mind]* **180**, *[Vert]* **235**, *[Head]* **377**, *[Eye]* **431**, *[Ear]* **495**, *[Face]* **595**, *[Teet]* **680**, *[Abdo]* **886**, *[Rect]* **934**, *[Male]* **1036**, *[Ches]* **1259**, *[Extr]* **1591**, *[Skin]* **1782**, *[Gene]* **1934**

rubbish *[Drea]* **1692**

rubs *[Nose]* **537**

rudeness *[Mind]* **180**

ruins *[Drea]* **1692**

rules *[Mind]* **180**

rumbling *[Stom]* **783**, *[Abdo]* **886**, *[Rect]* **934**, *[Ches]* **1259**, *[Back]* **1339**

run *[Visi]* **457**

runaround *[Extr]* **1591**

running *[Mind]* **180**, *[Head]* **377**, *[Coug]* **1157**, *[Back]* **1340**, *[Slee]* **1651**, *[Drea]* **1692**, *[Gene]* **1934**

running away *[Mind]* **180**

runs *[Mind]* **180**

rupia *[Skin]* **1782**

rupture *[Male]* **1036**

rush *[Ear]* **495**, *[Ches]* **1259**, *[Extr]* **1591**

rushing *[Ches]* **1259**

rusty *[Expe]* **1174**

S

sacral *[Back]* **1349**

sad *[Drea]* **1692**

sad news *[Chil]* **1710**

sad stories *[Mind]* **181**

saddle *[Face]* **596**

sadness *[Mind]* **181**, *[Vert]* **235**, *[Feve]* **1729**, *[Pers]* **1743**

sailing *[Drea]* **1692**

saliva *[Mout]* **640**

saliva-like *[Expe]* **1174**

Index of words

salivation *[Mout]* **641**

salmonellosis *[Rect]* **934**, *[Gene]* **1934**

salpingitis *[Fema]* **1087**

salt *[Teet]* **680**, *[Coug]* **1157**, *[Gene]* **1934**

salts *[Urin]* **1007**

salty *[Pers]* **1743**

sand *[Eye]* **431**, *[Thro]* **709**, *[Stom]* **783**, *[Stoo]* **946**, *[Extr]* **1591**, *[Gene]* **1934**

sanguineous *[Mind]* **186**

sarcasm *[Mind]* **186**

sarcocele *[Male]* **1036**

sarcoidosis *[Ches]* **1259**

sarcoma *[Head]* **240**, *[Eye]* **431**, **436**, *[Nose]* **542**, *[Back]* 1346, *[Gene]* 1807, **1934**, 1956

satiety *[Stom]* **783**

satyriasis *[Mind]* **186**, *[Male]* **1036**

saw *[Coug]* **1157**

sawing *[Resp]* **1132**

scab *[Thro]* **709**

scabies *[Extr]* 1387, 1392, *[Skin]* 1766

scabs *[Nose]* **537**, *[Mout]* **644**, *[Expe]* **1174**

scaly *[Skin]* **1782**

scanty *[Stoo]* **946**, *[Urin]* **1007**, *[Expe]* **1174**

scanty sweat *[Pers]* **1743**

scapegoat *[Mind]* **186**

scaphoid *[Abdo]* **888**

scared *[Mind]* **186**

scarlatina *[Ear]* **495**, *[Coug]* **1157**

scarlet *[Gene]* **1934**

scarlet fever *[Nose]* **537**, *[Feve]* **1729**

scars *[Skin]* **1782**

scattered *[Mind]* **186**

scenes *[Drea]* **1692**

scheuermann' *[Gene]* **1934**

schizophrenia *[Mind]* **186**

school *[Mind]* **186**

sciatica *[Extr]* **1591**

scientific *[Drea]* **1692**

scintillations *[Visi]* **457**

scirrhus *[Male]* **1036**

scleroderma *[Gene]* **1934**

sclerosis *[Head]* **377**, *[Ear]* **495**, *[Kidn]* **979**, *[Fema]* **1087**, *[Ches]* **1259**, *[Back]* **1340**, *[Skin]* **1782**, *[Gene]* **1935**

scoffing *[Mind]* **186**

scolding *[Mind]* **186**

scorbutic g *[Mout]* **644**

scorned *[Mind]* **186**

scorning *[Mind]* **186**

scotoma *[Head]* 272, 280, *[Visi]* **457**

scowl *[Mind]* **186**

scraping *[Nose]* **537**, *[Mout]* **644**, *[Thro]* **709**, *[Lary]* **1104**, *[Coug]* **1157**

scrapings *[Stoo]* **946**

scratch *[Pers]* **1743**

scratching *[Mind]* **186**, *[Vert]* **235**, *[Head]* **377**, *[Ear]* **495**, *[Mout]* **644**, *[Thro]* **709**, *[Fema]* **1087**, *[Lary]* **1104**, *[Coug]* **1158**, *[Extr]* **1591**, *[Chil]* **1710**, *[Gene]* **1935**

screaming *[Mind]* **186**, *[Coug]* **1158**

screeching *[Coug]* **1158**

scrofuloderma *[Skin]* **1782**

scrofulous *[Eye]* **431**, *[Gene]* **1935**

scrotum *[Male]* **1042**

scrupulous *[Mind]* **186**

scrutiny *[Mind]* **186**

scurf *[Male]* **1036**

scurfy *[Nose]* **537**

scurvy *[Gene]* **1935**

sea *[Coug]* **1158**, *[Drea]* **1692**, *[Gene]* **1935**

sea bathing *[Expe]* **1174**

searching *[Mind]* **186**, *[Drea]* **1692**

seasickness *[Gene]* **1935**

seaside *[Gene]* **1935**

seasons *[Mind]* **187**, *[Eye]* **431**, *[Nose]* **537**, *[Thro]* **709**, *[Abdo]* **888**, *[Resp]* **1132**, *[Coug]* **1158**, *[Feve]* **1729**, *[Skin]* **1782**, *[Gene]* **1935**

seborrhea *[Skin]* **1782**

secretive *[Mind]* **187**

secrets *[Mind]* **187**

secure *[Mind]* **187**

sedentary *[Mind]* 20, *[Head]* 283, *[Stom]* 752, *[Rect]* 901, 919, 933, *[Gene]* 1893, 1918, **1935**, 1971

sediment *[Urin]* **1007**

seducing *[Drea]* **1692**

seeing again *[Drea]* **1692**

seized *[Drea]* **1692**

self-absorbed *[Mind]* **187**

self-abuse *[Mind]* **187**

self-accusation *[Mind]* **187**

self-assertion *[Mind]* **187**

self-assured *[Mind]* **187**

self-blame *[Mind]* **187**

self-centered *[Mind]* **187**

self-conscious *[Mind]* **187**

self-contained *[Mind]* **187**

self-control *[Mind]* **187**
self-deception *[Mind]* **187**
self-denial *[Mind]* **187**
self-depreciation *[Mind]* **187**
self-destructive *[Mind]* **187**
self-discipline *[Mind]* **187**
self-distrust *[Mind]* **187**
self-esteem *[Mind]* **187**
self-indulgent *[Mind]* **187**
selfishness *[Mind]* **187**
selflessness *[Mind]* **187**
self-pity *[Mind]* **187**
self-righteous *[Mind]* **187**
self-satisfied *[Mind]* **187**
self-torture *[Mind]* **187**
semen *[Male]* **1036**
semi-conscious *[Slee]* **1651**
seminal *[Male]* **1036**
semisolid *[Stoo]* **946**
senile *[Ches]* **1259**
senile complaints *[Gene]* **1935**
senility *[Mind]* **187**
sensation *[Blad]* **959**, *[Uret]* **996**, *[Pers]* **1743**
senses *[Mind]* **187**
sensibility *[Ear]* **495**, *[Abdo]* **888**, *[Gene]* **1935**
sensible *[Drea]* **1692**
sensitive *[Mind]* **187**, *[Eye]* **431**, *[Ear]* **495**, *[Nose]* **537**, *[Face]* **596**, *[Mout]* **644**, *[Teet]* **680**, *[Thro]* **709**, *[Exte]* **720**, *[Abdo]* **888**, *[Rect]* **934**, *[Blad]* **959**, *[Uret]* **997**, *[Lary]* **1104**, *[Ches]* **1259**, *[Back]* **1340**, *[Extr]* **1591**
sensitiveness *[Head]* **377**, *[Stom]* **783**, *[Kidn]* **979**, *[Male]* **1036**, *[Fema]* **1087**, *[Skin]* **1782**, *[Gene]* **1935**
sensorium *[Mind]* **190**
sensual *[Mind]* **190**, *[Face]* **596**
sensuous *[Mind]* **190**
sentimental *[Mind]* **190**
separated *[Vert]* **235**, *[Head]* **378**, *[Ches]* **1259**, *[Extr]* **1591**
separation *[Mind]* **190**, *[Mout]* **644**
sepsis *[Mind]* **48**, *[Gene]* 1873, **1936**, 1965
sepsis puerperalis *[Fema]* **1088**
septic *[Thro]* 693, *[Abdo]* 822, *[Rect]* 910, 912, *[Urin]* 999, *[Fema]* 1068, 1086, *[Ches]* 1192, *[Slee]* 1656, *[Feve]* 1731, *[Gene]* 1815, 1819, 1870, 1871, 1875, 1979
septic fever *[Feve]* **1729**

septicemia *[Gene]* **1936**
sequelae *[Gene]* **1936**
serene *[Mind]* **190**
series *[Coug]* **1158**
serious *[Mind]* **190**
serious nature of *[Drea]* **1692**
serous *[Fema]* **1088**
serrated *[Teet]* **680**
servile *[Mind]* **191**
severe *[Coug]* **1158**
sewer *[Chil]* **1710**
sewer-gas *[Gene]* **1936**
sewing *[Vert]* **235**, *[Head]* **378**, *[Eye]* **431**, *[Gene]* **1936**
sexual *[Back]* **1340**, *[Pers]* **1743**
sexual aversion *[Male]* **1036**, *[Fema]* **1088**
sexual desire *[Mind]* **191**, *[Head]* **378**, *[Male]* **1036**, *[Fema]* **1088**, *[Gene]* **1936**
sexual development *[Gene]* **1937**
sexual excesses *[Mind]* **191**, *[Male]* **1038**, *[Gene]* **1937**
sexual excitement *[Male]* **1038**, *[Fema]* **1089**, *[Gene]* **1937**
sexual neurasthenia *[Male]* **1038**, *[Fema]* **1089**
sexual passion *[Male]* **1038**
shade *[Visi]* **457**
shadows *[Visi]* **457**
shaking *[Head]* **378**, *[Stom]* **783**, *[Abdo]* **888**, *[Coug]* **1158**, *[Ches]* **1259**, *[Extr]* **1591**, *[Chil]* **1710**
shaking palsy *[Gene]* **1937**
shaking the head *[Vert]* **235**, *[Head]* **378**
shallow *[Resp]* **1132**
shameful *[Mind]* **191**, *[Drea]* **1692**
shameless *[Mind]* **191**
sharp *[Teet]* **681**, *[Coug]* **1158**
sharper *[Visi]* **457**
shattering *[Coug]* **1158**
shaving *[Mind]* **191**, *[Vert]* **235**, *[Face]* **596**, *[Coug]* **1158**, *[Gene]* **1937**
shed *[Drea]* **1692**
sheep *[Stoo]* **946**
shining *[Mind]* **191**, *[Eye]* **431**, *[Stoo]* **946**, *[Extr]* **1592**, *[Skin]* **1783**, *[Gene]* **1937**
shining s *[Male]* **1039**
shiny *[Nose]* **537**, *[Face]* **596**, *[Mout]* **644**
shit *[Mind]* **191**
shivering *[Head]* **378**, *[Face]* **596**, *[Abdo]* **888**, *[Male]* **1039**, *[Ches]* **1259**, *[Back]* **1340**, *[Extr]*

Index of words

size *[Mind]* **194**, *[Visi]* **457**

sjögren's syndrome *[Gene]* **1939**

skating *[Drea]* **1693**

skeletons *[Drea]* **1693**

skeptical *[Mind]* **194**

skepticism *[Mind]* **194**

skin *[Visi]* **457**, *[Mout]* **644**, *[Lary]* **1104**, *[Expe]* **1174**

skullcap *[Head]* **379**

slaking *[Stom]* **784**

slander *[Mind]* **194**

slate colored *[Stoo]* **946**

slate-colored *[Expe]* **1174**

sleep *[Vert]* **235**, *[Head]* **379**, *[Mout]* **644**, *[Fema]* **1089**, *[Resp]* **1132**, *[Coug]* **1159**, *[Back]* **1341**, *[Chil]* **1712**, *[Feve]* **1729**, *[Pers]* **1743**, *[Gene]* **1939**

sleepiness *[Vert]* **235**, *[Slee]* **1652**

sleeping *[Drea]* **1693**

sleeplessness *[Slee]* **1658**

sleeps *[Slee]* **1667**

sleepy *[Eye]* **431**

sleigh-rides *[Drea]* **1693**

sliding down *[Gene]* **1940**

slight *[Chil]* **1712**

slime *[Teet]* **681**

slimy *[Face]* **596**, *[Mout]* **644**, *[Stoo]* **946**, *[Urin]* **1010**, *[Expe]* **1174**

slip *[Rect]* **934**

slippery *[Stoo]* **946**

slipping *[Drea]* **1693**

slipping p *[Extr]* **1593**

slips *[Expe]* **1174**

slovenly *[Mind]* **195**

slow *[Stom]* **784**, *[Rect]* **934**, *[Resp]* **1132**, *[Extr]* **1593**, *[Gene]* **1940**

slowness *[Mind]* **195**

sluggish *[Gene]* **1940**

sluggishness *[Mind]* **195**, *[Gene]* **1940**

slumber *[Slee]* **1667**

sly *[Mind]* **195**

smacking *[Face]* **596**, *[Mout]* **644**

small *[Visi]* **457**, *[Abdo]* **889**, *[Stoo]* **946**, *[Male]* **1039**, *[Fema]* **1089**, *[Ches]* **1260**, *[Extr]* **1593**, *[Skin]* **1783**

small face *[Face]* **596**

small ovaries *[Fema]* **1089**

small tongue *[Mout]* **644**

smaller *[Mind]* **195**, *[Head]* **379**, *[Eye]* **431**, *[Gene]* **1941**

smallpox *[Mind]* **48**, **111**, *[Head]* **252**, *[Eye]* **402**, **409**, *[Stom]* **780**, *[Rect]* **910**, *[Ches]* **1267**, *[Back]* **1275**, *[Slee]* **1657**, **1666**, *[Drea]* **1683**, **1693**, *[Feve]* **1724**, *[Skin]* **1756**, **1767**, **1768**, *[Gene]* **1815**, **1827**, **1874**, **1936**, **1958**

smarting *[Coug]* **1159**, *[Skin]* **1783**

smashed *[Ches]* **1260**

smeared *[Drea]* **1693**

smegma *[Male]* **1039**

smell *[Nose]* **538**, *[Pers]* **1743**

smelling *[Drea]* **1693**

smiling *[Mind]* **195**

smog *[Gene]* **1941**

smoke *[Eye]* **431**, *[Nose]* **538**, *[Lary]* **1104**, *[Coug]* **1159**, *[Ches]* **1260**, *[Gene]* **1941**

smoker' *[Extr]* **1593**

smokers *[Thro]* **709**

smoking *[Mind]* **195**, *[Vert]* **235**, *[Head]* **380**, *[Teet]* **681**, *[Thro]* **709**, *[Abdo]* **889**, *[Coug]* **1159**, *[Drea]* **1693**, *[Pers]* **1743**, *[Gene]* **1941**

smoky *[Visi]* **457**

smooth *[Mout]* **644**, *[Teet]* **681**, *[Gene]* **1941**

smoothness *[Extr]* **1593**

smothered *[Coug]* **1159**

smothering *[Coug]* **1159**

smuggled goods *[Drea]* **1693**

smuttiness *[Extr]* **1593**

smutty *[Face]* **596**

snake *[Visi]* **457**, *[Extr]* **1593**

snakes *[Drea]* **1693**

snapping *[Head]* **380**, *[Ches]* **1260**

snappish *[Mind]* **195**

snarling *[Mind]* **195**

sneering *[Mind]* **195**

sneezing *[Vert]* **235**, *[Head]* **380**, *[Eye]* **431**, *[Nose]* **538**, *[Thro]* **709**, *[Abdo]* **889**, *[Rect]* **934**, *[Resp]* **1132**, *[Coug]* **1159**, *[Ches]* **1260**, *[Back]* **1341**, *[Gene]* **1941**

snoring *[Resp]* **1133**, *[Coug]* **1159**

snow *[Eye]* **432**, *[Visi]* **457**, *[Drea]* **1693**, *[Gene]* **1941**

snow air *[Gene]* **1941**

snowfall *[Coug]* **1159**

snowy weather *[Gene]* **1941**

snub *[Mind]* **195**

snubbed *[Nose]* **541**

Index of words

snuffling *[Nose]* **541**
soaked *[Drea]* **1693**
soap-like *[Expe]* **1174**
soapsuds *[Stoo]* **946**, *[Expe]* **1174**
sobbing *[Mind]* **195**, *[Resp]* **1133**
soberness *[Mind]* **195**
sociability *[Mind]* **195**
social *[Mind]* **5, 85, 111, 132**
social meeting *[Mind]* **195**
society *[Mind]* **95, 111, 130, 131, 132, 148, 185, 195**
sodium *[Urin]* **1010**
sodomy *[Male]* **1039**
soft *[Head]* **380**, *[Mout]* **644**, *[Teet]* **681**, *[Abdo]* **889**, *[Stoo]* **946**, *[Fema]* **1089**, *[Extr]* **1593**, *[Skin]* **1783**, *[Gene]* **1941**
softening *[Head]* **380**, *[Mout]* **645**, *[Stom]* **784**, *[Male]* **1039**, *[Back]* **1341**, *[Extr]* **1593**, *[Gene]* **1941**
soiling *[Drea]* **1693**
solar plexus *[Abdo]* **896**
soldier *[Drea]* **1693**
soldier's heart *[Ches]* **1260**
soldier's heart *[Gene]* **1941**
solemn *[Mind]* **195**
solemnities *[Drea]* **1693**
soles *[Drea]* **1693**
solid *[Coug]* **1159**, *[Back]* **1341**
solitude *[Mind]* **195**
somber *[Mind]* **195**
somersaults *[Drea]* **1693**
somnambulism *[Mind]* **195**
somnambulistic *[Drea]* **1693**
somnolence *[Slee]* **1667**, *[Drea]* **1693**
sonorous *[Coug]* **1159**
sooty *[Nose]* **541**
sopor *[Mind]* **195**, *[Slee]* **1667**
sordes *[Face]* **596**, *[Mout]* **645**, *[Teet]* **681**
sore *[Skin]* **1783**
sore throat *[Thro]* **709**
soreness *[Nose]* **541**, *[Extr]* **1593**
sorrowful *[Mind]* **195**
soul *[Mind]* **74, 76, 82**
soundless *[Coug]* **1159**
sounds *[Ches]* **1260**
sour *[Head]* **380**, *[Expe]* **1174**
sour food *[Coug]* **1159**
sourness *[Gene]* **1941**

space *[Mind]* **195**
spaced-out *[Mind]* **195**
sparkling *[Eye]* **432**
sparks *[Eye]* **432**, *[Visi]* **457**, *[Nose]* **541**, *[Gene]* **1941**
spasm *[Blad]* **959**, *[Uret]* **997**, *[Coug]* **1160**, *[Extr]* **1593**
spasmodic *[Eye]* **432**, *[Blad]* **959**, *[Resp]* **1133**, *[Coug]* **1160**, *[Ches]* **1260**, *[Back]* **1341**
spasms *[Vert]* **235**, *[Eye]* **432**, *[Nose]* **541**, *[Face]* **596**, *[Mout]* **645**, *[Thro]* **709**, *[Exte]* **720**, *[Abdo]* **889**, *[Rect]* **934**, *[Fema]* **1089**, *[Lary]* **1104**, *[Ches]* **1260**, *[Back]* **1341**, *[Gene]* **1941**
speaking *[Coug]* **1160**
specific *[Urin]* **1010**
speech *[Mind]* **195**, *[Mout]* **645**, *[Drea]* **1693**
spermatic cords *[Male]* **1042**
sphincters *[Gene]* **1980**
spices *[Coug]* **1160**
spider *[Skin]* **1783**
spider web *[Face]* **596**
spiders *[Drea]* **1693**
spin *[Vert]* **235**
spina bifida *[Back]* **1341**
spina ventosa *[Extr]* **1593**
spinal irritation *[Back]* **1341**
spinal meningitis *[Back]* **1341**
spinal sclerosis *[Gene]* **1941**
spine *[Coug]* **1160**, *[Back]* **1349**
spineless *[Mind]* **197**
spinning *[Drea]* **1693**
spirit *[Mind]* **50, 62, 74, 77**
spirits *[Coug]* **1160**, *[Drea]* **1693**
spiteful *[Mind]* **197**
spitting *[Mind]* **197**, *[Mout]* **646**, *[Stom]* **784**, *[Gene]* **1941**
splashing *[Head]* **380**, *[Gene]* **1941**
spleen *[Abdo]* **896**, *[Coug]* **1160**
splendor *[Drea]* **1693**
splenomegaly *[Abdo]* **889**
splinter *[Skin]* **1783**, *[Gene]* **1941**
split *[Face]* **596**, *[Extr]* **1593**
splitting *[Coug]* **1160**
spoiled *[Mind]* **197**
spoiled food *[Abdo]* **889**
spoken *[Coug]* **1160**
spoken to *[Mind]* **197**
spondylitis *[Back]* **1341**

Index of words

spondylosis *[Back]* **1341**

sponge *[Abdo]* **889**, *[Extr]* **1593**

spongy *[Mout]* **646**, *[Teet]* **681**, *[Thro]* **710**, *[Fema]* **1089**, *[Gene]* **1941**

spoonerisms *[Mind]* **198**

spot *[Thro]* **710**, *[Stom]* **784**, *[Coug]* **1160**

spots *[Eye]* **432**, *[Visi]* **457**, *[Nose]* **541**, *[Face]* **596**, *[Thro]* **710**, *[Exte]* **720**, *[Abdo]* **889**, *[Male]* **1039**, *[Ches]* **1260**, *[Back]* **1341**, *[Pers]* **1743**, *[Skin]* **1783**, *[Gene]* **1941**

spotted *[Extr]* **1593**

sprained *[Exte]* **720**

sprains *[Extr]* **1593**, *[Gene]* **1941**

spread apart *[Extr]* **1593**

spring *[Vert]* **235**, *[Abdo]* **889**, *[Coug]* **1160**, *[Chil]* **1712**, *[Gene]* **1941**

springs *[Coug]* **1160**

spur calcaneal *[Extr]* **1593**

sputtering *[Stoo]* **947**

spying *[Mind]* **198**

squandering *[Mind]* **198**

square *[Stoo]* **947**

squatting *[Rect]* **933**, *[Fema]* **1055**, **1057**, *[Ches]* **1260**, *[Back]* **1323**, *[Extr]* **1504**, **1596**, **1606**, *[Gene]* **1941**

squeaking *[Nose]* **541**, *[Abdo]* **889**

squeezing *[Gene]* **1941**

squint *[Eye]* **432**

stab *[Drea]* **1693**

stabbed *[Drea]* **1693**

stabbing *[Mind]* **198**

stage fright *[Mind]* **198**

stages *[Chil]* **1712**, *[Feve]* **1729**, *[Pers]* **1743**

staggering *[Vert]* **235**, *[Extr]* **1593**

stagnated *[Gene]* **1941**

stagnation *[Head]* **380**, *[Stom]* **784**, *[Ches]* **1260**

stags *[Drea]* **1693**

staining *[Urin]* **1010**, *[Pers]* **1743**

stairs *[Drea]* **1693**

stamina *[Gene]* **1941**

stammering *[Mind]* **198**, *[Mout]* **646**

stamping feet *[Extr]* **1593**

standing *[Vert]* **235**, *[Abdo]* **889**, *[Rect]* **934**, *[Stoo]* **947**, *[Kidn]* **979**, *[Resp]* **1133**, *[Coug]* **1160**, *[Back]* **1341**, *[Extr]* **1593**, *[Feve]* **1729**, *[Gene]* **1941**

staphyloma *[Eye]* **432**

starch *[Stoo]* **947**, *[Expe]* **1174**

staring *[Mind]* **198**, *[Eye]* **432**

stars *[Vert]* **236**, *[Visi]* **458**, *[Drea]* **1693**

starting *[Mind]* **198**, *[Extr]* **1593**, *[Chil]* **1712**

startled *[Mind]* **200**

starving *[Gene]* **1942**

stasis *[Abdo]* **889**, *[Extr]* **1593**, *[Gene]* **1942**

stating *[Mind]* **200**

statue *[Mind]* **68**, **77**, **133**, **202**, **215**

stealing *[Mind]* **200**, *[Drea]* **1693**

steam *[Gene]* **1942**

steaming *[Pers]* **1743**

steatoma *[Ear]* **495**, **497**, *[Extr]* **1615**, *[Gene]* **1955**, **1956**

stein-leventhal *[Gene]* **1942**

stenocardia *[Ches]* **1260**

stenosis *[Ear]* **495**, *[Stom]* **784**, *[Fema]* **1071**, *[Ches]* **1260**, **1266**, *[Back]* **1341**

stepping *[Gene]* **1942**

stepping hard *[Head]* **380**, *[Ches]* **1260**

stereoscopic *[Visi]* **458**

stereotypic behavior *[Mind]* **200**

stereotypic movements *[Mind]* **200**

sterility *[Male]* **1039**, *[Fema]* **1089**

sternum *[Ches]* **1267**

stertorous *[Resp]* **1133**, *[Coug]* **1160**

stick *[Teet]* **681**

sticking *[Face]* **596**, *[Stoo]* **947**, *[Coug]* **1160**, *[Skin]* **1783**

sticks *[Mout]* **646**

sticky *[Eye]* **432**, *[Mout]* **646**, *[Teet]* **681**, *[Expe]* **1174**, *[Pers]* **1743**

stiff *[Mout]* **646**

stiffening *[Pers]* **1744**

stiffening out *[Gene]* **1942**

stiffness *[Head]* **380**, *[Eye]* **432**, *[Nose]* **541**, *[Face]* **596**, *[Thro]* **710**, *[Exte]* **720**, *[Abdo]* **889**, *[Ches]* **1260**, *[Back]* **1341**, *[Extr]* **1593**, *[Skin]* **1783**, *[Gene]* **1942**

stillness *[Mind]* **200**

stimulants *[Mind]* **200**, *[Coug]* **1161**

stinging *[Coug]* **1161**, *[Skin]* **1783**

stings *[Skin]* **1783**

stirred *[Head]* **380**

stitching *[Coug]* **1161**

stomacace *[Mout]* **646**

stomach *[Vert]* **236**, *[Head]* **380**, *[Coug]* **1161**

stomachache *[Stom]* **784**

stomatitis *[Mout]* **646**

Index of words

Index of words

sudden *[Vert]* **236**, *[Stoo]* **947**, *[Coug]* **1161**, *[Slee]* **1667**, *[Chil]* **1713**, *[Feve]* **1731**, *[Pers]* **1744**, *[Gene]* **1945**

suffering *[Drea]* **1693**

suffocation *[Drea]* **1693**

suffocative *[Thro]* **710**, *[Resp]* **1133**, *[Coug]* **1161**

suffused *[Eye]* **434**

sugar *[Abdo]* **889**, *[Urin]* **1010**, *[Coug]* **1161**

suggestible *[Mind]* **203**

suggestions *[Mind]* **203**, *[Drea]* **1694**

suggillations *[Eye]* **434**

suicidal *[Mind]* 11, 21, 26, 104, 128, 134, 149, 151, 172, 185, **203**, 209, *[Male]* **1038**, *[Fema]* **1089**, *[Gene]* 1844, 1895

suicide *[Mind]* 12, 77, 89, 112, 125, 186, 203, 204, 209, *[Drea]* **1694**

sulky *[Mind]* **204**

sullen *[Mind]* **204**

sulphur *[Thro]* **710**, *[Lary]* **1105**, *[Coug]* **1161**, *[Gene]* **1945**

summer *[Vert]* **236**, *[Stom]* **785**, *[Chil]* **1713**, *[Feve]* **1731**, *[Gene]* **1945**

summing up *[Mind]* **204**

sun *[Vert]* **236**, *[Head]* **380**, *[Coug]* **1162**, *[Feve]* **1731**, *[Gene]* **1945**

sunburn *[Face]* **596**, *[Gene]* 1945

sunken *[Eye]* **434**, *[Nose]* **541**, *[Face]* **596**, *[Abdo]* **889**, *[Gene]* **1945**

sunset *[Gene]* **1945**

sunshine *[Chil]* **1713**

sunstroke *[Mind]* 151, 153, 215, *[Head]* **380**, *[Eye]* **432**, *[Face]* 546, *[Mout]* 616, *[Extr]* 1625, *[Slee]* 1641, *[Gene]* 1819, 1843, **1945**, 1945, 1972

superficial *[Resp]* **1133**, *[Slee]* **1667**

superhuman *[Mind]* 78

supernatural *[Drea]* **1694**

superstitious *[Mind]* **204**

supper *[Coug]* **1162**

support *[Mind]* **204**, *[Coug]* **1162**, *[Gene]* **1945**

supporting *[Vert]* **236**, *[Lary]* **1105**

suppressed *[Mind]* **204**, *[Stoo]* **947**, *[Urin]* **1010**, *[Pers]* **1744**

suppressed complaints *[Gene]* **1945**

suppression *[Mind]* **204**, *[Kidn]* **980**, *[Feve]* **1731**

suppuration *[Ear]* **496**, *[Face]* **597**, *[Mout]* **647**, *[Thro]* **710**, *[Abdo]* **889**, *[Blad]* **960**, *[Kidn]* **980**, *[Pros]* **982**, *[Uret]* **997**, *[Male]* **1039**, *[Ches]* **1260**, *[Extr]* **1598**, *[Gene]* **1945**

surgery *[Gene]* **1945**

surging *[Head]* **381**, *[Ear]* **496**, *[Gene]* **1945**

surprise *[Mind]* 5, *[Head]* **245**, *[Stom]* **783**, *[Blad]* **966**, *[Coug]* **1162**, *[Ches]* **1255**, *[Extr]* **1625**, *[Gene]* 1843, 1954, 1972

surprises *[Mind]* 7, 112

suspended *[Ches]* **1260**

suspense *[Mind]* **204**

suspension *[Vert]* **236**

suspicious *[Mind]* **204**

swallow *[Thro]* **710**, *[Expe]* **1174**

swallowing *[Eye]* **434**, *[Ear]* **496**, *[Face]* **597**, *[Thro]* **710**, *[Exte]* **720**, *[Lary]* **1105**, *[Resp]* **1133**, *[Coug]* **1162**, *[Back]* **1344**, *[Drea]* **1694**, *[Chil]* **1713**, *[Gene]* **1945**

swashing *[Head]* **381**, *[Stom]* **785**, *[Abdo]* **889**, *[Gene]* **1946**

swaying *[Vert]* **236**, *[Extr]* **1598**

swear *[Drea]* **1694**

swearing *[Mind]* **204**

sweetmeats *[Coug]* **1162**

sweetness *[Mind]* **205**

sweets *[Teet]* **681**, *[Thro]* **712**, *[Abdo]* **889**, *[Coug]* **1162**

swelling *[Eye]* **434**, *[Ear]* **496**, *[Nose]* **541**, *[Face]* **597**, *[Mout]* **647**, *[Thro]* **712**, *[Exte]* **720**, *[Stom]* **785**, *[Abdo]* **889**, *[Rect]* **934**, *[Kidn]* **980**, *[Pros]* **982**, *[Uret]* **997**, *[Male]* **1039**, *[Lary]* **1105**, *[Coug]* **1162**, *[Ches]* **1260**, *[Back]* **1344**, *[Extr]* **1598**, *[Skin]* **1783**, *[Gene]* **1946**

swimming *[Mind]* **205**, *[Vert]* **236**, *[Visi]* **458**, *[Ches]* **1261**, *[Drea]* **1694**, *[Gene]* **1947**

swinging *[Vert]* **236**, *[Extr]* **1604**, *[Drea]* **1694**

swollen *[Head]* **381**, *[Eye]* **435**, *[Teet]* **681**, *[Abdo]* **890**, *[Blad]* **960**, *[Fema]* **1090**, *[Skin]* **1784**, *[Gene]* **1947**

swooning fits *[Mind]* **205**

sycosis *[Gene]* **1948**

symmetrical *[Mind]* 81, *[Head]* **240**, *[Face]* 561, 567, *[Mout]* 658, *[Exte]* 715, *[Extr]* 1399, *[Skin]* 1767, 1768, *[Gene]* 1816

sympathetic *[Mind]* **205**, *[Coug]* **1162**

sympathetic ophthalmia *[Eye]* **435**

sympathy *[Mind]* **205**

symphysiolysis *[Fema]* **1090**

symptoms *[Feve]* **1731**, *[Pers]* **1744**

synalgia *[Gene]* **1948**

synchronicity *[Gene]* **1948**

Index of words

synchronous *[Resp]* **1133**
syncope *[Vert]* **236**, *[Gene]* **1948**
syphilis *[Mind]* **205**, *[Abdo]* **890**, *[Gene]* **1948**
syphilitic *[Vert]* **236**, *[Nose]* **542**, *[Thro]* **713**
syringomyelia *[Back]* **1344**
syrup-like *[Expe]* **1174**

T

tabes *[Abdo]* **890**
tachycardia *[Ches]* **1261**
taciturn *[Mind]* **205**
taking *[Mind]* **205**
taking off *[Gene]* **1949**
talented *[Mind]* **205**
talk *[Head]* **381**
talkative *[Mind]* **205**
talking *[Mind]* **205**, *[Vert]* **236**, *[Head]* **381**, *[Ear]* **496**, *[Face]* **599**, *[Thro]* **713**, *[Stom]* **785**, *[Abdo]* **890**, *[Lary]* **1105**, *[Resp]* **1133**, *[Coug]* **1162**, *[Ches]* **1261**, *[Extr]* **1604**, *[Drea]* **1694**, *[Chil]* **1713**, *[Pers]* **1744**, *[Gene]* **1949**
tall *[Vert]* **236**, *[Coug]* **1162**, *[Drea]* **1694**, *[Gene]* **1949**
tallow *[Stoo]* **947**
taphephobia *[Mind]* **206**
tarry-looking *[Stoo]* **947**
tartar *[Teet]* **681**
task-oriented *[Mind]* **206**
taste *[Mout]* **648**, *[Expe]* **1174**, *[Pers]* **1744**
tastelessness *[Mind]* **207**
tea *[Vert]* **236**, *[Head]* **381**, *[Teet]* **681**, *[Coug]* **1162**
tearful *[Mind]* **207**
tearing *[Mind]* **207**, *[Coug]* **1162**, *[Skin]* **1784**
tearing out *[Gene]* **1949**
tears *[Eye]* **435**
teasing *[Mind]* **207**, *[Coug]* **1162**
tea-tasters *[Coug]* **1162**
tedious *[Coug]* **1162**
tedium *[Mind]* **207**
teeth *[Drea]* **1694**, *[Feve]* **1731**, *[Gene]* **1949**
teething *[Teet]* **681**
telling *[Mind]* **207**
temerity *[Mind]* **207**
temper tantrums *[Mind]* **207**
temperature *[Coug]* **1162**, *[Gene]* **1949**
temples *[Head]* **388**, *[Face]* **603**, *[Drea]* **1694**
temporomandibular joint syndrome *[Face]* **599**

tenacious *[Stoo]* **947**, *[Expe]* **1175**
tenderness *[Mind]* **207**, *[Nose]* **542**, *[Exte]* **720**, *[Ches]* **1261**, *[Extr]* **1604**, *[Gene]* **1949**
tendinous *[Stoo]* **947**
tendons *[Back]* **1289**, **1301**, *[Extr]* **1351**, **1365**, **1366**, **1367**, **1370**, **1400**, **1413**, **1415**, **1419**, **1425**, **1471**, **1473**, **1475**, **1476**, **1482**, **1488**, **1508**, **1510**, **1521**, **1528**, **1540**, **1588**, **1596**, **1597**, **1598**, **1601**, **1605**, **1606**, **1608**, **1614**, **1618**, **1620**, *[Gene]* **1816**, **1829**, **1876**, **1877**, **1879**, **1903**, **1918**, **1942**, **1947**
tenesmus *[Stom]* **778**, **796**, *[Abdo]* **845**, *[Rect]* **923**, **924**, **925**, **926**, **928**, **929**, **930**, **931**, **934**, *[Blad]* **955**, **960**, **962**, *[Kidn]* **976**, *[Uret]* **986**, **997**, *[Male]* **1027**, *[Fema]* **1043**, **1062**, **1067**, **1075**, *[Slee]* **1655**
tenonitis *[Eye]* **435**
tension *[Mind]* **207**, *[Head]* **381**, *[Eye]* **435**, *[Ear]* **496**, *[Nose]* **542**, *[Face]* **599**, *[Mout]* **656**, *[Teet]* **681**, *[Thro]* **713**, *[Exte]* **720**, *[Stom]* **785**, *[Abdo]* **890**, *[Rect]* **934**, *[Blad]* **960**, *[Kidn]* **980**, *[Pros]* **983**, *[Uret]* **997**, *[Male]* **1040**, *[Lary]* **1105**, *[Coug]* **1162**, *[Ches]* **1261**, *[Back]* **1344**, *[Extr]* **1604**, *[Skin]* **1784**, *[Gene]* **1949**
terrapin *[Drea]* **1694**
terrified *[Mind]* **207**
terror *[Mind]* **207**
tertian *[Chil]* **1713**
test *[Drea]* **1694**
testes *[Male]* **1042**
tetanus *[Gene]* **1950**
thalassemia *[Gene]* **1950**
thanatophobia *[Mind]* **207**
theater *[Drea]* **1694**
theft *[Drea]* **1694**
theorizing *[Mind]* **207**
thick *[Nose]* **542**, *[Face]* **600**, *[Mout]* **656**, *[Thro]* **713**, *[Urin]* **1010**, *[Expe]* **1175**, *[Extr]* **1608**, *[Skin]* **1784**
thickening *[Eye]* **436**, *[Ear]* **496**, *[Blad]* **960**, *[Male]* **1040**
thighs *[Extr]* **1637**, *[Pers]* **1744**
thin *[Head]* **381**, *[Face]* **600**, *[Stoo]* **947**, *[Male]* **1040**, *[Expe]* **1175**, *[Extr]* **1608**, *[Skin]* **1784**, *[Gene]* **1950**
things *[Lary]* **1105**, *[Drea]* **1694**
thinking *[Mind]* **207**, *[Vert]* **236**, *[Head]* **381**, *[Eye]* **436**, *[Coug]* **1162**, *[Chil]* **1713**
thinking of the pain *[Face]* **600**
thirst *[Stom]* **785**, *[Gene]* **1950**

Index of words

thirstless *[Stom]* **788**, *[Feve]* **1731**, *[Gene]* **1950**

thirsty *[Drea]* **1694**

thoughts *[Mind]* **207**

thread *[Eye]* **436**, *[Visi]* **458**, *[Mout]* **656**, *[Thro]* **713**, *[Ches]* **1261**

threads *[Head]* **381**, *[Extr]* **1608**, *[Gene]* **1950**

threatened *[Mind]* **210**

threatening *[Mind]* **210**

threats *[Drea]* **1694**

three *[Coug]* **1162**

thrill *[Male]* **1040**

thrilling *[Extr]* **1608**, *[Skin]* **1784**

throat *[Drea]* **1694**

throbbing *[Head]* **381**, *[Ear]* **497**, *[Nose]* **542**, *[Ches]* **1262**, *[Gene]* **1950**

thromboangitis *[Gene]* **1950**

thrombocytopenia *[Gene]* **1950**

thromboembolism *[Gene]* **1950**

thrombosis *[Head]* **381**, *[Eye]* **436**, *[Ches]* **1262**, *[Extr]* **1582**, **1608**, *[Gene]* **1950**

throwing *[Mind]* **210**, *[Head]* **381**, *[Drea]* **1694**

throwing back *[Ches]* **1262**

thrown *[Extr]* **1608**, *[Drea]* **1694**

throws *[Extr]* **1608**

thrush *[Mout]* **656**

thrusts *[Abdo]* **892**, *[Extr]* **1608**

thumb sucking *[Mout]* **656**

thumbs *[Extr]* **1637**

thunderstorm *[Mind]* **211**, *[Coug]* **1162**, *[Drea]* **1694**, *[Gene]* **1950**

thyroid gland *[Exte]* **721**

tic *[Face]* **600**

tic douloureux *[Face]* **600**

tickled *[Drea]* **1694**

tickling *[Head]* **381**, *[Eye]* **436**, *[Ear]* **497**, *[Nose]* **542**, *[Mout]* **656**, *[Teet]* **681**, *[Thro]* **713**, *[Exte]* **721**, *[Stom]* **789**, *[Rect]* **934**, *[Uret]* **997**, *[Male]* **1040**, *[Lary]* **1105**, *[Coug]* **1162**, *[Ches]* **1262**, *[Extr]* **1608**, *[Gene]* **1950**

ticklish *[Gene]* **1950**

ticklishness *[Mind]* **211**

tics *[Mind]* **211**, *[Gene]* **1950**

tidy *[Mind]* **211**

tied *[Head]* **381**, *[Male]* **1040**, *[Extr]* **1608**

tight *[Exte]* **721**, *[Stom]* **789**, *[Resp]* **1133**, *[Coug]* **1163**, *[Back]* **1345**

tightness *[Head]* **381**, *[Face]* **600**, *[Fema]* **1090**, *[Lary]* **1106**, *[Coug]* **1163**, *[Ches]* **1262**, *[Extr]* **1608**

time *[Mind]* **211**, *[Drea]* **1694**, *[Gene]* **1950**

timidity *[Mind]* **211**

tinea capitis *[Head]* **381**, *[Gene]* **1950**

tinea versicolor *[Skin]* **1784**, *[Gene]* **1950**

tingling *[Head]* **381**, *[Eye]* **436**, *[Ear]* **497**, *[Nose]* **542**, *[Face]* **600**, *[Mout]* **656**, *[Thro]* **713**, *[Exte]* **721**, *[Stom]* **789**, *[Abdo]* **892**, *[Rect]* **934**, *[Uret]* **997**, *[Male]* **1040**, *[Fema]* **1090**, *[Lary]* **1106**, *[Coug]* **1163**, *[Ches]* **1262**, *[Back]* **1346**, *[Extr]* **1608**, *[Skin]* **1784**, *[Gene]* **1950**

tinnitus *[Vert]* **236**, *[Ear]* **497**

tip *[Nose]* **543**

tipsy *[Mind]* **212**

tired *[Head]* **382**, *[Coug]* **1163**, *[Extr]* **1610**, *[Gene]* **1950**

tired expression *[Eye]* **436**

tired feeling *[Face]* **600**

tired sensation *[Eye]* **436**

tiring *[Drea]* **1694**

titillating *[Coug]* **1164**

toad *[Drea]* **1694**

tobacco *[Mind]* **21**, **67**, **79**, **116**, **169**, **186**, *[Vert]* **236**, *[Eye]* **390**, **436**, *[Visi]* **455**, *[Ear]* **488**, *[Nose]* **530**, **538**, *[Face]* **546**, **585**, *[Mout]* **609**, **634**, **636**, **648**, **650**, **651**, **652**, **653**, **655**, **656**, *[Teet]* **675**, *[Thro]* **709**, *[Stom]* **738**, **744**, **747**, **752**, **763**, **783**, *[Abdo]* **809**, **845**, *[Rect]* **901**, **910**, *[Pros]* **981**, *[Urin]* **1006**, *[Male]* **1019**, **1020**, *[Lary]* **1101**, **1105**, **1109**, *[Coug]* **1159**, **1164**, *[Expe]* **1175**, *[Ches]* **1179**, **1226**, **1253**, **1255**, **1262**, *[Extr]* **1613**, *[Slee]* **1666**, *[Feve]* **1731**, *[Gene]* **1827**, **1861**, **1893**, **1896**, **1950**, **1950**, **1951**, **1972**

tobacco poisoning *[Gene]* **1951**

toe *[Drea]* **1694**

toes *[Extr]* **1637**

toilets *[Drea]* **1694**

tolerant *[Mind]* **212**

toneless *[Coug]* **1164**

tongue *[Mout]* **659**, *[Drea]* **1694**

tongue-tie *[Mout]* **656**

tonsillitis *[Thro]* **713**, *[Gene]* **1951**

tonsils *[Thro]* **714**

toothache *[Teet]* **681**

tormented *[Mind]* **212**

tormenting *[Mind]* **212**, *[Coug]* **1164**

Index of words

torpor *[Mind]* **212**, *[Nose]* **542**, *[Teet]* **681**, *[Abdo]* **892**, *[Gene]* **1951**

torticollis *[Thro]* **686**, *[Exte]* **721**, 721

torturing *[Mind]* **212**

tossing *[Extr]* **1610**, *[Slee]* **1667**, *[Drea]* **1694**

tottering gait *[Extr]* **1610**

touch *[Vert]* **236**, *[Head]* **382**, *[Eye]* **436**, *[Face]* **600**, *[Teet]* **681**, *[Exte]* **721**, *[Stom]* **789**, *[Abdo]* **892**, *[Lary]* **1106**, *[Resp]* **1133**, *[Back]* **1346**, *[Extr]* **1611**, *[Chil]* **1713**, *[Skin]* **1784**, *[Gene]* **1951**

touched *[Mind]* **212**, *[Coug]* **1164**

touching *[Mind]* **212**, *[Chil]* **1713**, *[Gene]* **1952**

touchy *[Mind]* **212**

tough *[Mind]* **212**, *[Stoo]* **948**, *[Expe]* **1175**, *[Extr]* **1611**

tourette's *[Mind]* **212**

toys *[Mind]* **79**, 167

trachea *[Lary]* **1110**

trachoma *[Eye]* **436**

train *[Mind]* **20**, 21, 73, 79, *[Vert]* 234, *[Stom]* 761, *[Rect]* 910, *[Blad]* 966, *[Drea]* 1687, 1688, **1694**, 1694, *[Gene]* 1933

trance *[Mind]* **212**

tranquillity *[Mind]* **212**

transparent *[Teet]* **681**, *[Stoo]* **948**, *[Expe]* **1176**

transplant *[Gene]* **1952**

trapped *[Mind]* **212**

trauma *[Mind]* **212**

traumatic *[Feve]* **1731**

traumatism *[Extr]* **1611**

travelling *[Mind]* **212**, *[Drea]* **1694**, *[Gene]* **1952**

treatment *[Drea]* **1694**

trembling *[Vert]* **236**, *[Head]* **382**, *[Visi]* **458**, *[Ear]* **497**, *[Face]* **600**, *[Mout]* **656**, *[Teet]* **681**, *[Exte]* **721**, *[Stom]* **789**, *[Abdo]* **892**, *[Rect]* **934**, *[Ches]* **1262**, *[Back]* **1346**, *[Extr]* **1611**, *[Chil]* **1713**, *[Skin]* **1784**, *[Gene]* **1952**

tremulous *[Eye]* **436**, *[Nose]* **542**, *[Resp]* **1133**

tribadism *[Mind]* **212**

trichiasis *[Eye]* **436**

trickling *[Back]* **1346**, *[Gene]* **1954**

tricky *[Mind]* **212**

trifles *[Mind]* **9**, 10, 21, 25, 26, 28, 35, 40, 41, 47, 52, 85, 98, 113, 117, 121, 124, 128, 136, 137, 140, 141, 143, 145, 162, 170, 171, 172, 174, 186, 193, 194, 200, **212**, 215, 216, 217, 222, 223, *[Gene]* 1843, **1954**, 1972

trigeminal neuralgia *[Face]* **600**

triplopia *[Visi]* **458**

trismus *[Face]* **600**

triumph *[Drea]* **1694**

tropical *[Feve]* **1731**

trouble *[Drea]* **1694**

troubles *[Mind]* 26, 79, 113, 206, *[Resp]* 1129, *[Ches]* 1200, *[Skin]* 1770, *[Gene]* 1926

true *[Drea]* **1694**

true on waking *[Drea]* **1694**

trumpet-toned *[Coug]* **1164**

tube *[Resp]* **1133**, *[Coug]* **1164**, *[Gene]* **1954**

tubercle *[Ear]* **497**, *[Rect]* **934**

tubercles *[Mout]* **656**, *[Male]* **1040**, *[Fema]* **1090**, *[Expe]* **1176**, *[Back]* **1346**, *[Extr]* **1615**

tuberculosis *[Abdo]* **892**, *[Lary]* **1106**, *[Ches]* **1262**, *[Back]* **1346**, *[Extr]* **1615**, *[Gene]* **1954**

tuberculous *[Coug]* **1164**

tumor *[Head]* 321, 381, *[Eye]* 430, *[Nose]* **542**, *[Face]* **600**, 600, *[Stom]* **789**, *[Abdo]* 880, *[Uret]* 985, **997**, *[Male]* **1040**, *[Skin]* 1789

tumors *[Head]* **382**, *[Eye]* **436**, 436, *[Ear]* **497**, 497, *[Mout]* **656**, *[Exte]* **721**, *[Stom]* 730, 792, *[Abdo]* **892**, *[Blad]* **960**, *[Kidn]* **980**, *[Fema]* **1090**, *[Lary]* **1106**, *[Ches]* **1262**, *[Back]* **1346**, *[Extr]* 1398, **1615**, *[Pers]* **1740**, *[Skin]* **1784**, *[Gene]* 1822, 1871, **1955**

turbid *[Urin]* **1011**

turn *[Eye]* **436**, *[Drea]* **1694**

turned *[Vert]* **236**, *[Head]* **382**, *[Eye]* **436**

turning *[Vert]* **237**, *[Head]* **382**, *[Thro]* **713**, *[Stom]* **789**, *[Abdo]* **892**, *[Fema]* **1091**, *[Coug]* **1164**, *[Expe]* **1176**, *[Ches]* **1262**, *[Back]* **1346**, *[Extr]* **1615**, *[Chil]* **1713**, *[Gene]* **1956**

turning and twisting *[Head]* **382**

turning head *[Ear]* **497**, *[Lary]* **1106**

turning in bed *[Vert]* **237**

turning the eyes *[Eye]* **437**

turpentine *[Gene]* **1956**

twilight *[Mind]* **213**, *[Visi]* **458**, *[Gene]* **1956**

twisted *[Eye]* **437**, *[Teet]* **681**

twisting *[Head]* **382**, *[Stom]* **789**, *[Blad]* **960**, *[Extr]* **1615**

twitching *[Head]* **382**, *[Eye]* **437**, *[Ear]* **497**, *[Nose]* **542**, *[Face]* **601**, *[Mout]* **657**, *[Teet]* **681**, *[Thro]* **713**, *[Exte]* **721**, *[Stom]* **790**, *[Abdo]* **892**, *[Rect]* **934**, *[Blad]* **960**, *[Kidn]* **980**, *[Pros]* **983**, *[Uret]* **997**, *[Male]* **1040**, *[Fema]* **1091**, *[Coug]* **1164**,

Index of words

[Ches] **1262**, [Back] **1346**, [Extr] **1615**, [Gene] **1956**

two [Coug] **1164**
two-dimensional [Visi] **458**
tympanites [Abdo] **892**, [Gene] **1957**
tympanitic [Abdo] **892**
tympanitis [Ear] **497**, [Stom] **790**, [Gene] **1957**
tympanum [Ear] **499**
typhlitis [Abdo] **892**
typhoid fever [Feve] **1731**
typhus abdominalis [Gene] **1957**
typhus fever [Feve] **1732**

U

ulceration [Eye] **437**, [Ear] **497**, [Teet] **681**, [Rect] **934**, [Blad] **960**, [Uret] **997**, [Lary] **1106**, [Coug] **1164**
ulcerative p [Skin] **1784**
ulcers [Head] **383**, [Ear] **497**, [Nose] **542**, [Face] **601**, [Mout] **657**, [Thro] **713**, [Exte] **721**, [Stom] **790**, [Abdo] **892**, [Male] **1040**, [Fema] **1091**, [Ches] **1262**, [Back] **1346**, [Extr] **1620**, [Skin] **1784**, [Gene] **1957**
umbilicus [Abdo] **896**
unattractive [Mind] **213**
uncle [Drea] **1694**
uncleanliness [Gene] **1957**
unconcerned [Mind] **213**
unconscious [Extr] **1621**
unconsciousness [Mind] **213**, [Vert] **237**, [Coug] **1164**, [Drea] **1694**
uncoordinated [Extr] **1622**
uncover [Extr] **1622**
uncovered [Chil] **1713**, [Pers] **1745**
uncovering [Head] **383**, [Exte] **721**, [Abdo] **892**, [Coug] **1164**, [Ches] **1263**, [Back] **1346**, [Extr] **1622**, [Drea] **1694**, [Chil] **1713**, [Feve] **1732**, [Pers] **1744**, [Gene] **1957**
understanding [Mind] **215**
undertaking [Mind] **215**
undescended [Male] **1041**
undeveloped [Male] **1041**
undigested [Stoo] **948**
undignified [Mind] **215**
undressing [Mind] **215**, [Fema] **1091**, [Coug] **1164**, [Gene] **1958**
undulant [Feve] **1732**

undulation [Ches] **1263**
uneasiness [Mind] **215**, [Stom] **790**, [Abdo] **892**, [Blad] **960**, [Pros] **983**, [Extr] **1622**
uneasy [Nose] **543**
unfeeling [Mind] **215**
unforgiving [Mind] **216**
unfortunate [Mind] **216**
unfriendly [Mind] **216**
ungracious [Mind] **216**
ungrateful [Mind] **216**
unhappiness [Mind] **216**
unhealthy [Skin] **1789**
unhealthy skin [Extr] **1622**
unification [Mind] **216**
unimportant [Drea] **1695**
uninterrupted [Coug] **1164**
unlovable [Mind] **216**
unmarried [Gene] **1958**
unnatural [Hear] **504**
unnoticed [Rect] **935**
unobserving [Mind] **216**
unpleasant [Drea] **1695**
unpractical [Mind] **216**
unreal [Mind] **216**
unreasonable [Mind] **216**
unrefined [Mind] **216**
unrefreshing [Slee] **1667**
unreliable [Mind] **216**
unremembered [Drea] **1695**
unrequited sexual passion [Male] **1041**
unscrupulous [Mind] **216**
unsociable [Mind] **216**
unsteadiness [Extr] **1622**
unsteady [Head] **383**, [Eye] **438**
unsuccessful efforts [Drea] **1695**
unsympathetic [Mind] **216**
untidy [Mind] **216**
untruthful [Mind] **216**
unworthy [Mind] **216**
upheaval [Mind] **216**
upper [Chil] **1713**
upper arms [Extr] **1638**
upper limbs [Extr] **1638**
uptight [Mind] **216**
urate [Kidn] 980, [Urin] 1001, 1010
urea [Urin] **1011**

Index of words

uremia *[Mind]* 34, *[Kidn]* 974, **980**, *[Resp]* 1115, 1122, *[Ches]* 1265, *[Slee]* 1641, 1642, *[Gene]* 1802, **1958**

uremic *[Mind]* 215, *[Head]* 246, 306, *[Gene]* 1828

urethritis *[Uret]* **997**

urging *[Stom]* 790, *[Abdo]* **893**, *[Rect]* **935**, *[Uret]* **997**, *[Back]* **1346**, *[Gene]* **1958**

uric acid *[Kidn]* 980, *[Gene]* **1958**

urinary *[Blad]* **960**

urinating *[Mind]* 216, *[Drea]* **1695**

urination *[Vert]* 237, *[Head]* 383, *[Eye]* 438, *[Ear]* 497, *[Stom]* 790, *[Abdo]* **893**, *[Rect]* 936, *[Blad]* 960, *[Kidn]* 980, *[Pros]* 983, *[Uret]* 997, *[Male]* 1041, *[Fema]* 1091, *[Resp]* 1134, *[Ches]* 1263, *[Back]* **1346**, *[Extr]* 1622, *[Chil]* 1713, *[Pers]* **1744**, *[Gene]* **1958**

urine *[Uret]* 997, *[Drea]* **1695**

useful *[Mind]* 216

uterus *[Fema]* 1092

uveitis *[Eye]* **438**

uvula *[Thro]* 714

V

vacant *[Head]* 383, *[Eye]* **438**

vaccination *[Head]* 264, 306, 385, *[Eye]* 402, *[Ear]* 469, *[Face]* 561, *[Stom]* 763, 777, *[Rect]* 910, *[Resp]* 1116, 1118, *[Coug]* **1164**, *[Extr]* 1384, 1393, 1400, 1582, 1598, 1603, *[Slee]* 1651, 1667, *[Feve]* **1732**, *[Skin]* 1759, 1771, **1789**, *[Gene]* 1819, 1828, 1844, 1871, 1893, 1906, 1919, 1936, **1958**, 1958

vacillate *[Eye]* **438**

vacillation *[Mind]* 216

vagina *[Fema]* 1092

vaginismus *[Fema]* **1091**

vaginitis *[Fema]* **1091**

valve *[Ear]* **497**

valvular *[Ches]* **1267**

vampires *[Drea]* **1695**

vanishing *[Visi]* **458**

vanity *[Mind]* 216

vapor *[Thro]* **714**, *[Coug]* **1164**, *[Ches]* **1263**

varices *[Extr]* **1622**

varicocele *[Male]* **1041**

varicose *[Mind]* 134, *[Nose]* 521, *[Face]* **602**, 602, *[Mout]* **658**, *[Thro]* **714**, *[Abdo]* 893, *[Rect]* **936**, *[Extr]* 1353, 1421, 1608, 1615, 1620, 1621, *[Skin]* 1789, *[Gene]* **1958**

varicosities *[Extr]* **1623**

variegated *[Visi]* **458**

variola *[Coug]* **1164**

varnished *[Mout]* **658**

vaults *[Coug]* **1164**, *[Gene]* **1959**

vehement *[Mind]* **216**, *[Resp]* **1134**

vehicles *[Drea]* **1695**

veil *[Visi]* **458**

veins *[Mind]* 134, *[Head]* 240, 249, 256, 279, 381, *[Eye]* 396, 397, **438**, *[Ear]* 465, *[Nose]* 521, **543**, *[Face]* 551, **602**, 602, 603, *[Exte]* 720, *[Abdo]* **893**, *[Rect]* 917, *[Fema]* **1091**, *[Back]* 1344, *[Extr]* 1353, 1385, 1403, 1404, 1415, 1521, 1575, 1598, 1600, 1601, 1602, 1608, 1622, 1638, *[Slee]* 1647, 1662, *[Feve]* 1721, 1723, 1724, *[Skin]* 1749, *[Gene]* 1868, 1873, 1874, 1918, 1920, 1925, 1947, **1959**, 1980

velvet *[Mout]* **658**

velvety *[Lary]* **1106**, *[Ches]* **1263**

veneration *[Mind]* 216

venesection *[Gene]* **1959**

vengeance *[Drea]* **1695**

venous pulsations *[Gene]* **1959**

venous stasis *[Gene]* **1959**

veratrum *[Gene]* **1959**

verifying *[Mind]* 216

vermin *[Drea]* **1695**

verminosis *[Rect]* **936**

verses *[Mind]* **216**, *[Drea]* **1695**

vertebra *[Back]* 1273, 1300, 1301, 1314, 1315, 1318, 1346, *[Gene]* 1923

vertebrae *[Stom]* 802, *[Abdo]* 854, *[Back]* 1269, 1271, 1273, 1276, 1277, 1278, 1279, 1280, 1281, 1301, 1305, 1314, 1315, 1329, 1336, 1337, 1338, 1339, 1340, 1344, 1346, 1347, 1349, *[Extr]* 1528, *[Gene]* 1923

vertex *[Vert]* 237, *[Head]* **388**

vertigo *[Vert]* **225**, *[Head]* 383, *[Drea]* **1695**, *[Chil]* **1713**, *[Feve]* **1732**, *[Gene]* **1959**

vesicles *[Eye]* **438**, *[Mout]* **658**, *[Uret]* 997, *[Ches]* **1263**

vexation *[Mind]* 7, 21, 30, 40, 49, 80, 92, 104, 113, 130, 135, 141, 144, 145, 151, 154, 170, 186, 194, 211, **216**, 220, 222, 223, *[Vert]* 237, *[Head]* 262, 306, 324, 341, *[Visi]* 443, 449, *[Ear]* 488, *[Face]* 551, 554, 557, 558, 575, 585, *[Mout]* 646, 650, *[Teet]* 675, *[Stom]* 723, 728, 732, 738, 741, 752, 763, 777, 796, 797, 799, *[Abdo]* 823, 845, 868,

Index of words

880, *[Rect]* 901, 910, 930, *[Fema]* 1043, 1058, 1062, 1065, 1067, 1070, *[Resp]* 1118, 1127, *[Coug]* **1164**, *[Ches]* 1178, 1217, 1235, 1244, 1255, *[Back]* 1292, 1311, 1326, *[Extr]* 1361, 1410, 1412, 1493, 1515, 1526, 1530, 1538, 1573, 1614, 1616, **1623**, 1628, 1630, *[Slee]* 1651, 1667, *[Chil]* **1713**, *[Feve]* **1732**, *[Pers]* **1744**, *[Skin]* 1754, *[Gene]* 1824, 1828, 1896, 1911, 1926, 1927, 1954, 1972

vexatious *[Drea]* **1695**
vexed *[Mind]* **216**
vibrating *[Head]* **383**
vibration *[Visi]* **458**, *[Male]* **1041**, *[Ches]* **1263**, *[Back]* **1347**, *[Extr]* **1623**, *[Gene]* **1959**
vicarious *[Nose]* 523, *[Rect]* 916, *[Uret]* 988, *[Fema]* 1067, *[Ches]* 1194, *[Gene]* 1832, 1870
vice *[Exte]* **721**
vigor *[Gene]* **1959**
vindictive *[Mind]* **216**
vinegar *[Stom]* 790, *[Coug]* **1164**, *[Gene]* **1959**
violence *[Mind]* **216**, *[Drea]* **1695**
violent *[Mind]* **216**, *[Vert]* **237**, *[Coug]* **1164**, *[Chil]* **1713**, *[Feve]* **1732**
violent complaints *[Gene]* **1959**
violin *[Coug]* **1164**
virilism *[Fema]* **1091**
viscid *[Urin]* **1011**, *[Expe]* **1176**
viscous *[Pers]* **1744**
vision *[Vert]* **237**
visionary *[Drea]* **1695**
visions *[Mind]* **217**, *[Visi]* **458**
visits *[Drea]* **1695**
vital *[Mind]* **217**
vitality *[Gene]* **1960**
vitiligo *[Skin]* **1790**
vivacious *[Mind]* **217**
vivid *[Drea]* **1695**
voice *[Lary]* **1106**, *[Coug]* **1164**, *[Drea]* **1696**, *[Gene]* **1960**
voices *[Mind]* 11, 81, 113, 189, 200, *[Head]* 295, 369, *[Ear]* 479, *[Hear]* 501
volkmann' *[Gene]* **1960**
voluminous *[Stoo]* **948**
voluptuous *[Uret]* **997**, *[Male]* **1041**
voluptuous sensation *[Fema]* **1092**
vomiting *[Mind]* **217**, *[Vert]* **237**, *[Head]* **383**, *[Eye]* **438**, *[Abdo]* **893**, *[Rect]* **936**, *[Coug]* **1164**, *[Ches]*

1263, *[Slee]* **1668**, *[Drea]* **1696**, *[Chil]* **1713**, *[Feve]* **1732**, *[Pers]* **1744**, *[Gene]* **1960**

vomiting; type of *[Stom]* **796**
vulgar scenes *[Drea]* **1696**
vulnerable *[Mind]* **217**
vulva *[Abdo]* 813, *[Rect]* 921, 931, *[Fema]* 1044, 1046, 1048, 1050, 1051, 1052, 1059, 1071, 1084, 1085, 1089, 1090, 1091, *[Extr]* 1615, *[Gene]* 1831

W

wading *[Drea]* **1696**
wagons *[Drea]* **1696**
wailing *[Mind]* **217**
wakens *[Coug]* **1165**
waking *[Mind]* **217**, *[Vert]* **237**, *[Stoo]* **948**, *[Coug]* **1165**, *[Slee]* **1668**, *[Chil]* **1713**, *[Feve]* **1732**, *[Gene]* **1960**
walking *[Mind]* **217**, *[Vert]* **237**, *[Head]* **383**, *[Stom]* **801**, *[Abdo]* **893**, *[Rect]* **936**, *[Blad]* **971**, *[Kidn]* **980**, *[Pros]* **983**, *[Uret]* **997**, *[Male]* **1041**, *[Coug]* **1165**, *[Expe]* **1176**, *[Back]* **1347**, *[Extr]* **1623**, *[Slee]* **1671**, *[Drea]* **1696**, *[Chil]* **1714**, *[Feve]* **1732**, *[Pers]* **1744**, *[Gene]* **1960**
walls *[Vert]* **238**
walnut *[Abdo]* **893**
wandering *[Mind]* **217**, *[Eye]* **438**, *[Drea]* **1696**
want *[Drea]* **1696**
wanting *[Back]* **1347**
wants *[Mind]* **218**
war *[Drea]* **1696**
warbling *[Head]* **383**
warm *[Vert]* **238**, *[Head]* **383**, *[Eye]* **438**, *[Nose]* **543**, *[Mout]* **658**, *[Teet]* **681**, *[Abdo]* **893**, *[Fema]* **1092**, *[Coug]* **1165**, *[Ches]* **1263**, *[Back]* **1347**, *[Extr]* **1623**, *[Chil]* **1714**, *[Feve]* **1732**, *[Pers]* **1744**, *[Skin]* **1790**, *[Gene]* **1961**
warm ;becoming *[Coug]* **1165**
warm applications *[Rect]* **936**
warm in bed *[Pers]* **1745**
warm; becoming *[Gene]* **1963**
warmblooded *[Gene]* **1963**
warmth *[Vert]* **238**, *[Head]* **383**, *[Ear]* **497**, *[Nose]* **543**, *[Face]* **602**, *[Mout]* **658**, *[Teet]* **681**, *[Thro]* **714**, *[Stom]* **801**, *[Abdo]* **893**, *[Kidn]* **980**, *[Pros]* **983**, *[Uret]* **997**, *[Male]* **1041**, *[Fema]* **1092**, *[Lary]* **1110**, *[Coug]* **1165**, *[Ches]* **1263**, *[Back]* **1347**,

Index of words

[Extr] **1623**, [Chil] **1714**, [Feve] **1732**, [Skin] **1790**, [Gene] **1963**

wart [Thro] **714**

wart-like [Ear] **497**

warts [Mind] **82**, [Eye] **438**, [Nose] **543**, [Face] **602**, [Mout] **658**, [Exte] **721**, [Abdo] **893**, [Rect] **936**, [Male] **1041**, [Fema] **1092**, [Lary] **1110**, [Ches] **1263**, [Back] **1347**, [Extr] **1623**, 1637, [Drea] 1675, 1677, **1696**, 1696, [Skin] **1790**, 1790, [Gene] 1945

wash [Face] **602**

wash off [Pers] **1745**

washes [Extr] **1624**

washing [Mind] **218**, [Vert] **238**, [Head] **383**, [Extr] **1624**, [Feve] **1732**, [Pers] **1745**, [Skin] **1790**, [Gene] **1963**

wasps [Drea] **1696**

wasting [Mind] **218**, [Extr] **1624**

watched [Mind] **218**

watchfulness [Mind] **218**

watching [Vert] **238**

water [Mind] **218**, [Vert] **238**, [Head] **383**, [Ear] **497**, [Nose] **543**, [Teet] **681**, [Thro] **714**, [Stom] **801**, [Abdo] **893**, [Coug] **1165**, [Ches] **1263**, [Back] **1347**, [Extr] **1624**, [Drea] **1696**, [Chil] **1714**, [Feve] **1733**, [Gene] **1963**

water brash [Mout] **658**, [Stom] **801**

watery [Eye] **438**, [Mout] **658**, [Stoo] **948**, [Urin] **1011**, [Expe] **1176**

wavelike [Vert] **238**, [Back] **1347**, [Gene] **1963**

wavering [Visi] **458**

waves [Vert] **238**, [Drea] **1696**, [Chil] **1714**

waving [Head] **384**, [Visi] **458**

wax [Ear] **498**

waxy [Face] **602**, [Abdo] **893**, [Stoo] **949**, [Skin] **1790**

weak [Eye] **438**, [Visi] **458**

weak character [Mind] **218**

weakness [Mind] **218**, [Vert] **238**, [Head] **384**, [Face] **602**, [Mout] **658**, [Teet] **681**, [Thro] **714**, [Stom] **801**, [Abdo] **893**, [Rect] **936**, [Blad] **971**, [Kidn] **980**, [Male] **1041**, [Fema] **1092**, [Lary] **1110**, [Ches] **1263**, [Back] **1347**, [Extr] **1624**, [Drea] **1696**, [Gene] **1963**

weaning [Gene] **1973**

weariness [Kidn] **980**, [Gene] **1973**

wearisome [Mind] **218**

weary of life [Mind] **218**

weather [Mind] **218**, [Vert] **238**, [Head] **384**, [Nose] **543**, [Resp] **1134**, [Coug] **1165**, [Extr] **1632**, [Chil] **1715**, [Feve] **1733**, [Skin] **1790**, [Gene] **1975**

wedding [Drea] **1696**

wedge-shaped [Teet] **681**

weeping [Mind] **219**, [Coug] **1165**, [Drea] **1696**

wegener's granulomatosis [Gene] **1976**

weight [Head] **384**, [Nose] **543**, [Stom] **801**, [Abdo] **893**, [Rect] **937**, [Fema] **1092**, [Ches] **1264**, [Extr] **1632**, [Skin] **1790**, [Gene] **1976**

well [Mind] **223**, [Gene] **1976**

well-behaved [Mind] **223**

well-being [Mind] **223**

welling up [Gene] **1976**

wells [Drea] **1696**

wens [Head] **384**, [Eye] **436**, [Ear] **497**, **498**, [Extr] **1632**, [Skin] **1791**

wet [Nose] **543**, [Coug] **1165**, [Chil] **1715**, [Gene] **1976**

wet ;getting [Coug] **1165**

wet cloth [Back] **1348**

wet rooms [Feve] **1733**

wetting [Mout] **658**, [Extr] **1632**

wheezing [Resp] **1134**, [Coug] **1165**

whey [Stoo] **949**

whey like [Urin] **1011**

whimpering [Mind] **223**

whimsical [Mind] **223**

whining [Mind] **223**, [Coug] **1165**

whiplash [Back] **1348**

whipped [Drea] **1696**

whirling [Head] **384**, [Visi] **458**, [Stom] **801**, [Abdo] **893**, [Ches] **1264**, [Extr] **1632**

whispering [Coug] **1165**

whistling [Mind] **223**, [Nose] **543**, [Abdo] **893**, [Lary] **1110**, [Resp] **1134**, [Coug] **1165**

white [Visi] **458**, [Face] **602**, [Stoo] **949**, [Expe] **1176**

whiteness [Gene] **1977**

whitlow [Extr] **1632**

whizzing [Extr] **1632**

whooping [Coug] **1166**

whooping cough [Feve] **1733**, [Gene] **1977**

wicked [Mind] **223**

wild [Mind] **223**, [Head] **384**, [Eye] **439**, [Drea] **1696**

wildness [Mind] **223**

will [Mind] **6**, **11**, **12**, **17**, **23**, **28**, **32**, **37**, **39**, **40**, **41**, **44**, **51**, **52**, **53**, **54**, **55**, **57**, **58**, **60**, **61**, **62**, **63**, **64**,

Index of words

65, 66, 68, 69, 72, 74, 75, 76, 77, 78, 80, 82, 83, 102, 103, 104, 106, 107, 110, 111, 112, 113, 130, 133, 134, 147, 151, 168, 183, 192, 194, 209, **223**, 223, *[Vert]* **238**, *[Head]* 343, *[Eye]* 392, 410, *[Visi]* 450, *[Blad]* 958, 966, 967, 970, *[Fema]* 1063, *[Coug]* 1149, *[Ches]* 1180, 1203, *[Slee]* 1663, *[Drea]* 1693, *[Gene]* 1882

willful *[Mind]* **224**

wily *[Mind]* **224**

wimpy *[Mind]* **224**

wind *[Head]* **384**, *[Eye]* **439**, *[Ear]* **498**, *[Face]* **602**, *[Coug]* **1166**, *[Expe]* **1176**, *[Back]* **1348**, *[Extr]* **1632**, *[Chil]* **1715**, *[Pers]* **1745**, *[Skin]* **1791**, *[Gene]* **1977**

wind colic *[Drea]* **1696**

wind on chest agg *[Coug]* **1166**

window *[Mind]* **224**, *[Vert]* **238**, *[Drea]* **1696**

windshield *[Visi]* **459**

wine *[Vert]* **238**, *[Eye]* **439**, *[Visi]* **459**, *[Stom]* **801**, *[Kidn]* **980**, *[Coug]* **1166**, *[Ches]* **1264**, *[Feve]* **1733**, *[Pers]* **1745**, *[Gene]* **1977**

wings *[Nose]* **543**

winking *[Eye]* **439**

winter *[Nose]* **543**, *[Coug]* **1166**, *[Feve]* **1733**, *[Skin]* **1791**, *[Gene]* **1977**

wipe *[Eye]* **439**

wiping *[Eye]* **439**, *[Rect]* **937**, *[Gene]* **1977**

wiping the eyes *[Vert]* **238**

wire *[Head]* **384**

wisdom *[Teet]* **681**

witches *[Drea]* **1696**

withdrawal *[Mind]* **224**

withered *[Extr]* **1632**, *[Skin]* **1791**

withered t *[Mout]* **658**

witty *[Mind]* **224**

women *[Mind]* 3, 16, 20, 23, 24, 26, 32, 33, 82, 97, 98, 103, 114, 122, 124, 128, 131, 135, 141, 143, 151, 179, 180, 190, 217, **224**, 224, *[Head]* 248, 309, *[Eye]* 391, *[Nose]* 519, 523, *[Face]* 557, 560, 603, *[Mout]* 608, 625, 650, 651, *[Teet]* **681**, *[Stom]* 745, 752, 790, *[Abdo]* 806, 807, 808, 884, *[Rect]* 897, 901, 909, 916, 918, *[Blad]* 953, 961, 962, 965, 969, 970, 971, *[Kidn]* 978, *[Pros]* 981, *[Uret]* 996, 997, *[Urin]* 999, 1005, 1007, *[Male]* 1035, 1038, *[Fema]* 1043, 1049, 1054, 1056, 1057, 1058, 1059, 1061, 1062, 1066, 1067, 1070, 1072, 1088, 1091, *[Coug]* 1149, 1154, 1160, *[Ches]* 1189, 1199, 1201, 1232, 1252, 1254, *[Back]* 1293,

1294, 1330, 1333, *[Extr]* 1602, *[Slee]* 1667, *[Drea]* 1676, 1679, **1696**, 1696, *[Skin]* 1755, *[Gene]* 1815, 1816, 1817, 1840, 1864, 1882, 1894, 1895, 1931, 1935, 1967, 1968, 1969, 1970, 1971, 1973, 1975, **1977**

wonderful *[Drea]* **1696**

wood *[Mout]* **658**, *[Ches]* **1264**

wooden *[Extr]* **1632**, *[Gene]* **1977**

wool *[Skin]* **1791**, *[Gene]* **1977**

woozy *[Gene]* **1977**

word *[Mind]* **224**

work *[Mind]* **224**, *[Drea]* **1696**

world *[Drea]* **1697**

worm *[Mind]* 26, 114, 140, 142, 172, 201, *[Head]* 239, 269, 309, 318, 358, *[Teet]* **681**, *[Thro]* 686, **714**, *[Stom]* 731, 763, 769, 772, **801**, *[Abdo]* 825, *[Rect]* 915, *[Stoo]* 945, *[Blad]* **971**, *[Coug]* **1166**, *[Gene]* 1808, 1954, 1957

worm- *[Stoo]* **949**

worms *[Mind]* 52, 83, 114, 164, *[Vert]* 226, *[Eye]* 392, 433, *[Visi]* 445, *[Ear]* **498**, *[Nose]* 526, *[Mout]* 616, *[Teet]* 663, *[Stom]* 753, 778, 801, *[Abdo]* 823, 847, 881, *[Rect]* 899, 911, 921, 923, 932, **937**, 937, *[Blad]* 965, *[Male]* 1022, 1025, *[Fema]* 1052, 1089, **1092**, *[Coug]* **1167**, *[Ches]* 1256, *[Back]* 1276, *[Slee]* 1651, 1667, 1671, *[Drea]* 1696, **1697**, *[Feve]* **1733**, *[Skin]* 1774, **1791**, 1791, *[Gene]* 1811, 1821, 1824, 1828, 1892, 1893, 1973, **1977**, 1977

worn-out *[Skin]* **1791**

worries *[Drea]* **1697**

worry *[Mind]* **224**

worthless *[Mind]* **224**

wounded *[Drea]* **1697**

wounds *[Mind]* 26, *[Eye]* 402, 409, *[Mout]* 635, *[Extr]* 1351, 1415, **1632**, *[Drea]* 1680, **1697**, *[Skin]* 1773, **1791**, *[Gene]* 1803, 1815, 1827, 1843, 1870, 1874, 1918, 1946, **1977**, 1978, 1979

wrapped *[Head]* **384**

wrapping up head *[Head]* **384**

wraps *[Gene]* **1979**

wrath *[Mind]* **224**

wretched *[Mind]* **224**

wrinkled *[Eye]* **439**, *[Nose]* **543**, *[Face]* **602**, *[Mout]* **658**, *[Male]* **1041**, *[Back]* **1348**, *[Extr]* **1632**, *[Skin]* **1791**

wrinkling forehead *[Head]* **384**

wrist *[Extr]* **1638**

wrist-drop *[Extr]* **1632**
writer's *[Extr]* **1632**
writhing *[Gene]* **1979**
writing *[Mind]* **224**, *[Vert]* **238**, *[Head]* **384**, *[Eye]*
   439, *[Coug]* **1167**, *[Back]* **1348**, *[Extr]* **1632**, *[Drea]*
   1697, *[Chil]* **1715**, *[Pers]* **1745**
wrong *[Mind]* **224**
wrong; doing *[Drea]* **1697**

X

xenophobia *[Mind]* **224**
xerophthalmia *[Eye]* **439**
x-ray *[Gene]* **1979**

Y

yawning *[Mind]* **224**, *[Vert]* **238**, *[Head]* **384**, *[Eye]*
   439, *[Mout]* **659**, *[Stom]* **801**, *[Abdo]* **893**, *[Resp]*
   1134, *[Coug]* **1167**, *[Ches]* **1264**, *[Back]* **1348**,
   [Slee] **1671**, *[Chil]* **1715**, *[Gene]* **1979**
yeast *[Stoo]* **949**
yeast-like *[Urin]* **1011**
yellow *[Visi]* **459**, *[Nose]* **543**, *[Teet]* **681**, *[Stoo]*
   949, *[Expe]* **1176**, *[Feve]* **1733**, *[Gene]* **1979**
yellowness *[Eye]* **439**
yielding *[Mind]* **224**
youth *[Drea]* **1697**

Z

zealous *[Mind]* **224**
zigzag *[Gene]* **1979**
zigzags *[Visi]* **459**
zymotic fevers *[Feve]* **1733**

Dorsal region - Ribs - Below
Dorsal region - Scapulae
Dorsal region - Scapulae - Angles
Dorsal region - Scapulae - Angles - Below
Dorsal region - Scapulae - Angles - Inner
Dorsal region - Scapulae - Angles - Inner - left
Dorsal region - Scapulae - Angles - Inner - left - Margin
Dorsal region - Scapulae - Angles - Lower
Dorsal region - Scapulae - Angles - Upper
Dorsal region - Scapulae - Below
Dorsal region - Scapulae - Below - left
Dorsal region - Scapulae - Below - right
Dorsal region - Scapulae - Between
Dorsal region - Scapulae - Margins
Dorsal region - Scapulae - Margins - Inner
Dorsal region - Scapulae - Margins - Inner - right
Dorsal region - Scapulae - Margins - left
Dorsal region - Scapulae - Margins - Lower
Dorsal region - Scapulae - Margins - Lower - Inner
Dorsal region - Scapulae - Margins - Outer - right
Dorsal region - Scapulae - Spine
Dorsal region - Scapulae - Tips
Dorsal region - Scapulae - Upper part
Dorsal region - Scapulae - Vertebrae; near
Dorsal region - Spine
Dorsal region - Spine - Between scapula and spine
Dorsal region - Upper part
Dorsal region - Vertebrae - First
Dorsal region - Vertebrae - Near
Dorsal region - Vertebrae - Third
Lumbar region
Lumbar region - Flanks
Lumbar region - Hips; above
Lumbar region - Ilium
Lumbar region - Ilium - Attachment of muscles
Lumbar region - Ilium - Between ribs and ilium
Lumbar region - Ilium - Crest of ileum
Lumbar region - Ilium - Crest of ileum - right
Lumbar region - Kidneys; above
Lumbar region - Muscles
Lumbar region - Ribs - Last
Lumbar region - Ribs - Last; near
Lumbar region - Skin; below the
Lumbar region - Spine
Lumbar region - Vertebrae
Lumbar region - Vertebrae - Fourth
Lumbar region - Vertebrae - Last

Lumbosacral region
Lumbosacral region - Spine
Muscles
Muscles - Psoas muscles
Muscles - Tendons; and
Sacral region
Sacral region - Hips; and
Sacroiliac region
Sacroiliac symphyses
Sacrum
Sacrum - Coccyx; and
Sacrum - Hips; and
Sides
Spinal cord
Spine
Spine - Beside
Spine - Brain; base of
Spine - Joints of vertebrae
Spine - Lower part
Spine - Lumbar region - Above
Spine - Middle of spine
Spine - Upper part
Spine - Vertebrae
Spine - Whole

Bladder

Neck - Region of neck
Neck of bladder
Region of bladder
Sphincter

Chest

Anterior part
Axillae
Axillae - Below
Axillae - Glands
Axillae - Region of axillae
Clavicles
Clavicles - Above
Clavicles - Below
Clavicles - Region of clavicles
Costal cartilages
Costal cartilages - Between
Costal cartilages - False ribs; of
Costal cartilages - False ribs; of - Sternum; near
Costal cartilages - Fourth ribs; of
Costal cartilages - Last true ribs; of
Costal cartilages - Lower ribs; of

Costal cartilages - Third ribs; of
Diaphragm
Diaphragm - Region of diaphragm
External chest
Heart
Heart - Apex
Heart - Base
Heart - Below
Heart - Myocardium
Heart - Pericardium
Heart - Region of heart
Heart - Under the heart
Intercostal region
Intercostal region - Lower chest
Intercostal region - Muscles
Intercostal region - Nerves
Lower part
Lungs
Lungs - Anterior part
Lungs - Apex
Lungs - Apex - left
Lungs - Apex - right
Lungs - Behind
Lungs - Center - left
Lungs - Lower part
Lungs - Lower part - left
Lungs - Lower part - right
Lungs - Nipple; above - left
Lungs - Upper part
Mammae
Mammae - Above
Mammae - Between
Mammae - Nipples
Mammae - Nipples - Above - left
Mammae - Nipples - Behind - left
Mammae - Nipples - Below
Mammae - Nipples - Below - right
Mammae - Nipples - Lower half
Mammae - Nipples - Region of nipples
Mammae - Nipples - Under - left
Mammae - Nipples - Under - right
Mammae - Region of mammae
Mammae - Region of mammae - Under
Mammae - Under
Mammae - Under - left
Mammae - Under - right
Mammae - Upper part
Mammary glands; male

Mammary glands; male - Nipples
Mediastinum
Middle of chest
Muscles
Pectoral muscles
Pectoral muscles - Lower part
Pleura
Posterior part
Precordial region
Ribs
Ribs - Anterior part
Ribs - Between ribs
Ribs - Edges of ribs
Ribs - False ribs
Ribs - False ribs - Below - left
Ribs - Fourth
Ribs - Joints
Ribs - Last true rib
Ribs - Lower
Ribs - Lower - left
Ribs - Seventh
Ribs - Short - Below
Ribs - Sixth
Ribs - Third
Ribs - Third - Sternum; near
Ribs - Under
Ribs - Under - left
Sides
Sides - False ribs
Sides - left
Sides - left - Fourth rib
Sides - left - Fourth rib - Under
Sides - left - Heart; under
Sides - left - Lower part
Sides - left - Upper part
Sides - Lower part
Sides - right
Sides - right - Last rib
Sides - right - Lower part
Sides - right - Upper part
Sides - Upper part
Skin; below the
Sternum
Sternum - Above
Sternum - Behind
Sternum - Beside sternum
Sternum - Border
Sternum - left of sternum

Sternum - left side; along the
Sternum - Lower part
Sternum - Lower part - Under
Sternum - Over sternum
Sternum - Sternoclavicular joint
Sternum - Sternocostal joints
Sternum - Tip
Sternum - Under
Sternum - Upper part
Sternum - Xiphoid cartilage
Upper part

Ear

About the ears
About the ears - Bones
Above the ears
Antitragus
Base of ears; at the
Behind the ears
Below the ears
Bones - Petrous bone
Cartilages
Conchae
Conchae - Anterior part
Eustachian tubes
External ears
Front of ears; in
Inside
Lobes
Lobes - Behind the ear
Lobes - Hole of earring
Lobes - Under
Mastoid
Mastoid - Below
Mastoid - Region of mastoid
Meatus
Meatus - Inside
Middle ear
Nerves
Processus styloideus
Tragus
Tympanum

External throat

Blood vessels
Glands
Sides
Sternocleidomastoid muscles

Sternocleidomastoid muscles - Upper part
Submaxillary glands
Throat-pit
Thyroid cartilage
Thyroid gland

Extremities

Ankles
Ankles - Above
Ankles - Anterior part
Ankles - Below
Ankles - Bones
Ankles - Malleolus
Ankles - Malleolus - Inner
Ankles - Malleolus - Outer
Ankles - Malleolus - Outer - Behind
Ankles - Sides - Inner
Ankles - Sides - Outer
Ankles - Top
Bones
Bones - Condyles
Bones - Long bones
Bones - Long bones - Middle of long bones
Bones - Metatarsal
Bones - Periosteum
Cartilages
Elbows
Elbows - About the
Elbows - Bends of elbow
Elbows - Bones
Elbows - Condyles
Elbows - Olecranon
Elbows - Posterior surface
Elbows - Tips
Externally
Feet
Feet - Back of feet
Feet - Back of feet - left
Feet - Between toes
Feet - Bones
Feet - Bones - Metatarsal bones
Feet - Heels
Feet - Heels - Bones
Feet - Heels - Joints - Metatarsal
Feet - Heels - Periosteum
Feet - Joints
Feet - Periosteum
Feet - Sides

Legs - Calves
Legs - Calves - Above
Legs - Calves - Below
Legs - Calves - Internally
Legs - Calves - Middle of calves
Legs - Knees; below
Legs - Muscles
Legs - Muscles - Tibia; of
Legs - Periosteum
Legs - Sides - Inner
Legs - Tendo Achillis
Legs - Tendons
Legs - Veins
Legs - Veins - Saphenous
Lower limbs
Lower limbs - Bones
Lower limbs - Inner side
Lower limbs - Joints
Lower limbs - Muscles
Lower limbs - Periosteum
Lower limbs - Posterior part
Lower limbs - Sciatic nerve
Lower limbs - Skin
Lower limbs - Skin; below
Muscles
Muscles - Attachment of muscles
Muscles - Extensor muscles
Muscles - Flexor muscles
Muscles - Joints; near
Nails
Nails - Edges
Nails - Sides
Nails - Under
Nates
Nates - Between
Nates - Inner side
Nates - Tubera ischiadica
Scapulohumeral region
Shoulders
Shoulders - Acromion
Shoulders - Beneath
Shoulders - Between
Shoulders - Deltoid
Shoulders - Joints
Shoulders - Ligaments
Shoulders - Posterior part
Shoulders - Sides
Shoulders - Top of shoulders

Shoulders - Under
Tendons
Tendons - Attachments of tendons
Thighs
Thighs - Anterior part
Thighs - Anterior part - Inguinal region; near
Thighs - Anterior part - Lower part
Thighs - Anterior part - Upper part
Thighs - Back of thighs
Thighs - Bends of thighs
Thighs - Between
Thighs - Bones
Thighs - Crural nerves
Thighs - Crural nerves - Anterior
Thighs - Femur
Thighs - Genitalia; near
Thighs - Genitalia; near - Female
Thighs - Genitalia; near - Male
Thighs - Glands
Thighs - Hamstrings
Thighs - Inner side
Thighs - Inner side - Knees; above
Thighs - Inner side - Upper part
Thighs - Knees; above
Thighs - Lower part
Thighs - Lower part - Posterior part
Thighs - Middle
Thighs - Middle - Anterior part
Thighs - Middle - Internal part
Thighs - Middle - Posterior part
Thighs - Outer side
Thighs - Periosteum
Thighs - Posterior part
Thighs - Upper part
Thumbs
Thumbs - Balls
Thumbs - Bones
Thumbs - Extensor muscles
Thumbs - Joints
Thumbs - Joints - Carpometacarpal
Thumbs - Joints - Distal
Thumbs - Joints - Metacarpophalangeal
Thumbs - Joints - Metacarpophalangeal - left
Thumbs - Joints - Proximal
Thumbs - Nails
Thumbs - Nails - Roots of nails
Thumbs - Nails - Under
Thumbs - Phalanges

Thumbs - Phalanges - Distal
Thumbs - Phalanges - Proximal
Thumbs - sides
Thumbs - Sides - Inner
Thumbs - sides - Outer
Thumbs - Tips
Thumbs - Tips - right
Tips
Toes
Toes - Balls
Toes - Between
Toes - Bones
Toes - Fifth
Toes - Fifth - Balls
Toes - Fifth - Joints
Toes - First
Toes - First - Balls
Toes - First - Joints
Toes - First - Joints - Proximal
Toes - First - Nails
Toes - First - Nails - Roots of nails
Toes - First - Nails - Under
Toes - First - Tendons - Extensor tendons
Toes - First - Tips
Toes - Fourth
Toes - Joints
Toes - Joints - Small joints
Toes - Nails
Toes - Nails - Roots of nails
Toes - Nails - Under
Toes - Second
Toes - Second - Balls
Toes - Second - Joints
Toes - Second - Nails
Toes - Third
Toes - Third - Nails - Under
Toes - Tips
Toes - Under
Upper arms
Upper arms - Anterior part
Upper arms - Anterior surface
Upper arms - Biceps
Upper arms - Bones
Upper arms - Bones - Condyles
Upper arms - Bones - Condyles - External
Upper arms - Bones - Condyles - Internal
Upper arms - Bones - Elbow; near
Upper arms - Deltoid

Upper arms - Elbows; just above
Upper arms - Humerus
Upper arms - Inner side
Upper arms - Joints
Upper arms - Lower part
Upper arms - Muscles - Anterior
Upper arms - Muscles - Extensor muscles
Upper arms - Muscles - Flexor muscles
Upper arms - Outer side
Upper arms - Outer side - left
Upper arms - Posterior part
Upper arms - Side lain on
Upper arms - Skin
Upper arms - Triceps
Upper limbs
Upper limbs - Bones
Upper limbs - Brachial plexus
Upper limbs - Inner side
Upper limbs - Internally
Upper limbs - Joints
Upper limbs - Joints - Bones
Upper limbs - Joints - Joint to joint; from
Upper limbs - Joints - Side lain on
Upper limbs - Outer side
Upper limbs - Outer surface
Upper limbs - Part lain on
Upper limbs - Skin; below
Veins
Wrists
Wrists - Bones
Wrists - Dorsal side
Wrists - Palmar side
Wrists - Radial side
Wrists - Ulnar side

Eye

About the eyes
Around the eyes
Behind the eyes
Below the eyes
Below the eyes - left
Below the eyes - right
Between the eyes
Canthi
Canthi - Inner
Canthi - Inner - Above
Canthi - Outer
Caruncle

Chiasma
Ciliary body
Ciliary muscles
Conjunctiva
Conjunctiva - Under
Cornea
Eyeballs
Eyeballs - Center of eyeballs
Eyeballs - Inside
Eyeballs - Muscles
Eyebrows
Eyebrows - Above - left
Eyebrows - Between
Eyelashes
Eyes
Eyes; about
Infraorbital
Lachrymal ducts
Lachrymal glands
Lachrymal sacs
Lens
Lids
Lids - Behind
Lids - Inner side
Lids - Lower
Lids - Lower - Margins
Lids - Margins
Lids - Margins - Glands
Lids - nodules in the lids - Lower eyelids
Lids - Tarsi
Lids - Under
Lids - Under - right
Lids - Upper
Lids - Upper - Margins
Lids - Upper - right
Lids - Upper - Under
Lids - Upper - Under - left
Lids - Upper - Under - right
Optic nerve
Orbital arch
Orbits
Orbits - Around
Orbits - Below
Orbits - Bones
Orbits - Deep in
Orbits - Lower part
Orbits - Margins
Palpebral neuralgia

Papillae
Postorbital
Pupils
Sclera
Supraorbital

Face

Bones
Cheeks
Chin
Chin - Between the chin and lower lip
Chin - Skin
Chin - Under the chin
Eyes
Eyes - Around
Eyes - Below
Jaws
Jaws - Condyles
Jaws - Joints
Jaws - Joints - Behind
Jaws - Lower
Jaws - Lower - Angles
Jaws - Lower - Glands
Jaws - Lower - Middle
Jaws - Lower - Rami
Jaws - Point of jaws
Jaws - Upper
Jaws - Upper - Angles
Joints
Lips
Lips - Lower
Lips - Upper
Malar bones
Mouth - Around
Mouth - Corners of mouth
Muscles
Muscles - Masseter muscles
Nerves
Parotid glands
Sinuses
Sinuses - Ethmoidal
Sinuses - Frontal
Sinuses - Maxillary
Skin
Submaxillary glands
Temples
Temples - Skin
Trigeminus

Zygoma

Female genitalia/sex

Clitoris
Labia
Labia - Between
Meatus; region of
Mons veneris
Ovaries
Ovaries - Region of ovaries
Pubic bones
Pubic bones - Symphysis
Pubic region
Pudendum
Uterus
Uterus - Cervix
Uterus - Ligaments; broad
Uterus - Middle of uterus
Uterus - Os uteri
Vagina
Vagina - Around
Vulva

Generals

Affected parts
Blood vessels
Body; all over
Bones
Bones - Condyles
Bones - Epiphyses
Bones - Long bones
Bones - Marrow
Bones - Sutures; along
Cartilages
Distant parts
Distant parts; to
External parts
Externally
Externally - Affected parts
Fibrous tissue
Glands
Glands - Around
Internal parts
Internally
Joints
Joints - Small joints
Ligaments

Mucous membranes
Muscles
Muscles - Attachment of muscles
Muscles - Flexor muscles
Nerves
Paralyzed parts
Parts
Parts - Lain on
Periosteum
Single parts
Skin; below the
Tendons
Thorax
Upper part of body
Veins
Wounds

Head

Around
Arteries
Bones
Brain
Brain - Base of brain
Brain - Middle of brain
Brain - Side lain on
External head
Eyes - Behind
Eyes - Over the eyes
Forehead
Forehead - Above
Forehead - Across
Forehead - Behind eyes
Forehead - Bones
Forehead - Eminence; frontal
Forehead - Eminence; frontal - Above
Forehead - Eyebrows; above
Forehead - Eyes - Above
Forehead - Eyes - Above - Margin of orbits
Forehead - Eyes - Above - Muscles
Forehead - Eyes - Around
Forehead - Eyes - Behind
Forehead - Eyes - Between
Forehead - Frontal sinuses
Forehead - Lower part
Forehead - Margin of hair
Forehead - Meninges
Forehead - Middle
Forehead - Nose; above

Forehead - Sides
Forehead - Sides - right
Forehead - Upper part
Hair
Meninges
Occiput
Occiput - Bones
Occiput - Ears; behind
Occiput - Glands
Occiput - Protuberance; occipital
Occiput - Sides
Occiput - Suboccipital
Occiput and Forehead
Occiput and Vertex
Periosteum
Scalp
Sides
Sides - Brain
Sides - one side - Ear; behind the
Sides - right
Sides - Side lain on
Sinuses
Skin; below the
Skull
Sutures
Sutures - Along
Sutures - Coronal
Temples
Temples - Above
Temples - Side lain on
Temples - Sides
Upper half
Vertex
Vertex - Across
Vertex - Here and there

Kidneys

Kidneys
Region of kidneys
Ureters

Larynx and trachea

Air passages
Larynx
Larynx - Epiglottis
Throat-pit
Trachea

Male genitalia/sex

Penis - Glans
Penis - Glans - Behind
Penis - Prepuce
Penis - Prepuce - Margin of prepuce
Penis - Root
Penis - Tip
Scrotum
Scrotum - Sides
Scrotum - Thighs; between scrotum and
Spermatic cords
Spermatic cords; and
Testes
Testes - Epididymis

Mouth

Cheeks
Cheeks - Inner side
Gums
Gums - Cheeks; between gums and
Gums - Inner
Gums - Lower
Gums - Outer
Gums - Skin; below
Gums - Upper
Gums - Upper - Inner
Lips
Lips - Inner side
Lips - Inner side - Lower
Lips - Inner side - Upper
Lips - Lower
Lips - Upper
Palate
Palate - Arch
Palate - Hard palate
Palate - Sides
Palate - Soft palate
Palate - Velum
Salivary glands
Salivary glands - Orifices
Sublingual glands
Tongue
Tongue - Across
Tongue - Anterior part
Tongue - Below
Tongue - Below - Skin; below
Tongue - Border

Tongue - Center
Tongue - Edges
Tongue - Frenum
Tongue - Posterior part
Tongue - Root
Tongue - Root - Across
Tongue - Root - Below
Tongue - Sides
Tongue - Sides - Tip; near
Tongue - Surface of tongue; under
Tongue - Tip
Tongue - Transversely across

Nose

Above the nose
Around the nose
Behind the nose
Bones
Bones - Turbinated bones
Cartilage
Cartilage - Junction of cartilage
Corners of nose
Dorsum
Inside
Margins
Nostrils
Nostrils - Angle; anterior - left
Nostrils - Angle; interior - left
Nostrils - Inside
Outer part
Posterior nares
Root
Root - Behind
Root - Inside
Septum
Septum - Upper part
Sides
Sinuses
Sinuses - Maxillary
Skin
Tip
Upper part
Wings
Wings - Edges
Wings - Inner surface
Wings - left
Wings - right

Prostate

Region of prostate

Rectum

Anus
Anus - Skin; below the
Bladder; and
Glands - Anal
Glands - Circumanal
Glands - Perianal
Perineum
Perineum - Skin; below the
Rectum and anus

Skin

Below the skin
Mucocutaneous borders

Stomach

Below the stomach
Cardia
Cardiac opening
Cardiac region
Epigastrium
Epigastrium - Region of epigastrium
Epigastrium - Skin; below the
Pit of stomach
Posterior part
Pylorus
Transversely across

Teeth

Bicuspids
Bicuspids - Lower - First bicuspid
Bicuspids - Lower - Second bicuspid
Bicuspids - Upper
Bicuspids - Upper - right
Canines
Canines - Hollow
Canines - Lower
Canines - Upper
Canines - Upper - left
Canines - Upper - right
Hollow teeth
Hollow teeth - right

Throat

Urethra

A

About the ears → *ear*
About the ears - Bones → *ear*
About the eyes → *eye*
Above the ears → *ear*
Above the nose → *nose*
Affected parts → *gene*
Air passages → *lary*
Ankles → *extr*
Ankles - Above → *extr*
Ankles - Anterior part → *extr*
Ankles - Below → *extr*
Ankles - Bones → *extr*
Ankles - Malleolus → *extr*
Ankles - Malleolus - Inner → *extr*
Ankles - Malleolus - Outer → *extr*
Ankles - Malleolus - Outer - Behind → *extr*
Ankles - Sides - Inner → *extr*
Ankles - Sides - Outer → *extr*
Ankles - Top → *extr*
Anterior part → *abdo*
Anterior part → *ches*
Anterior part → *uret*
Antitragus → *ear*
Anus → *rect*
Anus - Skin; below the → *rect*
Appendix → *abdo*
Around the eyes → *eye*
Around the nose → *nose*
Around → *head*
Arteries → *head*
Axillae → *ches*
Axillae - Below → *ches*
Axillae - Glands → *ches*
Axillae - Region of axillae → *ches*

B

Base of ears; at the → *ear*
Behind the ears → *ear*
Behind the eyes → *eye*
Behind the nose → *nose*
Below the ears → *ear*
Below the eyes → *eye*
Below the eyes - left → *eye*
Below the eyes - right → *eye*
Below the skin → *skin*

Below the stomach → *stom*
Between the eyes → *eye*
Bicuspids → *teet*
Bicuspids - Lower - First bicuspid → *teet*
Bicuspids - Lower - Second bicuspid → *teet*
Bicuspids - Upper → *teet*
Bicuspids - Upper - right → *teet*
Bladder; and → *rect*
Blood vessels → *exte*
Blood vessels → *gene*
Body; all over → *gene*
Bones → *extr*
Bones → *face*
Bones → *gene*
Bones → *head*
Bones → *nose*
Bones - Condyles → *extr*
Bones - Condyles → *gene*
Bones - Epiphyses → *gene*
Bones - Long bones → *extr*
Bones - Long bones → *gene*
Bones - Long bones - Middle of long bones → *extr*
Bones - Marrow → *gene*
Bones - Metatarsal → *extr*
Bones - Periosteum → *extr*
Bones - Petrous bone → *ear*
Bones - Sutures; along → *gene*
Bones - Turbinated bones → *nose*
Brain → *head*
Brain - Base of brain → *head*
Brain - Middle of brain → *head*
Brain - Side lain on → *head*

C

Canines → *teet*
Canines - Hollow → *teet*
Canines - Lower → *teet*
Canines - Upper → *teet*
Canines - Upper - left → *teet*
Canines - Upper - right → *teet*
Canthi → *eye*
Canthi - Inner → *eye*
Canthi - Inner - Above → *eye*
Canthi - Outer → *eye*
Cardia → *stom*
Cardiac opening → *stom*
Cardiac region → *stom*
Cartilage → *nose*

Cartilage - Junction of cartilage → *nose*
Cartilages → *ear*
Cartilages → *extr*
Cartilages → *gene*
Caruncle → *eye*
Cecum → *abdo*
Cervical region → *back*
Cervical region - Nape of neck → *back*
Cervical region - Spine → *back*
Cervical region - Tendons → *back*
Cervical region - Vertebrae → *back*
Cervical region - Vertebrae - Fifth → *back*
Cervical region - Vertebrae - First → *back*
Cervical region - Vertebrae - Fourth → *back*
Cervical region - Vertebrae - Seventh → *back*
Cervical region - Vertebrae - Sixth → *back*
Cheeks → *face*
Cheeks → *mout*
Cheeks - Inner side → *mout*
Chiasma → *eye*
Chin → *face*
Chin - Between the chin and lower lip → *face*
Chin - Skin → *face*
Chin - Under the chin → *face*
Ciliary body → *eye*
Ciliary muscles → *eye*
Clavicles → *ches*
Clavicles - Above → *ches*
Clavicles - Below → *ches*
Clavicles - Region of clavicles → *ches*
Clitoris → *fema*
Coccyx → *back*
Coccyx - Skin; below the → *back*
Colon - Ascendens → *abdo*
Colon - Descendens → *abdo*
Colon - Transverse → *abdo*
Conchae → *ear*
Conchae - Anterior part → *ear*
Conjunctiva → *eye*
Conjunctiva - Under → *eye*
Cornea → *eye*
Corners of nose → *nose*
Costal cartilages → *ches*
Costal cartilages - Between → *ches*
Costal cartilages - False ribs; of → *ches*
Costal cartilages - False ribs; of - Sternum; near → *ches*
Costal cartilages - Fourth ribs; of → *ches*

Costal cartilages - Last true ribs; of → *ches*
Costal cartilages - Lower ribs; of → *ches*
Costal cartilages - Third ribs; of → *ches*

D

Diaphragm → *abdo*
Diaphragm → *ches*
Diaphragm - Region of diaphragm → *ches*
Distant parts → *gene*
Distant parts; to → *gene*
Dorsal region → *back*
Dorsal region - Lower part → *back*
Dorsal region - Middle part → *back*
Dorsal region - Muscles → *back*
Dorsal region - Ribs → *back*
Dorsal region - Ribs - Below → *back*
Dorsal region - Scapulae → *back*
Dorsal region - Scapulae - Angles → *back*
Dorsal region - Scapulae - Angles - Below → *back*
Dorsal region - Scapulae - Angles - Inner → *back*
Dorsal region - Scapulae - Angles - Inner - left → *back*
Dorsal region - Scapulae - Angles - Inner - left - Margin → *back*
Dorsal region - Scapulae - Angles - Lower → *back*
Dorsal region - Scapulae - Angles - Upper → *back*
Dorsal region - Scapulae - Below → *back*
Dorsal region - Scapulae - Below - left → *back*
Dorsal region - Scapulae - Below - right → *back*
Dorsal region - Scapulae - Between → *back*
Dorsal region - Scapulae - Margins → *back*
Dorsal region - Scapulae - Margins - Inner → *back*
Dorsal region - Scapulae - Margins - Inner - right → *back*
Dorsal region - Scapulae - Margins - Lower → *back*
Dorsal region - Scapulae - Margins - Lower - Inner → *back*
Dorsal region - Scapulae - Margins - Outer - right → *back*
Dorsal region - Scapulae - Margins - left → *back*
Dorsal region - Scapulae - Spine → *back*
Dorsal region - Scapulae - Tips → *back*
Dorsal region - Scapulae - Upper part → *back*
Dorsal region - Scapulae - Vertebrae; near → *back*
Dorsal region - Spine → *back*
Dorsal region - Spine - Between scapula and spine → *back*
Dorsal region - Upper part → *back*

Dorsal region - Vertebrae - First → *back*
Dorsal region - Vertebrae - Near → *back*
Dorsal region - Vertebrae - Third → *back*
Dorsum → *nose*
Duodenum → *abdo*

E

Elbows → *extr*
Elbows - About the → *extr*
Elbows - Bends of elbow → *extr*
Elbows - Bones → *extr*
Elbows - Condyles → *extr*
Elbows - Olecranon → *extr*
Elbows - Posterior surface → *extr*
Elbows - Tips → *extr*
Epigastrium → *stom*
Epigastrium - Region of epigastrium → *stom*
Epigastrium - Skin; below the → *stom*
Esophagus → *thro*
Esophagus - Cardiac orifice → *thro*
Eustachian tubes → *ear*
External abdomen → *abdo*
External chest → *ches*
External ears → *ear*
External head → *head*
External parts → *gene*
Externally → *extr*
Externally → *gene*
Externally - Affected parts → *gene*
Eyeballs → *eye*
Eyeballs - Center of eyeballs → *eye*
Eyeballs - Inside → *eye*
Eyeballs - Muscles → *eye*
Eyebrows → *eye*
Eyebrows - Above - left → *eye*
Eyebrows - Between → *eye*
Eyelashes → *eye*
Eyes → *eye*
Eyes → *face*
Eyes - Around → *face*
Eyes - Behind → *head*
Eyes - Below → *face*
Eyes - Over the eyes → *head*
Eyes; about → *eye*

F

Fauces → *thro*

Feet → *extr*
Feet - Back of feet → *extr*
Feet - Back of feet - left → *extr*
Feet - Between toes → *extr*
Feet - Bones → *extr*
Feet - Bones - Metatarsal bones → *extr*
Feet - Heels → *extr*
Feet - Heels - Bones → *extr*
Feet - Heels - Joints - Metatarsal → *extr*
Feet - Heels - Periosteum → *extr*
Feet - Joints → *extr*
Feet - Periosteum → *extr*
Feet - Sides → *extr*
Feet - Sides - Inner → *extr*
Feet - Sides - Outer → *extr*
Feet - Soles → *extr*
Feet - Soles - Balls → *extr*
Feet - Soles - Hollow → *extr*
Feet - Soles - Inner margins → *extr*
Feet - Soles - Outer margins → *extr*
Feet - Soles - right → *extr*
Fibrous tissue → *gene*
Fingers → *extr*
Fingers - Back of fingers → *extr*
Fingers - Balls → *extr*
Fingers - Between → *extr*
Fingers - Bones → *extr*
Fingers - Externally → *extr*
Fingers - First → *extr*
Fingers - First - Back of fingers → *extr*
Fingers - First - Balls → *extr*
Fingers - First - Bones → *extr*
Fingers - First - Externally → *extr*
Fingers - First - Joints → *extr*
Fingers - First - Joints - Distal → *extr*
Fingers - First - Joints - Middle → *extr*
Fingers - First - Joints - Proximal → *extr*
Fingers - First - Nails → *extr*
Fingers - First - Nails - Under → *extr*
Fingers - First - Phalanges - Distal → *extr*
Fingers - First - Phalanges - Middle → *extr*
Fingers - First - Phalanges - Proximal → *extr*
Fingers - First - Sides → *extr*
Fingers - First - Sides - Inner → *extr*
Fingers - First - Sides - Outer → *extr*
Fingers - First - Skin → *extr*
Fingers - First - Tendons → *extr*
Fingers - First - Tendons - Extensor tendons → *extr*

Fingers - First - Tips → *extr*
Fingers - Fourth → *extr*
Fingers - Fourth - Back of fingers → *extr*
Fingers - Fourth - Balls → *extr*
Fingers - Fourth - Bones → *extr*
Fingers - Fourth - Joints → *extr*
Fingers - Fourth - Joints - Distal → *extr*
Fingers - Fourth - Joints - Middle → *extr*
Fingers - Fourth - Joints - Proximal → *extr*
Fingers - Fourth - Sides - Inner → *extr*
Fingers - Fourth - Sides - Outer → *extr*
Fingers - Fourth - Tips → *extr*
Fingers - Joints → *extr*
Fingers - Joints - Distal → *extr*
Fingers - Joints - Metacarpophalangeal → *extr*
Fingers - Joints - Middle → *extr*
Fingers - Joints - Proximal → *extr*
Fingers - Muscles - Extensor muscles → *extr*
Fingers - Nails → *extr*
Fingers - Nails - Around → *extr*
Fingers - Nails - Roots → *extr*
Fingers - Nails - Under → *extr*
Fingers - Palmar surface of fingers → *extr*
Fingers - Periosteum → *extr*
Fingers - Phalanges - Distal → *extr*
Fingers - Second → *extr*
Fingers - Second - Back of fingers → *extr*
Fingers - Second - Balls → *extr*
Fingers - Second - Joints → *extr*
Fingers - Second - Joints - Distal → *extr*
Fingers - Second - Joints - Middle → *extr*
Fingers - Second - Joints - Proximal → *extr*
Fingers - Second - Nails → *extr*
Fingers - Second - Nails - Under → *extr*
Fingers - Second - Phalanges → *extr*
Fingers - Second - Phalanges - Distal → *extr*
Fingers - Second - Phalanges - Middle → *extr*
Fingers - Second - Phalanges - Proximal → *extr*
Fingers - Second - Sides - Inner → *extr*
Fingers - Second - Sides - Outer → *extr*
Fingers - Second - Tendons → *extr*
Fingers - Second - Tips → *extr*
Fingers - Sides → *extr*
Fingers - Sides - Inner → *extr*
Fingers - Tendons - Extensor tendons → *extr*
Fingers - Tendons - Flexor tendons → *extr*
Fingers - Third → *extr*
Fingers - Third - Joints → *extr*

Fingers - Third - Joints - Distal → *extr*
Fingers - Third - Joints - Middle → *extr*
Fingers - Third - Joints - Proximal → *extr*
Fingers - Third - Metacarpal → *extr*
Fingers - Third - Nails → *extr*
Fingers - Third - Nails - Behind → *extr*
Fingers - Third - Nails - inner border of → *extr*
Fingers - Third - Phalanges → *extr*
Fingers - Third - Phalanges - Distal → *extr*
Fingers - Third - Phalanges - Middle → *extr*
Fingers - Third - Phalanges - Proximal → *extr*
Fingers - Third - Sides - Inner → *extr*
Fingers - Third - Sides - Outer → *extr*
Fingers - Third - Tips → *extr*
Fingers - Tips → *extr*
Flexors → *extr*
Forearms → *extr*
Forearms - Anterior part → *extr*
Forearms - Bones → *extr*
Forearms - Bones - Between → *extr*
Forearms - Bones - Radius → *extr*
Forearms - Bones - Radius - Elbow; below → *extr*
Forearms - Bones - Radius - Periosteum → *extr*
Forearms - Bones - Ulna → *extr*
Forearms - Bones - Ulna - Elbow; near → *extr*
Forearms - Bones - Ulna - Lower part → *extr*
Forearms - Bones - Ulna - Middle → *extr*
Forearms - Bones - Ulna - Posterior part → *extr*
Forearms - Bones - Ulna - Wrist; near → *extr*
Forearms - Elbow; near → *extr*
Forearms - Extensor surface → *extr*
Forearms - Externally → *extr*
Forearms - Flexors → *extr*
Forearms - Lower part → *extr*
Forearms - Muscles - Extensor muscles → *extr*
Forearms - Muscles - Flexor muscles → *extr*
Forearms - Muscles - Flexor muscles - Radial side → *extr*
Forearms - Nerves - Ulnar → *extr*
Forearms - Posterior part → *extr*
Forearms - Radial side → *extr*
Forearms - Sides - Inner → *extr*
Forearms - Sides - Outer → *extr*
Forearms - Tendons → *extr*
Forearms - Ulnar side → *extr*
Forearms - Upper side → *extr*
Forearms - Wrist; near → *extr*
Forehead → *head*

Forehead - Above → *head*
Forehead - Across → *head*
Forehead - Behind eyes → *head*
Forehead - Bones → *head*
Forehead - Eminence; frontal → *head*
Forehead - Eminence; frontal - Above → *head*
Forehead - Eyebrows; above → *head*
Forehead - Eyes - Above → *head*
Forehead - Eyes - Above - Margin of orbits → *head*
Forehead - Eyes - Above - Muscles → *head*
Forehead - Eyes - Around → *head*
Forehead - Eyes - Behind → *head*
Forehead - Eyes - Between → *head*
Forehead - Frontal sinuses → *head*
Forehead - Lower part → *head*
Forehead - Margin of hair → *head*
Forehead - Meninges → *head*
Forehead - Middle → *head*
Forehead - Nose; above → *head*
Forehead - Sides → *head*
Forehead - Sides - right → *head*
Forehead - Upper part → *head*
Fossa navicularis → *uret*
Front of ears; in → *ear*

G

Gallbladder → *abdo*
Gallbladder - Region of gallbladder → *abdo*
Glands → *exte*
Glands → *gene*
Glands - Anal → *rect*
Glands - Around → *gene*
Glands - Circumanal → *rect*
Glands - Lymphatic → *abdo*
Glands - Perianal → *rect*
Glandular portion → *uret*
Gums → *mout*
Gums - Cheeks; between gums and → *mout*
Gums - Inner → *mout*
Gums - Lower → *mout*
Gums - Outer → *mout*
Gums - Skin; below → *mout*
Gums - Upper → *mout*
Gums - Upper - Inner → *mout*

H

Hair → *head*

Hands → *extr*
Hands - Back of hands → *extr*
Hands - Between fingers → *extr*
Hands - Between fingers - First → *extr*
Hands - Between fingers - First - Second; and → *extr*
Hands - Between fingers - First - Thumb; and → *extr*
Hands - Between fingers - Second - Third; and → *extr*
Hands - Between fingers - Third - Fourth; and → *extr*
Hands - Between wrist and knuckle of thumb → *extr*
Hands - Bones → *extr*
Hands - Bones - Metacarpal → *extr*
Hands - Bones - Metacarpal - First finger → *extr*
Hands - Bones - Metacarpal - Fourth finger → *extr*
Hands - Internally → *extr*
Hands - Joints → *extr*
Hands - Joints - Metacarpal → *extr*
Hands - Palms → *extr*
Hands - Palms - Balls → *extr*
Hands - Palms - Hypothenar → *extr*
Hands - Palms - Middle of hands → *extr*
Hands - Palms - Radial side → *extr*
Hands - Tendons → *extr*
Hands - Tendons - Extensor tendons → *extr*
Hands - Ulnar side → *extr*
Heart → *ches*
Heart - Apex → *ches*
Heart - Base → *ches*
Heart - Below → *ches*
Heart - Myocardium → *ches*
Heart - Pericardium → *ches*
Heart - Region of heart → *ches*
Heart - Under the heart → *ches*
Hips → *abdo*
Hips → *extr*
Hips - Above → *abdo*
Hips - Above → *extr*
Hips - Bones - Deep in → *extr*
Hips - Externally → *extr*
Hips - Gluteal muscles → *extr*
Hips - Gluteal region → *extr*
Hips - Joints → *extr*
Hips - Nerves; external sciatic → *extr*
Hips - Region of hips → *extr*
Hips - Trochanter → *extr*

Hips - Tubera ischiadica → *extr*
Hips; region of → *abdo*
Hollow teeth → *teet*
Hollow teeth - Sides of hollow teeth → *teet*
Hollow teeth - right → *teet*
Hypochondria → *abdo*
Hypogastrium → *abdo*
Hypogastrium - Across → *abdo*

I

Ileocecal region → *abdo*
Iliac fossa → *abdo*
Iliac region → *abdo*
Iliac region - Above → *abdo*
Iliac region - Muscles → *abdo*
Ilium → *abdo*
Ilium - Anterior superior spinous process → *abdo*
Ilium - Crest of ileum → *abdo*
Ilium - Crest of ileum - Above → *abdo*
Ilium - left → *abdo*
Incisors → *teet*
Incisors - Hollow → *teet*
Incisors - Lower → *teet*
Incisors - Lower - One → *teet*
Incisors - Lower - left → *teet*
Incisors - One → *teet*
Incisors - Roots → *teet*
Incisors - Upper → *teet*
Incisors - Upper - left → *teet*
Incisors - Upper - right → *teet*
Infraorbital → *eye*
Inguinal and pubic region → *abdo*
Inguinal region → *abdo*
Inguinal region - Glands → *abdo*
Inguinal region - Ring → *abdo*
Inside → *ear*
Inside → *nose*
Intercostal region → *ches*
Intercostal region - Lower chest → *ches*
Intercostal region - Muscles → *ches*
Intercostal region - Nerves → *ches*
Internal parts → *gene*
Internally → *gene*
Intestines → *abdo*
Intestines - Large → *abdo*
Intestines - Upper intestines → *abdo*
Ischium → *extr*

J

Jaws → *face*
Jaws - Condyles → *face*
Jaws - Joints → *face*
Jaws - Joints - Behind → *face*
Jaws - Lower → *face*
Jaws - Lower - Angles → *face*
Jaws - Lower - Glands → *face*
Jaws - Lower - Middle → *face*
Jaws - Lower - Rami → *face*
Jaws - Point of jaws → *face*
Jaws - Upper → *face*
Jaws - Upper - Angles → *face*
Joints → *extr*
Joints → *face*
Joints → *gene*
Joints - Side not lain on → *extr*
Joints - Small joints → *extr*
Joints - Small joints → *gene*

K

Kidneys → *kidn*
Knees → *extr*
Knees - Above → *extr*
Knees - Around → *extr*
Knees - Behind → *extr*
Knees - Below → *extr*
Knees - Bends of knees → *extr*
Knees - Front of knees → *extr*
Knees - Hollow of knees → *extr*
Knees - Hollow of knees - Outer side → *extr*
Knees - Hollow of knees - Tendons → *extr*
Knees - Hollow of knees - Tendons - Outer → *extr*
Knees - Joints → *extr*
Knees - Patella → *extr*
Knees - Patella - Below → *extr*
Knees - Patella - Tendon → *extr*
Knees - Sides → *extr*
Knees - Sides - Inner → *extr*
Knees - Sides - Outer → *extr*
Knees - Tendons → *extr*

L

Labia → *fema*
Labia - Between → *fema*
Lachrymal ducts → *eye*
Lachrymal glands → *eye*

Lachrymal sacs → *eye*
Larynx → *lary*
Larynx - Epiglottis → *lary*
Legs → *extr*
Legs - Anterior part → *extr*
Legs - Bones → *extr*
Legs - Bones - Tibia → *extr*
Legs - Bones - Tibia - Anterior border of tibia → *extr*
Legs - Bones - Tibia - Edges → *extr*
Legs - Calves → *extr*
Legs - Calves - Above → *extr*
Legs - Calves - Below → *extr*
Legs - Calves - Internally → *extr*
Legs - Calves - Middle of calves → *extr*
Legs - Knees; below → *extr*
Legs - Muscles → *extr*
Legs - Muscles - Tibia; of → *extr*
Legs - Periosteum → *extr*
Legs - Sides - Inner → *extr*
Legs - Tendo Achillis → *extr*
Legs - Tendons → *extr*
Legs - Veins → *extr*
Legs - Veins - Saphenous → *extr*
Lens → *eye*
Lids → *eye*
Lids - Behind → *eye*
Lids - Inner side → *eye*
Lids - Lower → *eye*
Lids - Lower - Margins → *eye*
Lids - Margins → *eye*
Lids - Margins - Glands → *eye*
Lids - Tarsi → *eye*
Lids - Under → *eye*
Lids - Under - right → *eye*
Lids - Upper → *eye*
Lids - Upper - Margins → *eye*
Lids - Upper - Under → *eye*
Lids - Upper - Under - left → *eye*
Lids - Upper - Under - right → *eye*
Lids - Upper - right → *eye*
Lids - nodules in the lids - Lower eyelids → *eye*
Ligaments → *gene*
Lips → *face*
Lips → *mout*
Lips - Inner side → *mout*
Lips - Inner side - Lower → *mout*
Lips - Inner side - Upper → *mout*

Lips - Lower → *face*
Lips - Lower → *mout*
Lips - Upper → *face*
Lips - Upper → *mout*
Liver → *abdo*
Liver - Below → *abdo*
Liver - Lobe → *abdo*
Liver - Region of liver → *abdo*
Lobes → *ear*
Lobes - Behind the ear → *ear*
Lobes - Hole of earring → *ear*
Lobes - Under → *ear*
Lower abdomen → *abdo*
Lower limbs → *extr*
Lower limbs - Bones → *extr*
Lower limbs - Inner side → *extr*
Lower limbs - Joints → *extr*
Lower limbs - Muscles → *extr*
Lower limbs - Periosteum → *extr*
Lower limbs - Posterior part → *extr*
Lower limbs - Sciatic nerve → *extr*
Lower limbs - Skin → *extr*
Lower limbs - Skin; below → *extr*
Lower part → *ches*
Lower teeth → *teet*
Lower teeth - Hollow → *teet*
Lower teeth - left → *teet*
Lower teeth - right → *teet*
Lumbar region → *back*
Lumbar region - Flanks → *back*
Lumbar region - Hips; above → *back*
Lumbar region - Ilium → *back*
Lumbar region - Ilium - Attachment of muscles → *back*
Lumbar region - Ilium - Between ribs and ilium → *back*
Lumbar region - Ilium - Crest of ileum → *back*
Lumbar region - Ilium - Crest of ileum - right → *back*
Lumbar region - Kidneys; above → *back*
Lumbar region - Muscles → *back*
Lumbar region - Ribs - Last → *back*
Lumbar region - Ribs - Last; near → *back*
Lumbar region - Skin; below the → *back*
Lumbar region - Spine → *back*
Lumbar region - Vertebrae → *back*
Lumbar region - Vertebrae - Fourth → *back*
Lumbar region - Vertebrae - Last → *back*

Lumbosacral region → *back*
Lumbosacral region - Spine → *back*
Lungs → *ches*
Lungs - Anterior part → *ches*
Lungs - Apex → *ches*
Lungs - Apex - left → *ches*
Lungs - Apex - right → *ches*
Lungs - Behind → *ches*
Lungs - Center - left → *ches*
Lungs - Lower part → *ches*
Lungs - Lower part - left → *ches*
Lungs - Lower part - right → *ches*
Lungs - Nipple; above - left → *ches*
Lungs - Upper part → *ches*

M

Malar bones → *face*
Mammae → *ches*
Mammae - Above → *ches*
Mammae - Between → *ches*
Mammae - Nipples → *ches*
Mammae - Nipples - Above - left → *ches*
Mammae - Nipples - Behind - left → *ches*
Mammae - Nipples - Below → *ches*
Mammae - Nipples - Below - right → *ches*
Mammae - Nipples - Lower half → *ches*
Mammae - Nipples - Region of nipples → *ches*
Mammae - Nipples - Under - left → *ches*
Mammae - Nipples - Under - right → *ches*
Mammae - Region of mammae → *ches*
Mammae - Region of mammae - Under → *ches*
Mammae - Under → *ches*
Mammae - Under - left → *ches*
Mammae - Under - right → *ches*
Mammae - Upper part → *ches*
Mammary glands; male → *ches*
Mammary glands; male - Nipples → *ches*
Margins → *nose*
Mastoid → *ear*
Mastoid - Below → *ear*
Mastoid - Region of mastoid → *ear*
Meatus → *ear*
Meatus → *uret*
Meatus - Inside → *ear*
Meatus; region of → *fema*
Mediastinum → *ches*
Meninges → *head*
Middle ear → *ear*

Middle of chest → *ches*
Molars → *teet*
Molars - Hollow → *teet*
Molars - Lower → *teet*
Molars - Lower - Hollow → *teet*
Molars - Lower - Hollow - right → *teet*
Molars - Lower - Roots → *teet*
Molars - Lower - Second molar → *teet*
Molars - Lower - left → *teet*
Molars - Lower - right → *teet*
Molars - Upper → *teet*
Molars - Upper - First - left → *teet*
Molars - Upper - Hollow → *teet*
Molars - Upper - left → *teet*
Molars - Upper - right → *teet*
Molars - left → *teet*
Molars - right → *teet*
Mons pubis → *abdo*
Mons veneris → *fema*
Mouth - Around → *face*
Mouth - Corners of mouth → *face*
Mucocutaneous borders → *skin*
Mucous membranes → *gene*
Muscles → *abdo*
Muscles → *back*
Muscles → *ches*
Muscles → *extr*
Muscles → *face*
Muscles → *gene*
Muscles - Attachment of muscles → *extr*
Muscles - Attachment of muscles → *gene*
Muscles - Extensor muscles → *extr*
Muscles - Flexor muscles → *extr*
Muscles - Flexor muscles → *gene*
Muscles - Joints; near → *extr*
Muscles - Masseter muscles → *face*
Muscles - Psoas muscles → *back*
Muscles - Tendons; and → *back*

N

Nails → *extr*
Nails - Edges → *extr*
Nails - Sides → *extr*
Nails - Under → *extr*
Nates → *extr*
Nates - Between → *extr*
Nates - Inner side → *extr*
Nates - Tubera ischiadica → *extr*

Neck of bladder → *blad*
Neck - Region of neck → *blad*
Nerves → *ear*
Nerves → *face*
Nerves → *gene*
Nostrils → *nose*
Nostrils - Angle; anterior - left → *nose*
Nostrils - Angle; interior - left → *nose*
Nostrils - Inside → *nose*

O

Occiput and Forehead → *head*
Occiput and Vertex → *head*
Occiput → *head*
Occiput - Bones → *head*
Occiput - Ears; behind → *head*
Occiput - Glands → *head*
Occiput - Protuberance; occipital → *head*
Occiput - Sides → *head*
Occiput - Suboccipital → *head*
Optic nerve → *eye*
Orbital arch → *eye*
Orbits → *eye*
Orbits - Around → *eye*
Orbits - Below → *eye*
Orbits - Bones → *eye*
Orbits - Deep in → *eye*
Orbits - Lower part → *eye*
Orbits - Margins → *eye*
Outer part → *nose*
Ovaries → *fema*
Ovaries - Region of ovaries → *fema*

P

Palate → *mout*
Palate - Arch → *mout*
Palate - Hard palate → *mout*
Palate - Sides → *mout*
Palate - Soft palate → *mout*
Palate - Velum → *mout*
Palpebral neuralgia → *eye*
Pancreas → *abdo*
Papillae → *eye*
Paralyzed parts → *gene*
Parotid glands → *face*
Parts → *gene*
Parts - Lain on → *gene*

Pectoral muscles → *ches*
Pectoral muscles - Lower part → *ches*
Pelvic region → *abdo*
Pelvis → *abdo*
Pelvis - Organs; pelvic → *abdo*
Penis - Glans → *male*
Penis - Glans - Behind → *male*
Penis - Prepuce → *male*
Penis - Prepuce - Margin of prepuce → *male*
Penis - Root → *male*
Penis - Tip → *male*
Perineum → *rect*
Perineum - Skin; below the → *rect*
Periosteum → *gene*
Periosteum → *head*
Peritoneum → *abdo*
Pharynx → *thro*
Pharynx - Lower part → *thro*
Pit of stomach → *stom*
Pleura → *ches*
Posterior nares → *nose*
Posterior part → *ches*
Posterior part → *stom*
Posterior part → *thro*
Posterior part → *uret*
Postorbital → *eye*
Precordial region → *ches*
Processus styloideus → *ear*
Pubic bones → *fema*
Pubic bones - Symphysis → *fema*
Pubic region → *abdo*
Pubic region → *fema*
Pubic region - Mons pubis → *abdo*
Pudendum → *fema*
Pupils → *eye*
Pylorus → *stom*

R

Rectum and anus → *rect*
Region of bladder → *blad*
Region of kidneys → *kidn*
Region of prostate → *Pros*
Ribs → *abdo*
Ribs → *ches*
Ribs - Anterior part → *ches*
Ribs - Below ribs → *abdo*
Ribs - Between ribs → *ches*
Ribs - Edges of ribs → *ches*

Ribs - False ribs → *abdo*
Ribs - False ribs → *ches*
Ribs - False ribs - Below → *abdo*
Ribs - False ribs - Below - left → *ches*
Ribs - Floating ribs → *abdo*
Ribs - Floating ribs - Below → *abdo*
Ribs - Floating ribs - left → *abdo*
Ribs - Fourth → *ches*
Ribs - Joints → *ches*
Ribs - Last true rib → *ches*
Ribs - Lower → *ches*
Ribs - Lower - left → *ches*
Ribs - Seventh → *ches*
Ribs - Short - Below → *ches*
Ribs - Sixth → *ches*
Ribs - Third → *ches*
Ribs - Third - Sternum; near → *ches*
Ribs - Under → *ches*
Ribs - Under - left → *ches*
Root → *nose*
Root - Behind → *nose*
Root - Inside → *nose*
Roots → *teet*
Roots - Sound teeth → *teet*

S

Sacral region → *back*
Sacral region - Hips; and → *back*
Sacroiliac region → *back*
Sacroiliac symphyses → *back*
Sacrum → *back*
Sacrum - Coccyx; and → *back*
Sacrum - Hips; and → *back*
Salivary glands → *mout*
Salivary glands - Orifices → *mout*
Scalp → *head*
Scapulohumeral region → *extr*
Sclera → *eye*
Scrotum → *male*
Scrotum - Sides → *male*
Scrotum - Thighs; between scrotum and → *male*
Septum → *nose*
Septum - Upper part → *nose*
Shoulders → *extr*
Shoulders - Acromion → *extr*
Shoulders - Beneath → *extr*
Shoulders - Between → *extr*
Shoulders - Deltoid → *extr*

Shoulders - Joints → *extr*
Shoulders - Ligaments → *extr*
Shoulders - Posterior part → *extr*
Shoulders - Sides → *extr*
Shoulders - Top of shoulders → *extr*
Shoulders - Under → *extr*
Sides → *abdo*
Sides → *back*
Sides → *ches*
Sides → *exte*
Sides → *head*
Sides → *nose*
Sides → *thro*
Sides - Brain → *head*
Sides - False ribs → *ches*
Sides - Flanks → *abdo*
Sides - Lower part → *ches*
Sides - Side lain on → *head*
Sides - Upper part → *ches*
Sides - left → *ches*
Sides - left - Fourth rib → *ches*
Sides - left - Fourth rib - Under → *ches*
Sides - left - Heart; under → *ches*
Sides - left - Lower part → *ches*
Sides - left - Ribs - Below → *abdo*
Sides - left - Upper part → *ches*
Sides - one side - Ear; behind the → *head*
Sides - right → *ches*
Sides - right → *head*
Sides - right - Last rib → *ches*
Sides - right - Lower part → *ches*
Sides - right - Ribs - Below → *abdo*
Sides - right - Ribs - Edge of ribs → *abdo*
Sides - right - Upper part → *ches*
Sigmoid flexure → *abdo*
Single parts → *gene*
Sinuses → *face*
Sinuses → *head*
Sinuses → *nose*
Sinuses - Ethmoidal → *face*
Sinuses - Frontal → *face*
Sinuses - Maxillary → *face*
Sinuses - Maxillary → *nose*
Skin → *face*
Skin → *nose*
Skin; below the → *abdo*
Skin; below the → *ches*
Skin; below the → *gene*

Skin; below the → *head*
Skull → *head*
Sockets → *teet*
Sockets - Absent teeth → *teet*
Solar plexus → *abdo*
Sound teeth → *teet*
Spermatic cords → *male*
Spermatic cords; and → *male*
Sphincter → *blad*
Spinal cord → *back*
Spine → *back*
Spine - Beside → *back*
Spine - Brain; base of → *back*
Spine - Joints of vertebrae → *back*
Spine - Lower part → *back*
Spine - Lumbar region - Above → *back*
Spine - Middle of spine → *back*
Spine - Upper part → *back*
Spine - Vertebrae → *back*
Spine - Whole → *back*
Spleen → *abdo*
Spleen - Region of spleen → *abdo*
Sternocleidomastoid muscles → *exte*
Sternocleidomastoid muscles - Upper part → *exte*
Sternum → *ches*
Sternum - Above → *ches*
Sternum - Behind → *ches*
Sternum - Beside sternum → *ches*
Sternum - Border → *ches*
Sternum - Lower part → *ches*
Sternum - Lower part - Under → *ches*
Sternum - Over sternum → *ches*
Sternum - Sternoclavicular joint → *ches*
Sternum - Sternocostal joints → *ches*
Sternum - Tip → *ches*
Sternum - Under → *ches*
Sternum - Upper part → *ches*
Sternum - Xiphoid cartilage → *ches*
Sternum - left of sternum → *ches*
Sternum - left side; along the → *ches*
Sublingual glands → *mout*
Submaxillary glands → *exte*
Submaxillary glands → *face*
Supraorbital → *eye*
Sutures → *head*
Sutures - Along → *head*
Sutures - Coronal → *head*
Symphysis → *abdo*

T

Teeth → *teet*
Temples → *face*
Temples → *head*
Temples - Above → *head*
Temples - Side lain on → *head*
Temples - Sides → *head*
Temples - Skin → *face*
Tendons → *extr*
Tendons → *gene*
Tendons - Attachments of tendons → *extr*
Testes → *male*
Testes - Epididymis → *male*
Thighs → *extr*
Thighs - Anterior part → *extr*
Thighs - Anterior part - Inguinal region; near → *extr*
Thighs - Anterior part - Lower part → *extr*
Thighs - Anterior part - Upper part → *extr*
Thighs - Back of thighs → *extr*
Thighs - Bends of thighs → *extr*
Thighs - Between → *extr*
Thighs - Bones → *extr*
Thighs - Crural nerves → *extr*
Thighs - Crural nerves - Anterior → *extr*
Thighs - Femur → *extr*
Thighs - Genitalia; near → *extr*
Thighs - Genitalia; near - Female → *extr*
Thighs - Genitalia; near - Male → *extr*
Thighs - Glands → *extr*
Thighs - Hamstrings → *extr*
Thighs - Inner side → *extr*
Thighs - Inner side - Knees; above → *extr*
Thighs - Inner side - Upper part → *extr*
Thighs - Knees; above → *extr*
Thighs - Lower part → *extr*
Thighs - Lower part - Posterior part → *extr*
Thighs - Middle → *extr*
Thighs - Middle - Anterior part → *extr*
Thighs - Middle - Internal part → *extr*
Thighs - Middle - Posterior part → *extr*
Thighs - Outer side → *extr*
Thighs - Periosteum → *extr*
Thighs - Posterior part → *extr*
Thighs - Upper part → *extr*
Thorax → *gene*
Throat-pit → *exte*
Throat-pit → *lary*

Thumbs → *extr*
Thumbs - Balls → *extr*
Thumbs - Bones → *extr*
Thumbs - Extensor muscles → *extr*
Thumbs - Joints → *extr*
Thumbs - Joints - Carpometacarpal → *extr*
Thumbs - Joints - Distal → *extr*
Thumbs - Joints - Metacarpophalangeal → *extr*
Thumbs - Joints - Metacarpophalangeal - left → *extr*
Thumbs - Joints - Proximal → *extr*
Thumbs - Nails → *extr*
Thumbs - Nails - Roots of nails → *extr*
Thumbs - Nails - Under → *extr*
Thumbs - Phalanges → *extr*
Thumbs - Phalanges - Distal → *extr*
Thumbs - Phalanges - Proximal → *extr*
Thumbs - Sides - Inner → *extr*
Thumbs - Tips → *extr*
Thumbs - Tips - right → *extr*
Thumbs - sides → *extr*
Thumbs - sides - Outer → *extr*
Thyroid cartilage → *exte*
Thyroid gland → *exte*
Tip → *nose*
Tips → *extr*
Toes → *extr*
Toes - Balls → *extr*
Toes - Between → *extr*
Toes - Bones → *extr*
Toes - Fifth → *extr*
Toes - Fifth - Balls → *extr*
Toes - Fifth - Joints → *extr*
Toes - First → *extr*
Toes - First - Balls → *extr*
Toes - First - Joints → *extr*
Toes - First - Joints - Proximal → *extr*
Toes - First - Nails → *extr*
Toes - First - Nails - Roots of nails → *extr*
Toes - First - Nails - Under → *extr*
Toes - First - Tendons - Extensor tendons → *extr*
Toes - First - Tips → *extr*
Toes - Fourth → *extr*
Toes - Joints → *extr*
Toes - Joints - Small joints → *extr*
Toes - Nails → *extr*
Toes - Nails - Roots of nails → *extr*
Toes - Nails - Under → *extr*
Toes - Second → *extr*

Toes - Second - Balls → *extr*
Toes - Second - Joints → *extr*
Toes - Second - Nails → *extr*
Toes - Third → *extr*
Toes - Third - Nails - Under → *extr*
Toes - Tips → *extr*
Toes - Under → *extr*
Tongue → *mout*
Tongue - Across → *mout*
Tongue - Anterior part → *mout*
Tongue - Below → *mout*
Tongue - Below - Skin; below → *mout*
Tongue - Border → *mout*
Tongue - Center → *mout*
Tongue - Edges → *mout*
Tongue - Frenum → *mout*
Tongue - Posterior part → *mout*
Tongue - Root → *mout*
Tongue - Root - Across → *mout*
Tongue - Root - Below → *mout*
Tongue - Sides → *mout*
Tongue - Sides - Tip; near → *mout*
Tongue - Surface of tongue; under → *mout*
Tongue - Tip → *mout*
Tongue - Transversely across → *mout*
Tonsils → *thro*
Trachea → *lary*
Tragus → *ear*
Transversely across → *stom*
Trigeminus → *face*
Tympanum → *ear*

U

Umbilicus → *abdo*
Umbilicus - Above → *abdo*
Umbilicus - Below → *abdo*
Umbilicus - Region of umbilicus → *abdo*
Umbilicus - Sides → *abdo*
Upper abdomen → *abdo*
Upper arms → *extr*
Upper arms - Anterior part → *extr*
Upper arms - Anterior surface → *extr*
Upper arms - Biceps → *extr*
Upper arms - Bones → *extr*
Upper arms - Bones - Condyles → *extr*
Upper arms - Bones - Condyles - External → *extr*
Upper arms - Bones - Condyles - Internal → *extr*
Upper arms - Bones - Elbow; near → *extr*

Upper arms - Deltoid → *extr*
Upper arms - Elbows; just above → *extr*
Upper arms - Humerus → *extr*
Upper arms - Inner side → *extr*
Upper arms - Joints → *extr*
Upper arms - Lower part → *extr*
Upper arms - Muscles - Anterior → *extr*
Upper arms - Muscles - Extensor muscles → *extr*
Upper arms - Muscles - Flexor muscles → *extr*
Upper arms - Outer side → *extr*
Upper arms - Outer side - left → *extr*
Upper arms - Posterior part → *extr*
Upper arms - Side lain on → *extr*
Upper arms - Skin → *extr*
Upper arms - Triceps → *extr*
Upper half → *head*
Upper limbs → *extr*
Upper limbs - Bones → *extr*
Upper limbs - Brachial plexus → *extr*
Upper limbs - Inner side → *extr*
Upper limbs - Internally → *extr*
Upper limbs - Joints → *extr*
Upper limbs - Joints - Bones → *extr*
Upper limbs - Joints - Joint to joint; from → *extr*
Upper limbs - Joints - Side lain on → *extr*
Upper limbs - Outer side → *extr*
Upper limbs - Outer surface → *extr*
Upper limbs - Part lain on → *extr*
Upper limbs - Skin; below → *extr*
Upper part of body → *gene*
Upper part → *ches*
Upper part → *nose*
Upper teeth → *teet*
Upper teeth - Hollow → *teet*
Upper teeth - left → *teet*
Upper teeth - right → *teet*
Ureters → *kidn*
Uterus → *fema*
Uterus - Cervix → *fema*
Uterus - Ligaments; broad → *fema*
Uterus - Middle of uterus → *fema*
Uterus - Os uteri → *fema*
Uvula → *thro*
Uvula - Behind → *thro*

V

Vagina → *fema*
Vagina - Around → *fema*

Veins → *extr*
Veins → *gene*
Vertex → *head*
Vertex - Across → *head*
Vertex - Here and there → *head*
Vulva → *fema*

W

Wall; abdominal → *abdo*
Wings → *nose*
Wings - Edges → *nose*
Wings - Inner surface → *nose*
Wings - left → *nose*
Wings - right → *nose*
Wisdom teeth → *teet*
Wisdom teeth - Lower - right → *teet*
Wounds → *gene*
Wrists → *extr*
Wrists - Bones → *extr*
Wrists - Dorsal side → *extr*
Wrists - Palmar side → *extr*
Wrists - Radial side → *extr*
Wrists - Ulnar side → *extr*

Z

Zygoma → *face*

History of
Kent's Repertory and Treasure

Ahmed Nooruddin Currim, M.D., Ph.D.

Introduction

In 1972, as a student of homeopathy, I had already realized that Kent's Repertory third American and later editions, had many printing mistakes, and it surprised me that these errors had not been rectified by Dr. Kent. On closer examination I realized that the publication of the Third Edition appeared in 1924, after June 5, 1916 (the date of Dr. Kent's death) and it occurred to me that Dr. Kent had never had the chance to correct these errors.

Logically, therefore, I tried to locate the second edition of the Repertory. I had spoken to Mr. Roger Ehrhart (the last of the Ehrhart family that owned the famous Homeopathic Pharmacy of Ehrhart and Karl-original publishers of Kent's Repertory Third, Fourth, Fifth, Sixth American Editions) in 1972 when he was still alive but he could not give me much help. It was not clear if the library of Ehrhart and Karl had this second edition (of Kent's own repertory or an uncovered one).

A paper in the January-February 1963 AIH Journal by Dr. K.C. Mittal was the first clue to the existence of Kent's own personal repertory and this repertory was in the possession of Dr. Schmidt of Geneva, Switzerland.

In June, 1972 I had the opportunity to be in Geneva, Switzerland and spoke to Dr. Pierre Schmidt about the errors I had observed in Kent's Repertory, the paper of Dr. Mittal, and asked for him to shed light on the matter. He informed me that Dr. Mittal had come to Geneva and diligently worked with Kent's own personal copy of the second edition of the repertory (abbreviated as "Treasure" from here on) and had copied carefully every correction from the Treasure into his own copy of the 6th American Edition 1957.

In addition, Dr. Mittal had also copied every correction from the two chapters "Mind and Generalities" into a copy of an Indian edition belonging to Dr. Pierre Schmidt which he showed me. This was a specially bound book (I believe this book had a green cover with special "spring" action separators between the various chapters). In it were very neatly copied corrections in a very symmetrical handwriting. A facsimile of one such page (Chapter of Mind) is printed in the so-called Kent's Final General Repertory. It is to be noted that the handwriting on this facsimile is completely different from Kent's signature also appearing in this book in the preface. The handwriting is probably Dr. Mittal's.

Dr. Pierre Schmidt informed me that, after carefully doing this work, Dr. Mittal had run away from Switzerland taking the Treasure with him as well as, of course, his own copy (6th American Edition of Kent's Repertory) in which he had made the corrections from the Treasure and that if this copy could be traced it would be as good as the Treasure. Dr. Mittal's copy will be referred to as MKR in what follows.

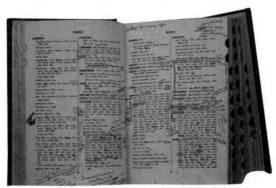

Fig 1.: Dr. Mittal's copy with handwritten additions
© Reinhard Rosé (Germany)

The Search

In 1973 I wound up my duties as Assistant Professor at a university in the USA to start the study of medicine at the University of Brussels. My motivation for giving up a previous profession as a mathematician lay in the inspiration I had received in the study of Kent's incredible Lectures in Homeopathic Philosophy, Materia Medica and Repertory. It was a dream and a deep intuitive feeling that Homeopathy could perhaps again triumph on the earth and regain its past glory in the healing of the nations; and that using the techniques of mathematics and computers I might play some role in the solution of medical problems. As a mathematician I had even written a working computer program in the Fortran language for such repertorization and diagnosis of diseases.

I was further inspired and encouraged by two wonderful friends, Mrs. Audrey Winthers (daughter of Dr. A.H. Grimmer, one of Kent's foremost student who had entrusted me with her father's original manuscripts-a work which appeared in 1996 as The Collected Works of Dr. A.H. Grimmer) and Joseph L. Kaplowe, M.D., of New Haven, Connecticut, also a homeopathic doctor, author of many papers in the Homeopathic Recorder, the foremost homeopathic journal in U.S.A.

During my years as a medical student I had many occasions to speak of the problem of Kent's repertory with Mme. Schmidt whose gracious help and encouragement in my days as a medical student really were instrumental in my success at completing my M.D.

In 1978 Mme. Schmidt wrote a letter to Dr. Mittal and gave it to me to present to him personally when I went for a 3 week vacation to India.

Mme. Schmidt told me that it was Dr. Eugene Alonzo Austin, beloved student of Kent who had passed on the Treasure to Dr. Pierre Schmidt in 1939, when the latter physician, had traveled to the U.S. to learn homeopathy with two of Kent's best students: Dr. Frederica Gladwin and Dr. Eugene Alonzo Austin.

Dr. Frederica Gladwin originally had acquired one of the three originally hand corrected (by Kent himself) 2nd Editions of Kent Repertories and had passed her copy to Dr. Austin or Dr. Schmidt.

It is not clear if Dr. Gladwin passed her copy directly to Dr. Schmidt or to Dr. Austin who subsequently passed it on to Dr. Schmidt, together with a ring belonging to Dr. Kent, which Dr. Schmidt wore for the rest of his life.

However, these corrections, which Dr. Austin had earnestly urged be incorporated, were never incorporated in the post-war editions of the repertory (Fourth, Fifth and Sixth American Editions).

The problem in finding Dr. Mittal was hard as he rarely stayed in one place, but after zig-zagging from Delhi to Lucknow to Delhi to Amrisar I finally located him and presented him with the letter from Mme Schmidt. This opened the doors of my search.

I spent one whole evening talking with Dr. Mittal. He told me that indeed he had taken the Treasure for many reasons. I had heard several of them but since they are not of immediate bearing in this discussion they need not be entertained for now. I still, to this day, have a 45 minute tape of part of this conversation with Dr. Mittal. It was agreed that every effort would be made by Dr. Mittal and myself to have these corrections incorporated. However I saw neither the Treasure nor Dr. Mittal's repertory (MKR).

Dr. Mittal informed me that he had been pursued by Dr. Schmidt and Dr. Chand who had called for the services of Interpol to retrieve the Treasure. He said that he had been constantly harassed and threatened and was fleeing from these people. The Treasure, however, was never found and, in fact, Dr. Mittal had cut up the Treasure into bits and pieces, some of which he currently carried on his person and some of which were hidden in a village.

Dr. Mittal informed me that his copy as well as the bits and pieces of the Treasure were kept in another town of which he would tell me at another occasion when I returned.

Fig 2.: Pieces of the Treasure
© Reinhard Rosé (Germany)

During this visit to India I also met with Dr. D. H. Chand at his home in Delhi, saw the Indian edition belonging to Dr. Pierre Schmidt mentioned in the introduction, and also several hundred bits of the Treasure and some pages of the Treasure.

The Return

After this first visit in February, 1978 there was sporadic correspondence between Dr. Mittal and myself.

In 1980 I had occasion to return to India for vacation and again, after considerable effort, I was able to locate Dr. Mittal. Together we traveled to a small village, Rampur, where he had told me he had hidden his copy of the repertory together with the remains of the Treasure. I endured the discomforts of a slow long train journey.

At Rampur the head of the family who had kept the MKR and cut up bits of the Treasure and Dr. Mittal conferred by themselves and then told me that I would have to return another time as the books were hidden in a small wood hut in the fields and the 14 mile trip by motorcycle was not possible at this time.

In vain I explained that I had limited time and that I had come so far from the U.S.A. However, after much persuasion they asked me to return in 7 days. It was with great discouragement I returned to my home in Bombay.

Despite my discouragement I vowed to try once more before returning to the U.S.A. I left Bombay and met Dr. Mittal in Delhi. We again journeyed to Rampur. This time Dr. Mittal asked the man to produce his books and after a lot of argument a large bundle wrapped in a large, dirty cloth was produced and the contents dumped out on the ground.

Among them was Dr. Mittal's copy of the repertory (MKR), another Indian edition of the repertory, a copy of the First Edition of Kent's Repertory published in 1899 and two volumes of Lectures on Materia Medica given by Kent in 1895 at the Hering Medical College and typed by his students. These Dr. Mittal bade me take with me to the U.S.A. In addition he entrusted me with thousands of pieces of the Treasure that had been cut up.

With this I departed for Delhi and from thence my flight to the U.S.A. At the stopover in Frankfurt I phoned Mme. Schmidt and, with joy, told her of the recovered treasures:

1. the MKR
2. the several thousand pieces of the Treasure
3. a copy of the First American Edition of Kent's Repertory
4. a set of 2 volume lecture notes on Materia Medica belonging to Mary Florence Taft with an inscription inside as being presented to Betty Prescott Dolbease and Louis Prescott Dolbease
5. a typed paper written by Dr. K.C. Mittal entitled The Importance of Kent's Repertory in the Clinic and Practice delivered at the International Congress for Homeopathic Medicine, (LIGA) in Dusseldorf, Germany, Sept., 1962.

Examination

For two years I reviewed the material entrusted to me by Dr. Mittal. There were several thousand pieces of the Treasure (in Kent's own handwriting) that were cut up.

I spent several hundred hours identifying several hundreds of these to see where they fit in the Third and later American Editions and then compared these with the MKR.
I found that the MKR had the exact corrections of these several hundred bits (a slide of several of these bits has been shown in the past).

There are also 44 almost complete pages (22 double sided sheets) of the Treasure, easily identifiable as being from the Chapter on Extremities. One easily recognizes the handwriting of Dr. J.T. Kent in these and it is clear that this is quite different from that appearing in the 1980 Indian Edition (in Dr. Harish Chand's Office) .The handwriting therein seems to be that of Dr. Mittal.

The agreement of the bits of the Treasure as well as of the 44 almost complete pages with MKR therefore leads to the conclusion that the MKR (Dr. K.C. Mittal's copy of the 6 th American Edition of Kent's Repertory) is a true and correct version of the Treasure (Dr. Kent's personal copy of the Second Revised Edition).

The identification of the bits of the Treasure is difficult, not only because only a part of the rubric is visible, but because the bits of the treasure are from the Second Edition while the comparison is made with a Third or Fourth or Fifth or Sixth American Edition, (with different pagination). It is of course clear that the back of each Second Edition bit will be either 1 or 3 consecutive columns ahead or behind where it appears in the Third Edition.

Conclusion

I am very indebted to Dr. Mittal for making these works available to enable the repertory of Kent to be completed as Dr. Kent had himself envisioned.

In 1980, in India, a revision of Kent's repertory was published under a new title, "Kent's Final General Repertory" instead of the original title. "Repertory of the Homeopathic Materia Medica." This book was "Revised, corrected, Augmented and Edited" by Dr. Pierre Schmidt and Dr. Diwan Harish Chand.

Several errors are inherently present in this version of the repertory.
1. The book that Dr. D.H. Chand used to publish his edited version was a copy of another person, Mr. Shindoo. Apparently Dr. Mittal often visited this person for a few days at a time, when Mr. Shindoo would copy whatever information he could from the MKR into his copy. It is not clear whether Mr. Shindoo really carefully copied all of the MKR. Dr. D. H. Chand had purchased this copy. A repertory shows errors from the MKR. It is highly probable that many inaccuracies crept up in such transcribing, done under such conditions.
2. In addition, MKR contained not only the corrections from the Treasure but also Dr. Mittal had added remedies from Kent's own copy of Hering's 10 volumes of Guiding Symptoms (also in Dr. Pierre Schmidt's office). These remedies he had, however, marked separately with the initials KHG (Kent's Hering Guiding Symptoms). These Mr. Shindoo copied without noting their origin. Therefore, remedies not in the Treasure have in this way been added into this new repertory.

241

It is of course possible that Dr. Kent would have agreed they belonged there since he had written them himself in his own copy of Hering Guiding Symptoms.

Slides of examples of this were shown in my presentation of this paper at the 1987 Liga meeting, together with a slide of a letter from Dr. Mittal. The "purchase of the mutilated copy of the treasure" as mentioned in the preface (pg. xiv) by Dr. D. H. Chand is only partial and has not been compared with the Shindoo copy in the manner that the author has compared the MKR copy with the bits and almost complete pages of the Treasure.

In late 1984 Mrs. D. H. Chand visited her daughter in Norwalk, CT. and joined me and my family for a pleasant evening. I discussed with Mrs. D. H. Chand about my findings. In view of the difficulty of communicating with Dr. Mittal in India some discussion was entertained about bringing the information (that I had strived to uncover) before the Homeopathic profession.

In 1985, before the Washington meeting of the National Center of Homeopathy, Dr. D. H. Chand was in my home and he took back with him a xerox copy of the MKR with the promise that he and I would work together to bring out a true version of the repertory to completion. However I never again heard from Dr. D. H. Chand regarding this matter.

The original MKR copy is kept secure, to this day. With the aid of modern computers, Frederik Schroyens, and the wonderful people at Archibel, the publishing of these additions/corrections have now been accomplished with perfect accuracy. Essential Synthesis has now been published, just as Dr. Kent had wished.

These are the words that Dr. Gladwin wrote about Dr. Kent: "This accomplished master in the science and art of homeopathic medicine has bequeathed to us his imperishable works, thanks to his tireless labor and exceptional qualities. But in addition, he showed the example of infinite patience, constant kindness, and led our halting steps in the world of homeopathic truths, sparing neither time nor effort to explain every step of the way we had to travel, constantly correcting us and putting us back on the right road when through ignorance, clumsiness or negligence, we strayed from the path of truth." In grave and difficult cases presented to Kent he always gave competent help.

The help Kent gave was so kind and affable, so rich in practical teaching, that they considered him a spiritual father or elder brother. Everybody loved and respected him.

"Things will grow brighter as minds are brought together and men think harmoniously. The more we keep together the better, and the more we think as one the better. It is a pity that differences should arise among us when we have so perfect a truth to bind us together." So said Dr. Kent in the first paragraph of his last lecture (Lecture XXXVII) of his inspiring "Lectures on Homeopathic Philosophy."

Dear fellow homeopaths, let us rejoice at the loving kindness of our Heavenly Father and the soul of James Tyler Kent for giving us ways to heal ourselves, and the nations, with the guidance of Hahnemann's spirit; in particular with Frederik Schroyens and the team at Archibel, who deserve our heartfelt thanks.

Ahmed N. Currim, MD, PhD

Notes

Notes

Notes

Notes

Notes